TRANSESOPHAGEAL ECHOCARDIOGRAPHY

IN CLINICAL PRACTICE

Rotterdam Postgraduate School of Cardiology

A slide atlas of *Transesophageal Echocardiography in
Clinical Practice*, based on the contents of this book, is
available. In the slide atlas format, the material is split into
volumes, each of which is presented in a binder together
with numbered 35mm slides of each illustration. Each
slide atlas volume also contains a list of abbreviated slide
captions for easy reference when using the slides. Further
information can be obtained from:

Gower Medical Publishing
Middlesex House
34–42 Cleveland Street
London W1P 5FB

Gower Medical Publishing
101 5th Avenue
New York, NY. 10003
USA

TRANSESOPHAGEAL ECHOCARDIOGRAPHY

IN CLINICAL PRACTICE

George R Sutherland FRCP FESC
Consultant Cardiologist
Western General Hospital
Edinburgh, UK

Jos RTC Roelandt MD, FESC, FACC
Professor of Cardiology
Academisch Ziekenhuis Dijkzigt
and Erasmus University Rotterdam
Rotterdam, The Netherlands

Alan G Fraser BSc MB ChB MRCP
Senior Registrar in Cardiology
University Hospital of Wales
Cardiff, UK

Robert H Anderson BSc MD FRCPath
Professor in Paediatric Cardiac Morphology
National Heart and Lung Institute
London, UK

Gower Medical Publishing • London • New York

Distributed in the USA and Canada by:
J B Lippincott Company
East Washington Square
Philadelphia
PA 19105
USA

Distributed in the UK and Continental Europe by:
Gower Medical Publishing
Middlesex House
34–42 Cleveland Street
London W1P 5FB
UK

Distributed in Australia and New Zealand by:
Harper and Row (Australia) Pte Ltd
PO Box 226
Artarmon
NSW 2064
AUSTRALIA

Distributed in Southeast Asia, Hong Kong, India and Pakistan by:
Harper and Row (Asia) Pty Ltd
37 Jalan Pemimpin 02–01
Singapore 2057

Distributed in Japan by:
Nankodo Co Ltd
42–6 Hongo 3-chome
Bunkyo-ku
Tokyo 113
JAPAN

British Library Cataloguing in Publication Data:
Sutherland GR, Roelandt JRTC, Fraser AG and Anderson RH
Transesophageal echocardiography in clinical practice.
1. Man. Heart. Diagnosis. Transesophageal echocardiography.
I. Title
616.1207543

Library of Congress Cataloging in Publication Data:
Transesophageal echocardiography in clinical practice/George
Sutherland ... [et al.].
p. cm.
Includes index.
1. Transesophageal echocardiography. I. Sutherland,
George R., MB.
[DNLM: 1. Arrhythmia—diagnosis. 2. Echocardiography.
3. Electrocardiography. 4. Heart Diseases—diagnosis. WG
141.5.E2
T7725]
RC683.5.T83T734 1991
616.1'207543—dc20
DNLM/DLC
for Library of Congress

ISBN: 0–397–44640–3

Project Manager:	Saba Zafar
Designer:	Anne–Marie Woodruff
Illustrations:	Jane Brown
Line artist:	Dereck Johnson
Production:	Susan Bishop
Publisher:	Fiona Foley

Text set in New Baskerville
Originated in Hong Kong by Bright Arts
Produced by Mandarin Offset
Printed in Hong Kong

CONTRIBUTORS

Robert H Anderson
Joseph Levy Foundation Professor in Paediatric
  Cardiac Morphology
Department of Paediatrics
National Heart and Lung Institute
London, UK

Marc E R M van Daele
Research Fellow
Interuniversity Cardiology Institute
  of The Netherlands, and
Thoraxcentre, Academisch Ziekenhuis Dijkzigt
Rotterdam, The Netherlands

Alan G Fraser
British Heart Foundation Fellow
Department of Cardiology
Thoraxcentre, Academisch Ziekenhuis Dijkzigt
Rotterdam, The Netherlands
Present address:
Department of Cardiology
University Hospital of Wales
Cardiff, UK

Heinz Lambertz
Assistant Professor
Department of Cardiology
Klinikum of the Rheinische Westfälische
Technische Hochshule — Klinikum
Aachen, Germany
Present address:
Department of Cardiology
German Diagnostic Centre
Wiesbaden, Federal Republic of Germany

Massimo Pozzoli
Research Fellow
Department of Cardiology
Thoraxcentre, Academisch Ziekenhuis Dijkzigt
Rotterdam, The Netherlands
Present address:
Divisione di Cardiologia
Centro Medico di Montescano
Montescano, Pavia, Italy

Jos R T C Roelandt
Professor of Cardiology and Head
Thoraxcentre, Academisch Ziekenhuis Dijkzigt
  and Erasmus University Rotterdam
Rotterdam, The Netherlands

John H Symllie
Research Fellow
Department of Cardiology
Thoraxcentre, Academisch Ziekenhuis Dijkzigt
Rotterdam, The Netherlands
Present address:
Department of Cardiology
Leeds General Infirmary
Leeds, UK

Oliver F W Stümper
Research Fellow
Department of Cardiology
Thoraxcentre, Academisch Ziekenhuis Dijkzigt
Rotterdam, The Netherlands
Present address:
Department of Paediatric Cardiology
Royal Hospital for Sick Children
Sciennes Road
Edinburgh, UK

George R Sutherland
Director of Clinical Echocardiography
Thoraxcentre, Academisch Ziekenhuis Dijkzigt
Rotterdam, The Netherlands
Present address:
Department of Cardiology
Western General Hospital
Edinburgh, UK

Meindert A Taams
Cardiologist
Department of Cardiology
Thoraxcentre, Academisch Ziekenhuis Dijkzigt
Rotterdam, The Netherlands

Bernardino Tuccillo
Research Fellow
Department of Cardiology
Thoraxcentre, Academisch Ziekenhuis Dijkzigt
Rotterdam, The Netherlands
Present address:
II Policlinico
Cattedra di Cardiologia
Universita di Napoli
Napoli, Italy

ABBREVIATIONS

Certain common abbreviations are used throughout this book, especially in the figures and tables. These are listed below and therefore not explained in the legends to the figures. The meanings of other, uncommon or infrequent abbreviations are given in the relevant legends to particular figures.

A	anterior wall of left ventricle
AAVC	absent atrioventricular connexion
AML	anterior (aortic) mitral leaflet
AO	aorta
AR	aortic regurgitation
Asc	ascending
AV	aortic valve
AVR	aortic valve replacement
CS	coronary sinus
CX	circumflex (coronary artery)
Desc	descending
ECG	electrocardiogram
FL	false lumen (of an aortic dissection)
HV	hepatic vein
I	inferior wall of left ventricle
IAS	interatrial septum
ICV	inferior caval vein (inferior vena cava)
IVS	interventricular septum
L	lateral wall of left ventricle
LA	left atrium
LAA	left atrial appendage
LAD	left anterior descending (coronary artery)
LCA	left coronary artery
LCC	left coronary cusp (leaflet) of the aortic valve, or left coronary sinus
LCX	left circumflex (coronary artery)
LLPV	left lower pulmonary vein
LPA	left pulmonary artery
LUPV	left upper pulmonary vein
LV	left ventricle
LVOT	left ventricular outflow tract

MRI	magnetic resonance image/imaging
MV	mitral valve
MVR	mitral valve replacement
NCC	noncoronary cusp (leaflet) of the aortic valve, or noncoronary sinus
OE	oesophagus
PCG	phonocardiogram
PM	papillary muscle
PML	posterior (mural) mitral leaflet
PSA	pseudoaneurysm
PT	pulmonary trunk
PV	pulmonary valve
PVA	pulmonary venous atrium
RA	right atrium
RAA	right atrial appendage
RCA	right coronary artery
RCC	right coronary cusp (leaflet) of the aortic valve, or right coronary sinus
RCX	right circumflex
RLPV	right lower pulmonary vein
RPA	right pulmonary artery
RUPV	right upper pulmonary vein
RV	right ventricle
RVOT	right ventricular outflow tract
S	ventricular septum
SCV/SVC	superior caval vein (superior vena cava)
SVA	systemic venous atrium
TL	true lumen (of an aortic dissection)
TV	tricuspid valve
VA	ventricular arterial
VSD	ventricular septal defect

ORIENTATION OF IMAGES

Abbreviations

A	anterior	**P**	posterior
AL	anterolateral	**PI**	posteroinferior
AS	anterosuperior	**PM**	posteromedial
I	inferior	**R**	right
L	left	**S**	superior

Most of the echocardiographic images reproduced in this book were obtained using single plane (transverse) transesophageal probes. These illustrations are displayed in the conventional manner, with the posterior aspect of the heart (or the inferior aspect, for transgastric images) at the top of the echocardiographic image, as follows:

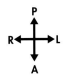

Since this orientation is standard, it is not explained or illustrated on every figure; if there is no indication to the contrary, it can be assumed to apply to all images obtained with a transverse transoesophageal transducer. Where the orientation of an echocardiographic illustration or anatomical section is unusual or unfamiliar, however, it is stated in the legend to the figure, or illustrated with a compass. This applies particularly to those images obtained with a longitudinal transoesophageal transducer.

CONTENTS

1

Introduction

George R Sutherland
Jos R T C Roelandt
Alan G Fraser
Robert H Anderson

Within only a few years, transoesophageal echocardiography has become established as an important new imaging technique in cardiology. It was introduced in Europe in 1981 for diagnosis, and was subsequently applied in the USA for monitoring during anaesthesia. The oesophageal approach came of age as a diagnostic technique in 1985, when transoesophageal probes that were capable of imaging with high resolution were introduced. Since this major improvement in the quality of the images, and with the later addition of colour flow mapping, the transoesophageal approach has been adopted in many cardiac centres, initially in Europe and latterly in North America, as a diagnostic method that is applicable to a wide variety of clinical situations, both in the out-patient clinic and for the needs of in-patients.

The advantages of imaging from the oesophagus have been demonstrated for a wide spectrum of cardiac lesions in adults. The major indications for its use include acute or chronic disease of the thoracic aorta, native and prosthetic valvar endocarditis, and dysfunction of prosthetic mitral valves, as well as the investigation of possible intracardiac sources of emboli, and the evaluation of adolescents and adults with complex congenital heart disease. New and unique insights have been gained into the morphology and haemodynamic disturbances found in each of these clinical settings. The information that transoesophageal echocardiography now provides is likely to have a major influence on the way in which these conditions are investigated and managed.

Recently, small transoesophageal probes have been developed for use in children. Imaging is now being performed in anaesthetized children, and the technique has been found to be a valuable adjunct to the precordial approach in both the diagnosis and follow-up of certain aspects of complex congenital heart disease. Other technological developments have led to the introduction of biplane probes, probes with integrated continuous wave Doppler, and probes with a combined facility for atrial pacing, which can be used in stress-echo applications. In the near future, probes with a single array of elements, which can be rotated or angled in order to image multiple planes, will be introduced. These have the potential to provide three-dimensional reconstructions of cardiac morphology.

Since the introduction of high-resolution imaging and colour flow mapping, the applications of transoesophageal echocardiography have extended into cardiac surgery. The technique is now used in the operating room, not only for monitoring ventricular function and volume, but also increasingly for monitoring the results of surgery such as valvar reconstruction or replacement, and the repair of congenital defects. Indeed, some surgeons now aim for the 'perfect echocardiographic repair'. In general surgery, transoesophageal echocardiography is used to monitor left ventricular function in elderly patients undergoing a

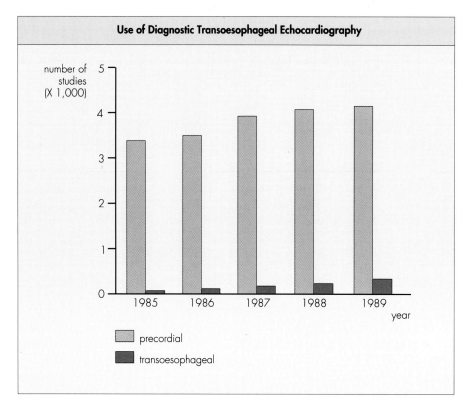

Fig.1.1 The increasing use of diagnostic transoesophageal echocardiography in the out-patient clinic of the Thoraxcentre between 1985 and 1989. Note that the ratio of diagnostic transoesophageal studies to routine precordial studies has increased progressively. During 1989, 1 in 13 of all diagnostic ultrasound studies was carried out using the oesophageal approach. In 1990, the ratio was 1 in 8. This marked increase in the proportion of transoesophageal studies reflects our cumulative clinical experience with the technique, and the important diagnostic role which it now has in our centre.

variety of general surgical procedures who are at risk of perioperative myocardial ischaemia or infarction. These practices are not yet widespread, but are likely to become so as more surgeons and anaesthetists become aware of the potential benefits of transoesophageal echocardiography.

Transoesophageal echocardiography has now been available in the Thoraxcentre for five years, and has been used for all the clinical applications described above (Figs. 1.1–1.5). It seemed appropriate to us, therefore, to review our experience in order to clarify, both for ourselves and others, the value of the technique in the out-patient clinic, the operating room, and the in-patient service. In producing this book (based on our clinical experience as well as our research interests), it is inevitable that it is, to some extent, a sum of our opinions rather than a comprehensive account of all possible applications of the technique. Inevitably, while attempting to keep the book to manageable proportions, we have not been able to cover all subjects. We have tried, nonetheless, to evaluate the role of transoesophageal imaging accurately over the whole range of its current clinical applications, while also indicating what are likely to be the important future developments.

This book is intended primarily for those who are learning the technique of transoesophageal echocardiography so that they can introduce it into their clinical practice. We hope that it will prove to be of value, not only to all cardiologists (both adult and paediatric),

but also to anaesthetists and cardiac surgeons who are interested in the potential applications of the technique in the operating room. It may also be of interest to internists who refer patients for noninvasive cardiological investigations, and to radiologists who assess cardiac patients.

The experience reflected in this book is the result of multidisciplinary collaboration, and we should like to express our warm thanks to the many colleagues who have helped us. Professor Klaas Bom, Dr Charles Lancée, Dr Elma Gussenhoven, and their colleagues in the Division of Experimental Echocardiography and the Department of Bioengineering of the Erasmus University Rotterdam, developed the high-resolution transoesophageal probe that was used for the initial clinical studies that began in 1985. This probe has since been produced commercially, and it is now in widespread use. More recently, Pieter Brommersma has collaborated in the development of a prototype transoesophageal probe for use in children. Many studies were performed by clinical colleagues, including Dr Rene Geuskens, Dr Jos Saelman, Dr Folkert ten Cate, and Dr Anton de Porto. Our cardiac surgeons, including Professor Egbert Bos, Professor Jan Quaegebeur, Dr Lex van Herwerden, Dr Bas Mochtar, and Dr Ad Bogers, have been enthusiastic colleagues in the operating room. The cardiac anaesthetists, including Dr Omar Prakash, Dr Evert Rulf, Dr Eddy Cruz, Dr Ronald Schepp, Dr Dries van de Woerd, Dr Yvon Deryck, Dr King Siphanto, and visitors Dr Michael Cahalan and Dr

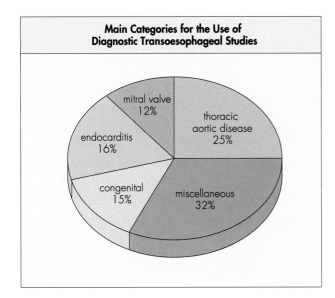

Fig. 1.2 A summary of the main categories of patients referred for a diagnostic transoesophageal study during the period 1985–1989. The most common reason for requesting a study was suspected pathology of the thoracic aorta. Suspected infective endocarditis was the second most common reason, pathology of the mitral valve (including suspected mitral prosthetic dysfunction), the third, and complex congenital heart disease in adolescents and adults, the fourth. In this last group, the number and complexity of studies has increased markedly in the past three years as we became aware of the unique diagnostic role of transoesophageal echocardiography in these patients.

Transoesophageal Echocardiography in Adult Cardiology Indications: 1990	
Established	thoracic aortic pathology
	infective endocarditis
	prosthetic valve malfunction
	systemic embolism — ? cardiac source
	native mitral valvar disease
	intraoperative mitral valvar surgery
	suspected atrial abnormality (tumours etc.)
	adults and adolescents with congenital heart disease
Uncertain	transient ischaemic attacks
	ischaemic heart disease
Evolving	intraoperative monitoring in cardiac surgery
	intraoperative monitoring in general surgery
Potential	stress echocardiography (combined with atrial pacing)

Fig. 1.4 A summary of our perspective of the main clinical indications for a transoesophageal study in adults — 1990.

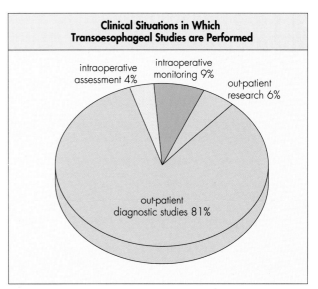

Fig. 1.3 The differing clinical situations in which the studies were performed. As well as routine out-patient diagnostic studies, research studies were performed in specific patient groups. In addition, transoesophageal echocardiography was introduced into the operating room in 1988 for monitoring surgical repairs, particularly for mitral regurgitation or congenital heart disease.

Transoesophageal Echocardiography in Paediatric Cardiology Indications: 1990	
Diagnostic	abnormalities of venous drainage
	atrial morphology (especially atrial septal defects)
	atrial baffle function
	Fontan circulation
	complex atrioventricular junctional morphology
	postatrioventricular valve repair/replacement
	subaortic obstruction
Monitoring	intraoperative
	intensive care
	interventional catherization

Fig. 1.5 A summary of the main indications for a transoesophageal study in children — 1990.

Mark Mitchell, have greatly assisted with routine and research studies in the operating room. Professor John Hess, Dr Nynke Elzenga, and Dr Renate Kaulitz helped with many of the transoesophageal studies in children. Invaluable assistance was provided by our ultrasonographers for all out-patient studies.

We also acknowledge the valuable help of other colleagues in the preparation of illustrations for this book. Many anatomical sections were prepared or photographed by Professor Michael Davies and Dr Louis

Chow at St George's Hospital Medical School, London, and by Dr Siew Yen Ho at the National Heart and Lung Institute, London. We are particularly grateful to Professor Michael Davies for his permission to publish Figs. 3.15, 3.42, 3.45, and 3.50. Dr Robert Jan van Suylen of the Erasmus University Rotterdam and Professor Adriana Gittenberger-de Groot of the University of Leiden also provided specimens and support. The nuclear magnetic-resonance images were obtained by Dr Wim Koops of the Department of Radiology, Academisch Ziekenhuis Rotterdam-Dijkzigt, with the assistance of Dr Michael Scheffer and Dr Jan Heyn Cornel.

Although we owe a great debt to all our colleagues and, indeed, could not have completed this book without their help, the final responsibility is ours. We would also like to thank Gower for their help and understanding in completing this project. Saba Zafar, Fiona Foley, and Anne–Marie Woodruff have dealt with us kindly and have, at all times, coped with the whims of the authors with merely a raised eyebrow or a quizzical smile. If there are deficiencies, which undoubtedly there are, they are of our making and will, hopefully, be corrected should our book come to a second edition.

2

History, development, and technical features

Jos R T C Roelandt

INTRODUCTION

In the early days of echocardiography, difficulties in obtaining good-quality ultrasonic signals through the chest wall stimulated many investigators to search for alternative approaches. Interestingly, most investigators directed their initial efforts towards developing ultrasonic systems for intravascular imaging. As early as 1960, Cieszynski mounted a single element on a catheter to be introduced into the jugular vein. Echoes in the amplitude mode were obtained from cardiac structures in dogs (1). Three years later, Omoto *et al* (2) obtained static cross-sectional images in patients, with a slowly rotating single-element transducer mounted at the tip of a sonde that was introduced into the right atrium via the femoral or jugular vein. A device to monitor the dynamic behaviour of intracardiac dimensions, using a single element at the tip of a catheter capable of scanning in all directions, was reported in 1968 by Carleton and Clark (3). In 1970, Eggleton constructed a catheter with four elements at its tip (4), and produced cross-sectional images of intracardiac structures. The images were reconstructed by computer using slow rotation and electrocardiographic triggering. Two years later, Bom *et al* (5) from the Thoraxcentre of the Erasmus University in Rotterdam described a real-time intracardiac scanner using an electronically phased circular array of 32 elements at the tip of a 9-F catheter.

Problems in manufacturing catheter systems that al-

lowed rapid acquisition in real time of cross-sectional images with good resolution, led to the fading of interest in these innovative approaches. The original impetus and indication for their development also became less important since there were marked improvements in the quality of images obtained by transthoracic echocardiography.

In 1968, a new generation of gastroscopes with a steerable tip became available, which allowed direct contact between the oesophageal wall and an ultrasonic transducer mounted at the tip. The first cardiac investigations with ultrasound via the oesophagus using such a gastroscope were reported by Side and Gosling in 1971 (6). They used a dual-element construction mounted on a standard gastroscope to obtain continuous wave Doppler information about the velocity of cardiac blood flow. Olson and Shelton in 1972 (7,8) measured displacement of the walls of the thoracic aorta and pulmonary artery. Pulsed wave Doppler interrogation from within the oesophagus was described by Daigle *et al* in 1975 (9).

Transoesophageal echocardiography was introduced by Frazin *et al* in 1976 (10). They, and others (26), recorded M-mode echocardiograms of the left ventricle, and used changes in dimensions to monitor its function (Fig. 2.1). Their work did not attract the attention of clinicians because of problems associated with swallowing the probe in conscious patients, and this slowed its development. Since this was less of a

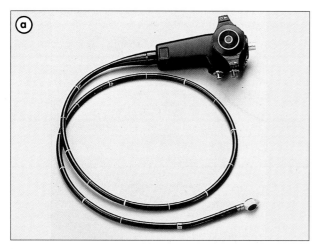

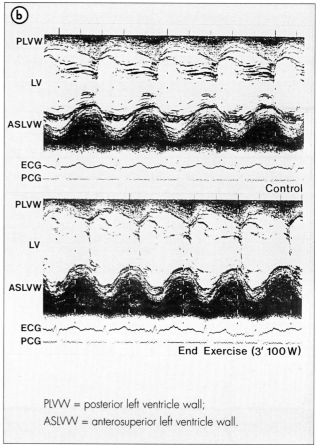

Fig. 2.1 (a) The original transoesophageal M-mode echo transducer system that was developed in Hamburg. (b) M-mode echocardiogram of the left ventricle. The upper-right tracing shows the control M-mode recorded at rest, and the lower panel shows the ventricular dimensions and pattern of contraction at the end of a three-minute period of exercise at a 100-W workload. (Reproduced with permission of Matsumoto M, Hanrath P, Kremer P *et al*. The evaluation of left ventricular function by transoesophageal M-mode exercise echocardiography. In: Hanrath P, Bleifeld W, Souquet J, eds. *Cardiovascular diagnosis by ultrasound*. Martinus Nijhoff Publishers, 1982:227–36).

PLVW = posterior left ventricle wall;
ASLVW = anterosuperior left ventricle wall.

problem for anaesthetists, further research was directed towards the intraoperative monitoring of left ventricular performance. This work was undertaken mainly by Japanese investigators and particularly by Matsumoto and colleagues (11).

Cross-sectional real-time imaging was first reported in 1977 by Hisanaga *et al* (12). They constructed a scanning device that consisted of a rotating single element in an oil-filled balloon mounted at the tip of a gastroscope. Much later, in 1984, a similar system was described by Bertini *et al* (13). One year after their first report, Hisanaga *et al* also described a linear mechanical scanner that was suitable for transoesophageal echocardiographic studies (14). A single element was moved parallel to the long axis of the gastroscope, and 8–20 images/s were obtained.

The introduction of electronic scanners marked the next, and most important step in the development of transoesophageal echocardiography. DiMagno *et al* (1980) constructed a high-frequency (10MHz) linear array that was originally designed for scanning the gastrointestinal tract (15). The electronic phased-array transducer introduced by Souquet *et al* in Hamburg in 1982 represented the definitive breakthrough for the

transoesophageal approach (16), since the frequency of this phased-array transducer was equal to that of standard precordial transducers (2.25MHz).

The initial applications in the USA were the intraoperative monitoring of regional myocardial function in high-risk noncardiac surgical patients, and the recognition of intracardiac air during neurosurgical procedures (17), while European investigators used the system for the diagnosis of cardiac disease in the out-patient clinic (18). The technique rapidly became integrated into diagnostic practice because of its unique advantages over conventional precordial echocardiography (Fig. 2.2).

Subsequently, specific clinical applications evolved which stimulated the production of newer transducers having higher resolution. At the Thoraxcentre, the first phased-array transducer for use via the oesophagus was constructed in 1982. Improvements in micro-miniature cutting and bonding technology resulted in the production of a series of transducers that progressively provided better-quality images. The final design was an array of 64 elements with a frequency of 5.6MHz, which exhibited an extremely low level of artefacts (grating lobes) combined with superior lateral resolution (Figs.

Advantages of Transoesophageal Echocardiography Over Precordial Echocardiography
No obstruction to ultrasound by chest-wall (or intracardiac) structures or lung tissue
Different imaging planes allow visualization of structures not seen from the precordium (for example, thoracic aorta, left atrial appendage)
Improved signal-to-noise ratio allows detection of poor echo-reflective structures (intracardiac tumour, thrombus)
Higher ultrasonic frequencies can be used, providing higher resolution and more detailed images
Reduced target range for pulsed Doppler, and higher sensitivity of colour flow imaging, when studying posterior cardiac structures

Fig. 2.2 Advantages of transoesophageal echocardiography over precordial echocardiography.

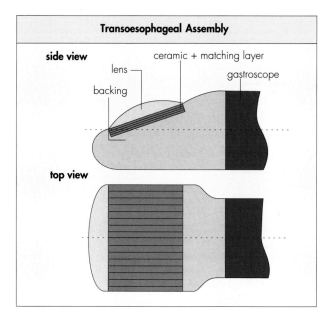

Fig. 2.3 A schematic diagram of a transoesophageal assembly. The lateral view shows the different parts. A transverse beam and a silicon rubber lens are positioned in front of the ceramic transducer elements in order to allow focusing.

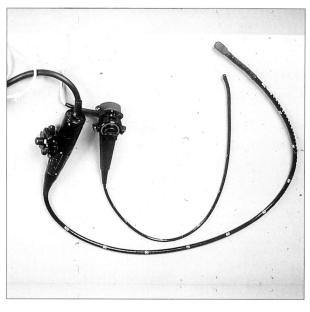

Fig. 2.4 Two different transoesophageal transducer systems. The outer probe is the standard adult probe and the inner probe is a newly developed paediatric probe. The external controls for flexion-extension and sideways movement can be seen.

2.3 and 2.4) (19). Of the wide range of transducers commercially available, this is now the most widely used.

Another important breakthrough occurred in 1987 with the widespread introduction of colour flow mapping combined with high-resolution imaging. This combination led to an explosive and worldwide increase in the application of transoesophageal echocardiography. Later developments have included mechanically driven high-frequency transducers with an annular array, providing both high resolution and the capability for continuous wave Doppler interrogation, a combination not available with systems using phased-array transducers (20,21).

Recently, Omoto *et al* (22) have introduced a bi-plane transoesophageal probe in an attempt to overcome the lack of versatility associated with imaging structures only in transverse planes. Two phased-array transducers, one imaging in transverse and one in longitudinal planes, are mounted side-by-side at the tip of the gastroscope (Fig. 2.5). Each transducer has 32 elements and operates at 5MHz. Cross-sectional images from each transducer are sampled in sequence and stored in memory, and then both cine loops are re-played simultaneously on the monitor screen. The distance between the centres of the two transducers is 1cm. As a consequence, minimal re-positioning of one transducer is required if they are to be used to visualize exactly the same cardiac segment. To overcome the problem of re-positioning, a phased-array matrix is being developed which will allow orthogonal biplane scanning from one transducer kept at a constant position.

The size of standard transoesophageal transducers and gastroscopes is a major limitation to the application of transoesophageal echocardiography in paediatric cardiology, especially in infants. It also limits the use of the technique for prolonged monitoring of patients in intensive care. Thus, efforts have been directed towards the further miniaturization of phased-array transducers and the provision of higher frequencies for improved resolution, so that probes can be used in small children and infants (see *Fig. 2.4*). These systems will extend the range of clinical applications of transoesophageal echocardiography (23). It is possible to use standard adult transoesophageal probes in children more than 20kg in weight if they are anaesthetized, but only small probes can be used safely in children below this weight. Paediatric probes will also influence other applications of echocardiography, such as the development of miniature finger-tip transducers for intraoperative imaging from the epicardial surface.

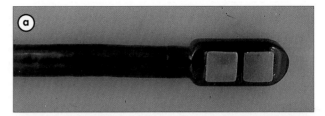

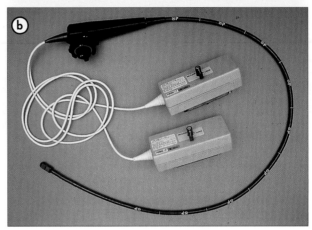

Fig. 2.5 (a) The tip of a biplane imaging system currently in use. Two transducers are mounted: the more distal tranducer images in the transverse plane and the proximal one in the longitudinal plane. (b) The biplane probe. Note the two sets of connectors to the ultrasound machine. Biplane real-time imaging is currently not possible, but this may be simulated by recording one plane into the cine loop and subsequently displaying this in a side-by-side manner with the second plane using a split-screen format. Dual-matrix arrays may be developed, which will make this feasible.

Fig. 2.6 Transoesophageal echocardiographic systems —1990.

Transoesophageal Echocardiographic Systems — 1990					
Manufacturer transducer/ gastroscope	Frequency (MHz)	Elements (n)	Scanhead width/thickness/ length (mm)	Gastroscope diameter (mm)	length (cm)
Acuson/acmi	5	64	14/11/28	10,5	110
Aloka/Olympus	5	48	14/12/19	9	100
	5*	48	7/7.5/16	6,8	100
biplane	5	32 X 2	10.5/14/48	9	100
ATL/acmi	4.8	48	14/10/30	9,5	100
biplane	4.8	48 X 2	—/12/—	10	110
Hewlett-Packard/acmi	5	64	14/11/27	10,5	
Siemens/acmi	5	64	14/11/16	10,5	100
Toshiba/Mashida	3, 7	48	10/12/48	10 (+fibreoptics)	105
	5, 6	64	14/11/16	10,5	100
Vingmed/shott †	5	—	13/13	11	100
	5–7, 5*		11/11	9	100
			11/11	6	100

acmi = American cystoscopic makers, inc.
* = paediatric probes
† = mechanical annular phased array — facilities for pulsed and continuous wave Doppler

The most recent development has been the modification of oesophageal probes so that they incorporate a series of electrodes which can be used for atrial pacing. Left ventricular wall motion can be monitored during the onset of ischaemia induced by pacing (see *Chapter 10*).

CHARACTERISTICS OF TRANSOESOPHAGEAL SYSTEMS

The basic construction of all transoesophageal transducers is similar. A commercially available gastroscope or bronchoscope is adapted by fitting a phased-array transducer at its tip for imaging in the transverse axis. The fibreoptics, together with the channels used for suction and biopsy, are removed to provide space for the electronic connections for the transducer, but the normal guidance controls are retained, giving the tip at least 90° of anteroposterior mobility and up to 70° of lateral mobility in each direction. In one probe (Toshiba/Mashida), the fibreoptics and channel for insufflating air are retained, so that the transducer can be positioned under direct endoscopic control. The probe cannot be used for simultaneous upper gastrointestinal endoscopy since it has no channels for suction or for taking biopsies. Most investigators agree, however, that fibreoptics are unnecessary when performing transoesophageal echocardiography.

Most transducers provide images with a sector of 90°. The number of elements varies, but the operating frequency is typically centered around 5MHz. The characteristics of the different systems that are available commercially are listed in Fig. 2.6, and some of the probes are illustrated in Fig. 2.7. In the Vingmed system, an annular phased-array transducer and a miniature motor for its mechanical rotation are both incorporated into the tip of the gastroscope. Annular phased-array transducers are capable of providing frequencies of up to 7.5MHz and continuous wave Doppler (21). This feature is not available at present from linear phased-array systems.

At present, there are three types of paediatric probes: the Aloka probe, the experimental design produced by the Thoraxcentre, and the mechanical probe made by Vingmed. The two phased-array probes are mounted on paediatric fibreoptic bronchoscopes that allow angulation of the tip only anteriorly or posteriorly, but experience in small children has shown that this is sufficient to obtain all standard imaging planes, particularly since small children seem to have a relatively larger oesophageal window than adults.

The length of adult gastroscopes varies between 70 and 110cm. The shaft is marked at intervals of 10cm. A longer cable is desirable when the probe is being used for intraoperative monitoring or in the intensive care unit, so that access to the patient for other purposes is not impeded by the echocardiographic machine.

TRANSOESOPHAGEAL COLOUR FLOW MAPPING

The basic advantages of the use of the transoesophageal approach include a reduced target range for many structures when compared with the transthoracic approach. This results in an improvement in the sensitivity of colour flow mapping and in the ability to encode a wider range of velocities, without causing aliasing. Within this range, however, the same limitations apply as are present during colour flow mapping from the precordium (24). Since there are constraints on the time available for processing the signals from the transducer, a compromise has to be made between the frame rate, the density of the scan lines, the frequency of resolution, and the depth of scanning. Thus, to obtain the optimal colour flow maps of a particular area of interest, the depth of scanning should be reduced to the minimum required to include that area, and the sector of the colour encoding should be kept narrow, if possible.

More detailed information about the optimization of colour flow maps is available in other published textbooks (25). Other specific technical points are discussed throughout this book when appropriate.

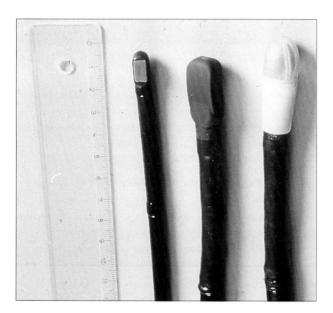

Fig. 2.7 Three of the currently available transoesophageal probes. Left: A mechanical probe (Vingmed). Centre: A standard adult transverse-plane phased-array probe (Hewlett-Packard). Right: One of the paediatric probes that is currently used (Aloka). For the dimensions of these probes, see *Fig. 2.6*.

SAFETY CONSIDERATIONS

Considerations for safety include the control of electrical hazards and temperature. Internationally accepted standards prescribe a leakage of current of less than 50mA at 50MHz and 220V. Both trauma (cuts and bites) and chemical agents used in cleaning the probe can cause deterioration and breaks in the coating of insulating material. Such breaks may not be apparent on simple visual inspection. Thus, recommendations made by the manufacturer, both for cleaning the probe and for checking it regularly for electrical leakage, must be adhered to rigorously. A thermocouple has been added at the tip of some transducers to monitor temperature, especially during periods of prolonged use for monitoring. Its necessity, however, has not been generally accepted. A reasonable recommendation would be that the transducer should be switched off when there is an increase of 2 or 3°C, or more, in the temperature at the tip of the probe relative to the patient's temperature.

REFERENCES

1. Cieszynski T. Intracardiac method for the investigation of the structure of the heart with the aid of ultrasonics. *Arch Immum Ter Dosw* 1960;**8**:551–7.

2. Omoto R, Atsumi K, Suma K *et al.* Ultrasonic intravenous sonde — 2nd report. *Med Ultrason (Jpn)* 1963;**1**:11.

3. Carleton RA, Clark JG. Measurements of left ventricular diameter in the dog by cardiac catheterization. Validation and physiologic meaningfulness of an ultrasonic technique. *Circ Res* 1968;**22**:545–8.

4. Eggleton RC, Townsend C, Herrick J *et al.* Ultrasonic visualization of left ventricular dynamics. *Ultrasonics* 1970;**17**:143–53.

5. Bom N, Lancée CT, Van Egmond FC *et al.* An ultrasonic intracardiac scanner. *Ultrasonics* 1972;**10**:72–6.

6. Side CG, Gosling RG. Non-surgical assessment of cardiac function. *Nature* 1971;**232**:335.

7. Olson RM, Shelton DK. A nondestructive technique to measure wall displacement in the thoracic aorta. *J Appl Physiol* 1972;**32**:147–51.

8. Shelton DK, Olson RM. A nondestructive technique to measure pulmonary artery diameter and its pulsatile variations. *J Appl Physiol* 1972;**33**:542–4.

9. Daigle RE, Miller CW, Histand MB *et al.* Nontraumatic aortic blood flow sensing using an ultrasonic eosophageal probe. *J Appl Physiol* 1975;**38**:6.

10. Frazin L, Talan JV, Stephanides L *et al.* Esophageal echocardiography [Abstract]. *Circulation* 1976;**54**:102.

11. Matsumoto M, Oka Y, Strom J *et al.* Application of transesophageal echocardiography to continuous intraoperative monitoring of left ventricular performance. *Am J Cardiol* 1980;**46**:95–105.

12. Hisanaga K, Hisanaga A, Nagata K, Yoshida S. A new transesophageal real-time two-dimensional echocardiographic system using a flexible tube and its clinical application. *Proc Jpn Soc of Ultrasonics in Med* 1977;**32**:43–4.

13. Bertini A, Masotti L, Zuppiroli A, Cecchi F. Rotating probe for transoesophageal cross-sectional echocardiography. *J Nucl Med Allied Sci* 1984;**28**:115–21.

14. Hisanaga K, Hisanaga A, Ichie Y. A new transesophageal real-time linear scanner and initial clinical results. *Proc Jpn Soc of Ultrasonics in Med* 1978;**35**:115–6.

15. DiMagno EP, Buxton JL, Regan PT *et al.* Ultrasonic endoscope. *Lancet* 1980;**i**:629.

16. Souquet J, Hanrath P, Zitelli L *et al.* Transesophageal phased array for imaging the heart. *IEEE Trans Biomed Engineer* 1982;**29**:707.

17. Kremer P, Schwartz L, Cahalan MK *et al.* Intraoperative monitoring of left ventricular performance by transesophageal M-mode and 2-D echocardiography [Abstract]. *Am J Cardiol* 1982;**49**:956.

18. Hanrath P, Kremer P, Langenstein BA *et al.* Transösophageale Echokardiographie: Ein neues Verfahren zur dynamischen Ventrikelfunktionsanalyse. *Dtsch Med Wochenschr* 1981;**106**:523–5.

19. Lancée CT, De Jong N, Bom N. Design and construction of an esophageal phased array probe. *Med Prog Technol* 1988;**13**:139–48.

20. Angelsen BAJ, Hoem H, Dorum S *et al.* High-frequency annular array transesophageal probe for high-resolution imaging and continuous wave Doppler measurements. In: Erbel R *et al*, eds. *Transesophageal Echocardiography.* Heidelberg, Berlin: Springer–Verlag, 1989:13–20.

21. Chapman JV, Vandenbogaerde J, Everaert JA, Angelsen BAJ. The initial clinical evaluation of a transesophageal system with pulsed Doppler, continuous wave Doppler, and color flow imaging based on an annular array technology. *Int J Cardiac Imaging* 1989;**5**:9–16.

22. Omoto R, Kyo S, Matsumura M *et al.* Recent technological progress in transesophageal color Doppler flow imaging with special reference to newly developed biplane and pediatric probes. In: Erbel R *et al*, eds. *Transesophageal Echocardiography.* Heidelberg, Berlin: Springer–Verlag, 1989:21–26.

23. Stümper OFW, Elzenga NJ, Hess J, Sutherland GR. Transoesophageal echocardiography in children with congenital heart disease — an initial experience. *J Am Coll Cardiol* 1990;**16**(2):433–41.

24. Omoto R. *Colour atlas of real-time two-dimensional Doppler echocardiography (2nd edition).* Tokyo: Shinan-To Chiryo Co. Ltd, 1987.

25. Kisslo J, Adams DB, Belkin RN. *Doppler color flow imaging.* New York: Churchill Livingstone, 1988.

The normal examination: technique, imaging planes, and anatomical features

Alan G Fraser
Robert H Anderson

INTRODUCTION

Transoesophageal echocardiography is a semi-invasive investigation that can be performed quickly and with minimal risk, even in seriously ill patients. Occasionally, however, it may cause considerable discomfort or distress, particularly if the operator is inexperienced. In order to ensure that the investigation is performed safely, and for appropriate indications, it should only be carried out by cardiologists or other doctors who have had adequate training and experience in both cardiac ultrasound and upper gastrointestinal endoscopy. A sound understanding of the potential and limitations of the technique, and a precise knowledge of the anatomy of the heart and great vessels, are required in order to appreciate when it is likely that clinically useful information will be obtained. Transoesophageal echocardiography demonstrates many of the features of the heart and great vessels in much greater anatomical detail than is possible with conventional transthoracic imaging, because of the proximity of the oesophagus to these structures. It is essential, therefore, to understand the normal variations in anatomy, as well as the appearances in disease.

Before undertaking transoesophageal echocardiographic studies independently, an operator should have performed endoscopies under the guidance of a skilled endoscopist; at the Thoraxcentre, we recommend a total of 50 studies. This is most useful for learning the techniques of atraumatic intubation of the oesophagus, and for acquiring expertise in the manipulation of endoscopic probes. In addition, it is useful for a transoesophageal echocardiographer to have experience of the range and appearance of disease in the oesophagus and stomach in order to appreciate the possible dangers of manipulating the probe with excessive force, and the types of abnormalities that may be encountered at the gastroesophageal junction. In particular, effective manipulation of the probe within the gastric fundus in order to retain good contact between the surface of the transducer and the mucosa, and to produce high-quality images, is easier when the operator has a clear mental image of the stomach and the manipulation of a probe within it. The purpose of this chapter is to provide the necessary anatomic background for transoesophageal echocardiography, together with details of equipment and technique, thereby supplementing and expanding the anatomical–echocardiographic correlations already performed (1–3).

PERSONNEL AND EQUIPMENT

Transoesophageal echocardiographic studies should only be performed by a qualified physician. A nurse or trained assistant should be available to help with the

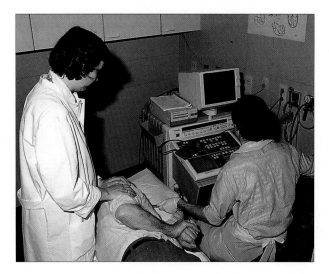

Fig. 3.1 An out-patient study in progress at the Thoraxcentre. The doctor has access to the controls of the ultrasound machine, and is assisted by a trained echocardiographer. Piped suction facilities are on the wall next to the machine.

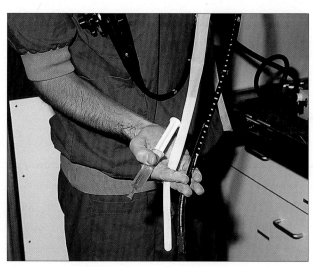

Fig. 3.2 Equipment used for a transoesophageal study. The long rubber sheath contains ultrasound gel, and after it has been placed over the probe, its surface is lubricated with sterile anaesthetic gel.

care of the patient. It is also helpful if an ultrasound technician can operate the controls of the ultrasound machine. Facilities for suction should be immediately available (Fig. 3.1), and access to resuscitation equipment should be rapid.

Before each study is carried out, the guidance controls of the probe should be checked. The normal full range of movement of the tip of the probe is 125° of forward flexion, 95° of extension from a neutral central position, and 95° of lateral tilt in either direction. Between studies, the probe should be cleaned thoroughly and washed in detergent, and then sterilized according to the manufacturer's guidelines, similar to the practice for standard nonimmersible endoscopes (4). This usually consists of immersion of the shaft of the probe in a 2% solution of glutaraldehyde for four minutes. Care should be taken since glutaraldehyde solution is allergenic. The room in which the probe is sterilized should be well ventilated in order to prevent the sensitization of staff to glutaraldehyde. The handle and steering controls of the probe should be wiped with a 70% solution of alcohol since they cannot be immersed. Alcohol should not be applied to the tip of the probe because it may penetrate the rubber seals and damage the transducer. Transoesophageal probes that combine endoscopic imaging with echocardiographic facilities must be cleaned more thoroughly since they contain a channel for the insufflation of air.

An alternative method of using a transoesophageal probe is to insert it into a long rubber sheath that contains some ultrasound gel at its tip (Fig. 3.2). If this procedure is followed, disinfection of the probe between successive examinations may not be required, although, to our knowledge, no detailed bacteriological or virological studies of the efficacy of this method for protecting the probe have yet been performed. The probe should still be cleaned and washed between examinations, and disinfection is advisable as a precaution at the end of each day. If any holes are found in the sheath when the probe is withdrawn after an examination, then the shaft of the probe should be sterilized.

There is no reason why transoesophageal echocardiography cannot be performed, if required for an important clinical indication, in a patient with AIDS or antibodies to the human immunodeficiency virus or to hepatitis B. The human immunodeficiency virus is inactivated by the commonly used disinfectants (5), and nowadays, the same procedures are recommended for cleaning endoscopic probes after all patients, on the assumption that it is not possible to identify, in advance, patients who are infectious (4). The recommendations for cleaning and disinfecting a transoesophageal probe should always be followed scrupulously; risks of cross infection, however, appear to be very low.

PREPARATION OF THE PATIENT

When transoesophageal echocardiography is planned in a conscious patient, he or she should be fasted for four hours beforehand in order to reduce the risk of vomiting and aspiration. The procedure should be explained in detail, and reassurance should be given in advance about the possibility of breathing normally while the probe is in place. Informed consent should be obtained.

Transoesophageal echocardiography can be performed without sedation but, in our experience, most patients opt to have sedation if it is offered routinely. It is particularly important to use sedation in younger and less-stoical patients, and when it is anticipated that the examination may last longer than normal or that subsequent serial studies may be indicated. A short-acting benzodiazepine, such as midazolam (0.05mg/kg, usual dose 2.5–5mg), may be given intravenously; larger doses may cause unconsciousness, although they also produce anterograde amnesia. Midazolam has a half-life of three hours (6) compared with approximately 20 hours for diazepam, and it is twice as potent. Paradoxically, however, its effects may wear off more slowly than those of diazepam (7,8), and so patients should be advised to rest and not to drive for at least four hours afterwards. Midazolam may cause a reduction in minute volume (7), and it has a slight hypotensive effect (9).

Many patients develop a marked response of the sympathetic nervous system to a transoesophageal investigation, and so it is important to use sedation to try to prevent this in patients who might be at risk from any sudden haemodynamic changes; obvious examples include patients with acute aortic dissection (in whom an increase in blood pressure might lead to an extension of the dissection) (10) and patients with heart failure (in whom excessive sedation and hypotension need to be avoided).

Copious secretion of saliva may occur during a transoesophageal study. In order to prevent this, some investigators advocate that an anticholinergic agent such as glycopyrrolate, should also be given. In our experience, this is rarely necessary as long as the patient is positioned during the study so that any saliva that accumulates in the mouth can trickle out, and as long as suction is used when this is not sufficient. If patients ask for treatment to dry up their saliva, the usual dose that is administered intravenously is 0.2mg, or 0.5µg/kg. Glycopyrrolate is more effective than atropine in drying salivary secretions, and it has fewer subjective side effects and no significant haemodynamic effects (11).

The mucosal surfaces of the soft palate, the posterior half of the tongue, and the hypopharynx, should all be anaesthetized topically by the administration of lignocaine (lidocaine) spray (1–2%). Between three and five puffs are usually sufficient. Peak effects occur within 2–5 minutes, and the duration of anaesthesia is between 30 and 45 minutes (12). It should be remembered that good topical anaesthesia will not alleviate pain or discomfort caused by pressure and distortion of adjacent structures.

There is no standard practice for antibiotic prophylaxis. No cases of infective endocarditis attributable to transoesophageal echocardiography have yet been reported, but this remains a theoretical risk. One case of clinically apparent bacteraemia after transoesophageal echocardiography has been reported (13), but the chance of bacteraemia or septicaemia occurring is probably less than that after an upper gastrointestinal study in which the duodenum is entered and biopsies are taken — which is low (14). Nevertheless, mucosal trauma can occur during an echocardiographic study, and occasionally there may be streaks of blood on the probe when it is removed. In addition, haematomas have been observed around the posterior pharynx following a technically difficult introduction of a transoesophageal echocardiographic probe. It has been reported recently that bacteraemia may be provoked by transoesophageal echocardiography in between 7% (7/100) and 17% (4/24) of patients (15,16), most commonly involving organisms that are commensal in the mouth and pharynx. It seems reasonable, therefore, to recommend that antibiotic prophylaxis should be given, at least to all high-risk patients (those with prosthetic heart valves or other foreign material in the circulation, those with a history of infective endocarditis, and those with a compromised immune response). The current guidelines recommend intravenous or intramuscular amoxycillin or vancomycin (17). It is less clear, however, what should be done in patients who are investigated for suspected endocarditis, for example involving a prosthetic valve, especially if they have a fever but negative blood cultures. At present, we do not give such patients antibiotics.

Artificial teeth and any other dental appliances should be removed before the study. Patients with their own teeth should be given a biteguard to place between their teeth so that the probe is protected. Endoscopic control systems are very responsive but not very robust, so they are likely to break down if the probe is not looked after properly, or if it is subjected to excessive stress. Manufacturers recommend that probes should be kept hanging up when not in use.

SAFETY AND COMPLICATIONS

Transoesophageal echocardiography has been performed for approximately 10 years, and thousands of studies have been completed, virtually all of them without significant complications. In our experience at the Thoraxcentre, of the first 1,100 patients to be studied, there were no serious complications (18).

A small proportion of patients cannot tolerate the

study and either gag so much that the probe cannot be inserted or else forcibly remove the probe before the study has been completed. These problems can be minimized if there is careful and sympathetic explanation before the start of the study about the sensations to be expected, if careful and good local anaesthesia is applied, and if intravenous sedation is used. The option always remains of performing transoesophageal echocardiography under heavy sedation or even under general anaesthesia, if it is deemed essential for the management of a particular patient.

Experience of the procedure in 10,419 patients has been reviewed in a co-operative study involving 15 European centres (19). The investigation was impossible in 201 patients (1.9%) because the probe could not be inserted. It was incomplete in a further 90 patients (0.9%) because the study had to be terminated prematurely after the development of complications. These complications included intolerance of the procedure (65 patients), bronchospasm (6 patients), tachyarrhythmias (6 patients), vomiting (5 patients), hypoxia (2 patients), complete heart block (1 patient), angina (1 patient), and pharyngeal bleeding (1 patient). There was one death when a patient with an oesophageal tumour developed haematemesis and mediastinitis after oesophageal perforation. Outside Europe, other serious complications have occurred, but in general, the procedure is very safe (20). Nevertheless, a careful history concerning upper gastrointestinal problems should be taken in all patients when consent is sought. If symptoms that are suggestive of severe oesophagitis, hiatus hernia, or oesophageal diverticulum, are reported, the opinion of a gastroenterologist should be requested before the investigation is carried out. Oesophageal varices and oesophageal stricture are contraindications to transoesophageal echocardiography, and an investigation should be postponed in patients who have a severe infection of the upper respiratory tract. Since arrhythmias can occur (21), electrocardiographic monitoring is mandatory. A transoesophageal echocardiographic probe should never be inserted with force, and it should not be advanced while maintained in extreme flexion, extension, or lateral tilt. The guidance controls on the probe should always be unlocked when the probe is being inserted. The tip of the probe should never be maintained in an imaging position with extreme force, since contact pressures of up to 60mmHg can be produced (22) and these might damage the oesophageal or gastric mucosa. The usual contact pressure, however, is much less.

There is no evidence that the ultrasonic output of a transoesophageal transducer causes any local injury to adjacent tissue. Several commercially available probes monitor temperature at their tip so that if the temperature rises above a preset cut-off level (usually 39°C), the probe is either switched off automatically or the operator is warned. In order to minimize any possible thermal injury to the oesophagus, the probe should be switched off when it is not in use and it is left in position for any period of time, for example in the operating room. These problems are not normally encountered during a standard out-patient study, which should be completed within 10 or 15 minutes.

THE NORMAL EXAMINATION

The patient should lie on his or her left side, with the operator opposite (see *Fig. 3.1*). The probe is best introduced under active steering (Fig. 3.3) but with the lateral tilt control locked to avoid deviation into the lateral (piriform) recesses of the pharynx. Free flexion and extension of the probe should be allowed. The tip of the probe is flexed as it reaches the posterior wall of the nasopharynx to direct it downwards, and then immediately hyperextended as it is advanced further, so that it is directed preferentially backwards towards the oesophagus and away from the glottis and trachea (Fig. 3.4). Resistance is felt once the tip reaches the cricopharyngeus (the upper oesophageal sphincter). The probe should then be kept in a constant position with gentle pressure being maintained against the resistance while the patient is asked to swallow voluntarily; this relaxes the cricopharyngeus, and when this occurs, the probe slips forward easily and without resistance into the oesophagus. The lateral guidance system of the probe should then be unlocked and, thereafter, further passage of the probe is possible without difficulty or undue discomfort, although it may be helpful if the patient swallows again while the probe is being advanced more deeply. Some patients become distressed soon after the endoscope has been introduced. It is therefore helpful to pause for several minutes without attempting to advance the probe, while the patient becomes tolerant of it and settles to a regular pattern of breathing through the nose. This is easier if the patient's neck is fully flexed.

The gastroesophageal junction (the cardia) is reached at approximately 40cm from the teeth. Passage of the tip of the probe beyond this level, and its manipulation in the stomach, may cause subjective discomfort, while manipulation within the oesophagus itself rarely causes any symptoms. If the patient is comfortable, the probe may first be advanced to the stomach. All the standard transoesophageal echocardiographic imaging planes can then be obtained as the probe is gradually

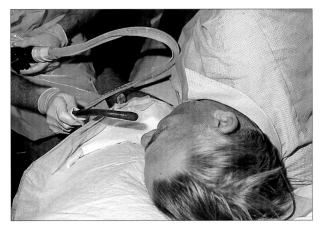

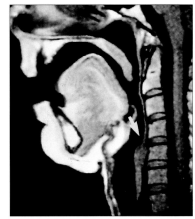

Fig. 3.4 Magnetic-resonance image of a midline sagittal section through the nasopharynx and upper neck. The upper end of the oesophagus, just above the sphincter, is indicated by the arrow.

Fig. 3.3 The probe, flexed before it is introduced.

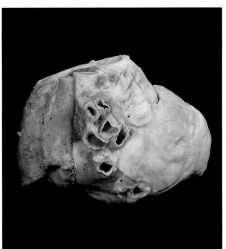

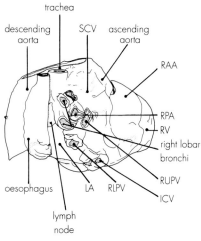

trachea
descending aorta
SCV
ascending aorta
RAA
RPA
RV
right lobar bronchi
RUPV
ICV
oesophagus
LA
RLPV
lymph node

Fig. 3.5 The posterior aspect of the heart viewed from behind and slightly to the right. The tissue around the oesophagus has been dissected to show its relationship to the posterior surface of the left atrium, and the descending thoracic aorta. Part of the surface of the left atrium is concealed behind a large lymph node that is lying beneath the carina.

withdrawn. In patients who are distressed, however, it is advisable to carry out the recording of the transgastric images and the study of the distal descending thoracic aorta, at the end of the investigation, and to concentrate initially on what is most important for answering the clinical question that led to the examination.

A conventional transoesophageal echocardiographic probe has a single phased-array ultrasonic transducer mounted at its tip to produce images in the transverse plane with an arc of 90°; these images are orientated at right angles to the shaft of the probe. As the oesophagus passes through the middle mediastinum, it is directly related to the posterior aspect of the left atrium (Fig. 3.5). The stomach is separated from the ventricular mass only by the diaphragm (Fig. 3.6). Images obtained from the oesophagus as it passes behind the left atrium are similar to basal short-axis imaging planes obtained from a left parasternal approach during a precordial echocardiographic study. From the fundus of the stomach, short-axis views are obtained through

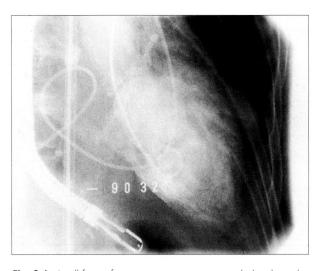

Fig. 3.6 A still frame from a cineangiogram recorded in the right anterior oblique projection, during left ventriculography in a patient who was undergoing balloon aortic valvotomy. The tip of the probe is positioned in the fundus of the stomach (using lateral tilt as well as flexion), at the site from which a clear transgastric image of the left ventricle was obtained.

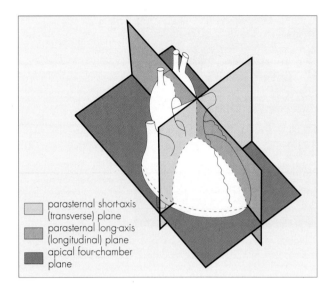

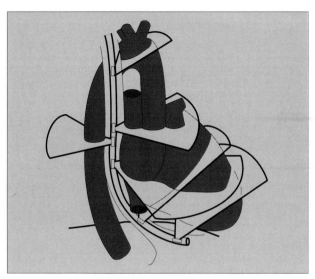

Fig. 3.7 Diagram of the heart with the three standard orthogonal imaging planes. Transoesophageal echocardiography with a transverse planar transducer provides images in the short-axis and four-chamber planes, but not in the long-axis (parasternal) plane.

Fig. 3.8 Schematic representation of the heart, great vessels, and oesophagus, with the positions of the transoesophageal transducer from which the five main series of imaging planes are obtained.

the ventricles. The proximity of the probe to the heart and great vessels, and the absence of restrictions to imaging caused by the sternum and ribs, allows images of much greater quality and definition to be produced, together with images of structures that are inaccessible from precordial windows. Considerable downwards angulation of the transducer from a site posterior to the left atrium produces images that are similar to apical four-chamber views, but approached from the opposite side of the heart. From these three basic positions, a standard transoesophageal echocardiographic probe can therefore view the heart in imaging planes corresponding to two of the usual three approaches from the precordium (Fig. 3.7). Images corresponding to the normal parasternal long-axis planes cannot be produced. This is, however, now possible with the biplane transoesophageal probes.

The standard imaging planes obtained with a conventional single transducer (mounted to image transverse planes), and their anatomical correlations, are discussed initially. The manipulation of the probe is described for an operator who is facing the patient. The standard longitudinal plane cross-sectional images obtained with a biplane probe are subsequently reviewed.

The transducer is positioned at five main sites during a transoesophageal study, to obtain the standard views (Fig. 3.8). These positions are the fundus of the stomach, the distal oesophagus near the gastroesophageal junction, the midoesophagus opposite the middle of the left atrium (for four-chamber views) and

opposite the upper left atrium (for basal planes through the great vessels), and posteriorly and laterally directed positions from which to study the thoracic aorta.

TRANSGASTRIC IMAGES OF THE VENTRICLES

Passage of the tip of the probe beyond the gastroesophageal junction is usually recognized by the appearance of echoes from the liver. If the probe is advanced slightly further, ultrasonic images may be lost as the tip becomes free in the stomach. Images can be restored by flexing the tip considerably and withdrawing it slightly to bring its surface back into contact with the mucosa in the fundus. Anticlockwise rotation usually brings the heart into view (position I, Fig. 3.8). The colon and other intra-abdominal organs may also be identified. Since the heart lies predominantly over the left hemidiaphragm, and is orientated from posteromedial to anterolateral, additional tilt of the tip of the transoesophageal probe is often required to produce a true short-axis image with a circular cross section of the left ventricle. In such a cross section, the papillary muscles supporting the mitral valve are demonstrated, with the posteromedial one at the top of the image as it is displayed on the screen, and the anterolateral one to the right (Figs. 3.9 and 3.10). The arc of circle between them is often shown as 90°, although it is much greater than this (130°) in reality. Such a cross-sectional image demonstrates components of the left ventricular

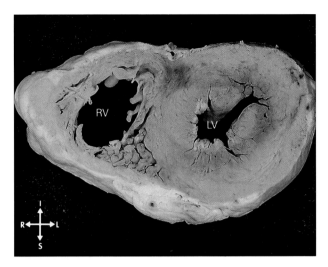

Fig. 3.9 Transverse section through the ventricles, orientated as it is imaged from the stomach. The inferior wall of the left ventricle and the posteromedial papillary muscle lie at the top of the image, and the anterior wall is displayed at the bottom of the image. The left ventricle is hypertrophied.

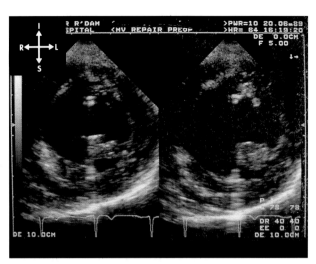

Fig. 3.10 Transgastric images of a normal left ventricle, in systole (on the left) and diastole.

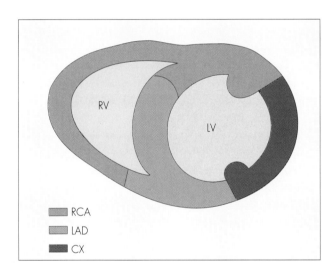

Fig. 3.11 Diagram of the ventricles as imaged from the stomach, demonstrating the areas of myocardium that are supplied by the three major coronary arteries when there is a normal, dominant right coronary artery.

myocardium supplied by all three major coronary arteries (Fig. 3.11). The septum and anterior wall (including the anterolateral papillary muscle) are supplied by the left anterior descending (interventricular) artery. The lateral wall is supplied by the circumflex artery. The posterior wall, part of the posterior ventricular septum, and the posteromedial papillary muscle are supplied by the right coronary artery when this is dominant (as in 90% or more of normal subjects). When the left coronary artery is dominant, it supplies these latter structures through the terminal branches of the circumflex artery. The endocardium is usually seen very clearly, and the epicardium can also be identified, so these views are excellent for analysing left ventricular function. Both regional wall motion and thickening can be studied, as described in *Chapter 12*.

With experience and considerable manipulation, it may be possible, from the stomach, to scan the left ventricle in serial cross sections down to the apex, although it becomes increasingly difficult to maintain good contact of the probe, and these attempts may cause discomfort. It is even possible, on rare occasions, when the tip of the probe is advanced to the apex and flexed maximally, to obtain an apical four-chamber view during a transoesophageal echocardiographic study. While the probe is in the fundus, it may also be possible to demonstrate the inlet and body of the right ventricle, by applying considerable lateral angulation of the probe towards the right, and some clockwise rotation (Fig. 3.12). These, however, are both unconventional imaging planes, and since even with experience they can only be obtained in a minority of patients, it is not recommended that time is spent in trying to reproduce them. The apical plane in particular has no inherent advantages over its precordial equivalent which can usually be produced with much less trouble.

Since the quality of the images of the ventricles is very high, minor variations in anatomy may be appreciated more readily during transoesophageal studies than precordial ones. These variations include the presence

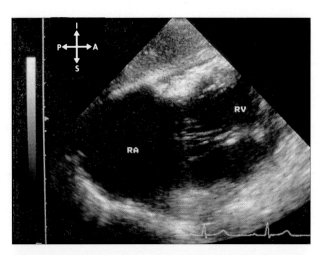

Fig. 3.12 Long-axis image of the right ventricle obtained with a transverse transducer from the stomach. The liver is traversed at the top of the image, and the diaphragmatic surface of the right ventricle is seen. The leaflets of the tricuspid valve are the inferior (at the top) and anterosuperior ones.

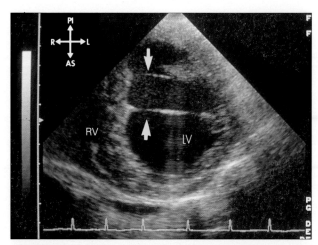

Fig. 3.13 Oblique section through the left ventricle obtained when the transducer was positioned near the gastroesophageal junction. Two false tendons are shown (arrowed), stretching across the left ventricular cavity.

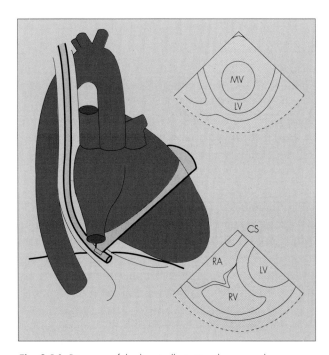

Fig. 3.14 Diagram of the heart, illustrating the general orientation of the imaging planes that can be studied when the transducer is in the lower oesophagus.

of left ventricular false tendons (Fig. 3.13) and the observation of insignificant variations in the positions of the papillary muscles.

When the transducer is positioned fairly high in the stomach with some anticlockwise rotation, the left ventricular outflow tract and the proximal ascending aorta may be identified. This is the best transoesophageal view in which to interrogate the outflow tract with pulsed Doppler or colour flow mapping.

DISTAL OESOPHAGEAL VIEWS

The orientation of distal oesophageal views is indicated in Fig. 13.14.

The coronary sinus and tricuspid valve

As the probe is pulled back from the fundus of the stomach to the level of the gastroesophageal junction, the coronary sinus becomes visible in the posterior atrioventricular groove. In order to demonstrate the coronary sinus most clearly along its length, and also to show its orifice, some tilt of the tip of the probe towards the right side of the patient may be required. These scan planes usually include the left atrium and the right heart in the region of the tricuspid valve but, since the coronary sinus lies on the outer surface of the heart, they may exclude the left ventricle (Fig. 3.15). Movement of the heart with respiration may temporarily take the coronary sinus out of the scan plane, particularly if the sinus is not enlarged, but often a position can be maintained that is stable enough for pulsed Doppler signals to be recorded from within the sinus (Fig. 3.16).

This view is also one of the best for imaging the tricuspid valve. It is difficult with transoesophageal imaging in the transverse plane to study all three leaflets and to interrogate their zone of coaptation, but usually, the function of the tricuspid valve can be assessed quite well. The septal and anterosuperior leaflets are seen in the planes in which the coronary sinus is demonstrated (Fig. 3.17).

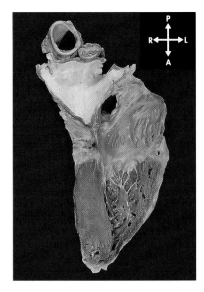

Fig. 3.15 Anatomical section in a transverse plane that passes through the orifice of the coronary sinus. Only the inferior surface of the left atrium is seen on the left side of the heart. This section also demonstrates the junction of the inferior caval vein within the right atrium.

The basal views through the right atrium are also the best for studying venous inflow from the inferior caval vein (see *Fig. 3.15*). Although it is hard to image its exact site of entry, it is possible to scan from the vein into the right atrium and assess abnormalities of flow through it. It is quite common to identify a flap of tissue producing a valve-like structure. This is a remnant of the Eustachian valve which, during fetal life, directs oxygenated blood that is returning from the placenta via the inferior caval vein preferentially across the oval foramen. It is seen in the floor of the right atrium near the orifice of the inferior caval vein (Fig. 3.18).

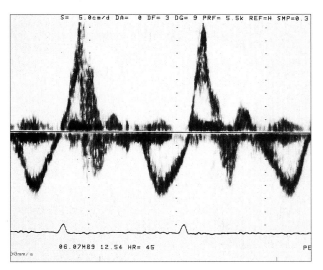

Fig. 3.16 Pulsed Doppler recording of flow within the coronary sinus in a patient who had severe tricuspid regurgitation. There is retrograde regurgitant flow into the coronary sinus (towards the transducer) during ventricular systole, so that normal forward drainage only occurs during diastole.

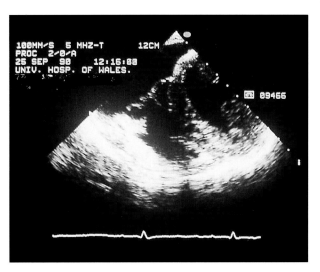

Fig. 3.17 Image of the distal coronary sinus, the right atrium, and the tricuspid inlet. This plane demonstrates the septal and anterosuperior leaflets of the tricuspid valve, and the left ventricle in short axis.

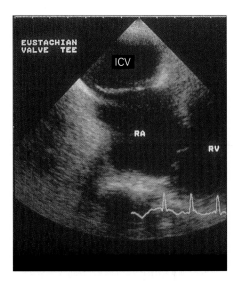

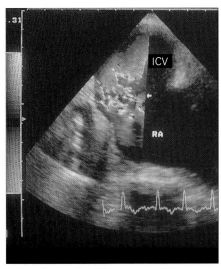

Fig. 3.18 The Eustachian valve is seen as a large, thin, and mobile flap around the margin of the inferior caval vein, where it communicates with the cavity of the right atrium. In this patient, the valve was large enough to cause turbulence of venous inflow, but there was no obstruction, and this pattern was a normal variant. Compare with *Fig. 3.15*.

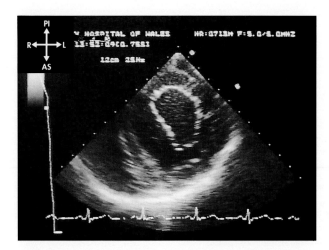

Fig. 3.19 Image through the mitral valve in short axis near its orifice. The tip of the probe is opposite the coronary sinus.

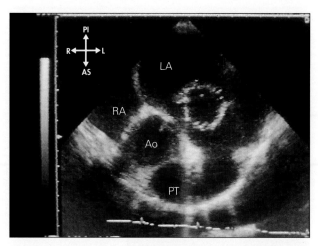

Fig. 3.21 Cross-sectional image through the 'floor' of the left atrium, obtained by tilting the transducer upwards from a position low in the oesophagus. The sewing ring of a prosthetic mitral valve is seen in profile, and anterosuperiorly, the left atrial appendage is imaged. The colour flow map that was obtained in this patient in a similar imaging plane, is shown in *Fig. 8.9b.*

The short axis of the mitral valve/floor of the left atrium

If the tip of the probe is pulled back a little and rotated slightly in an anticlockwise direction from the view that images the coronary sinus, and then flexed anteriorly, it is possible to image the orifice of the mitral valve (Fig. 3.19) or to examine the floor of the left atrium just above the orifice (Fig. 3.20). These views approximate to the standard short-axis images obtained from the left parasternal approach during a precordial study. They are particularly useful for studying prosthetic valvar function since it may be possible to view the whole of a prosthetic valve ring in profile as it projects into the left atrium (Fig. 3.21) and thereby identify the exact location and number of any paraprosthetic leaks.

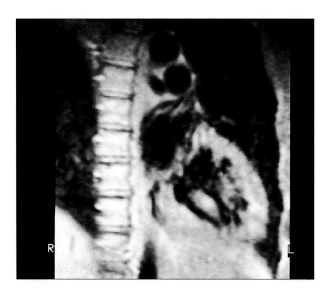

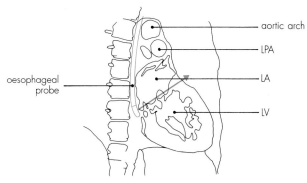

aortic arch

LPA

LA

LV

oesophageal probe

Fig. 3.20 Magnetic-resonance image of the left heart seen in a right anterior oblique projection. The diagram demonstrates where the ultrasonic beam is directed, in order to image the left atrium just above the orifice of the mitral valve. This view cannot be obtained in all patients because the lung may be interposed between the lower oesophagus and the left atrium, but it can almost always be studied when the left atrium is enlarged.

VIEWS FROM THE POSTERIOR TO THE LEFT ATRIUM

As discussed above, the oesophagus runs vertically down the middle of the posterior wall of the left atrium, the two structures being closely apposed over a distance of several centimetres (Fig. 3.22). This region is the echocardiographic window from which the majority of transoesophageal views are obtained (Fig. 3.23). It is relatively short, however, in relation to the size of the heart. Much of the skill involved in performing a good and comprehensive transoesophageal echocardiographic study, therefore, lies in the subtle manipulation of the probe over this relatively short distance.

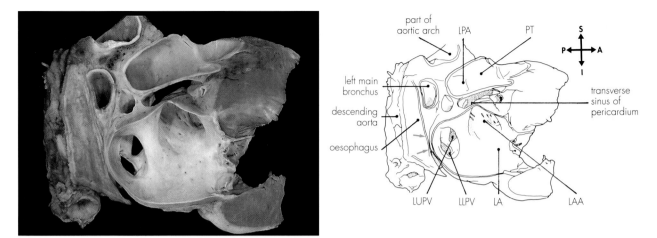

Fig. 3.22 Longitudinal section through the oesophagus and left atrium, which shows that these two structures are in direct contact over a distance of only a few centimetres. This is the oesophageal window (between the blue arrows) from which all the four-chamber views and views of the left ventricular outflow tract and the aortic valve have to be obtained.

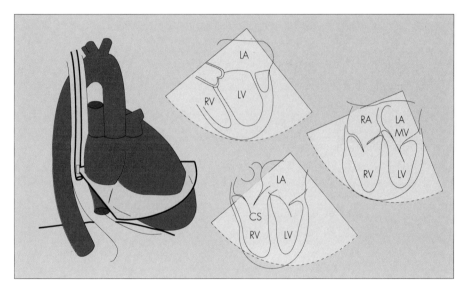

Fig. 3.23 Diagrammatic summary of the four-chamber views obtained when the transducer is positioned in the midoesophagus.

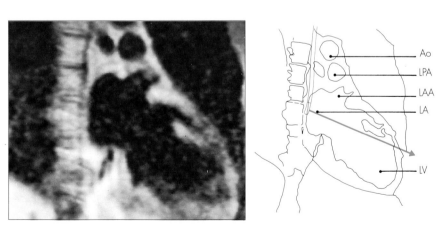

Fig. 3.24 Magnetic-resonance image of the left heart, in a right anterior oblique projection, with the diagram displaying how the transoesophageal image of the left ventricular cavity, which is obtained from behind the left atrium, is foreshortened and does not include the true cardiac apex.

Four-chamber views and the mitral valve

When the probe is pulled back to the level of the middle of the left atrium, the view obtained with the transverse plane of the transducer in a neutral position is a very foreshortened section through the ventricles, as illustrated in Fig. 3.24. In order to obtain the transoeophageal equivalent of a four-chamber view, considerable extension

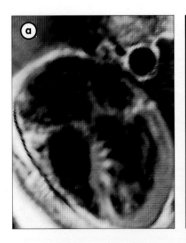

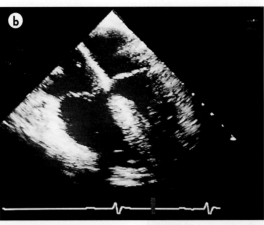

Fig. 3.25 (a) Magnetic-resonance image prepared to illustrate the four-chamber view. This is orientated to mimic the appearance obtained when the transducer is rotated towards the left. (b) A comparable transoesophageal image showing good definition of the atrial and ventricular septums and the atrioventricular valves, but poor definition of the apical part of the left ventricle.

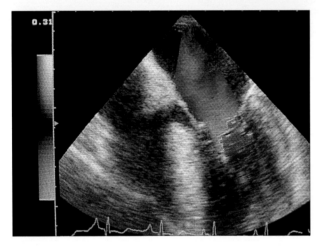

Fig. 3.26 Echocardiographic cross section through the mitral valve with colour flow mapping during diastole. The dropout of echoes from the upper (membranous) ventricular septum is artefactual and caused by the septum lying almost exactly parallel to the ultrasonic beams. This phenomenon is normal and does not imply that the patient has a ventricular septal defect.

Fig. 3.27 Image of the mitral valve near the middle point of the closure line in a patient with apparent prolapse of both leaflets. The primary and secondary cords are clearly seen, inserting into the edges of the leaflets and the middle of the bodies of the leaflets, respectively.

(retroflexion) of the tip of the probe is required. This manoeuvre often results in the loss of good contact between the transducer and the oesophageal wall, so that the quality of the image becomes very poor. This problem can usually be overcome by advancing the probe again towards the cardia, and then extending the tip before withdrawing the probe until the image is obtained.

Even with such adjustments, it is difficult during a transoesophageal echocardiographic study to obtain an image through the true anatomical long axis of the ventricle that passes through the apex (Figs. 3.25 and 3.26). This is because it is very difficult to maintain good contact from the probe after applying the considerable angulation that is required. The apex and the distal muscular ventricular septum, therefore, are not well demonstrated with transoesophageal echocardiography.

In comparison, the middle portion of the muscular ventricular septum and the atrioventricular septum are better demonstrated, but there may be artefactual discontinuity of the membranous portion of the ventricular septum when it is imaged parallel to the beams of ultrasound (Fig. 3.26). The components of the mitral valve, including its subvalvar apparatus, are usually visualized in considerable detail; for example, the primary and secondary tendinous cords (chordae tendineae) can readily be distinguished (Fig. 3.27). As previously mentioned, the leaflets of the tricuspid valve cannot be analysed in such detail. The four-chamber planes, however, are well aligned for colour mapping of flow across both atrioventricular valves. Regurgitation across the mitral (23) or across the tricuspid valve may be detected in healthy subjects. Although transoesophageal studies of many normal subjects have not been reported,

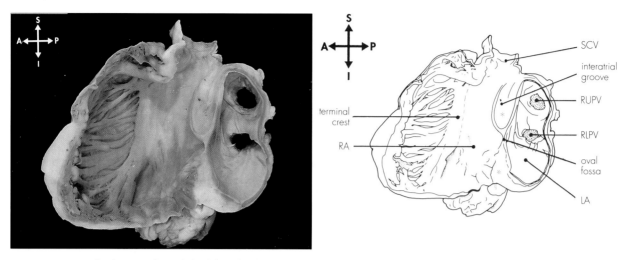

Fig. 3.28 Longitudinal section through the left and right atria viewed from the left side. The oval fossa in the middle of the atrial septum is a thin structure, while the thickened segments above and below the fossa are caused by fat in the interatrial groove (*).

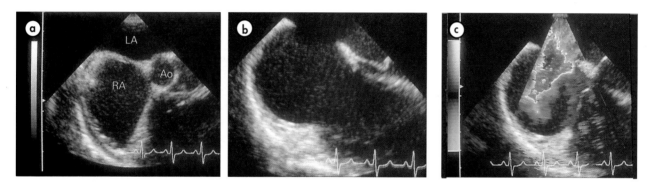

Fig. 3.29 (a) This rather high section shows both atria and an apparently intact atrial septum. There is a small pericardial effusion. When the probe is inserted more deeply to the level of the true interatrial septum, however, further imaging (b) and colour flow mapping (c) in the same patient, demonstrate that there is an atrial septal defect within the oval fossa.

previous investigations using colour flow mapping from the precordium have shown a very high prevalence of mitral and tricuspid regurgitation, which increases with age (24–26).

The normal appearances of the mitral valve in the four-chamber plane seen from the oesophagus have not yet been defined; for example, exact criteria for mitral valve prolapse have not been reported. On precordial imaging, a higher rate of prolapse is observed from the apex than on parasternal imaging in the long axis, because the annulus of the valve is not planar (27). Since the transoesophageal view is analogous to the apical view, except that the valve is imaged from the opposite side of the heart, a high rate of prolapse might be expected. Preliminary transoesophageal observations appear to confirm this (28,29). Thus, it would be unsafe to report a diagnosis of mitral valve prolapse on the basis of a transoesophageal examination unless the

prolapse was considerable. Minor degrees of 'prolapse' are probably normal. The anatomy of the mitral valve as imaged on transoesophageal echocardiography, is discussed in more detail in *Chapter 6.*

The atrial septum and the atria

Scanning from the left towards the right atrium in successive four-chamber views, with adjustment of the depth of the probe, is an excellent technique for studying the atrial septum. The floor of the oval fossa is clearly seen as the thinnest and central part of the septum (Fig. 3.28); this makes searching for atrial septal defects relatively easy to perform. When using a transverse transoesophageal transducer, the integrity of the septum must be checked at many levels (Fig. 3.29). Similarly, it may not be possible to demonstrate the

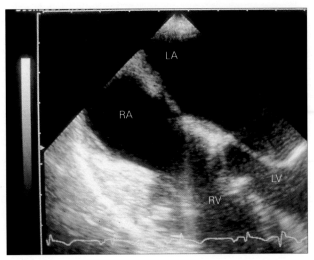

Fig. 3.30 A small fluid-filled space is seen, separating the thinner primary atrial septum from the secondary septum (arrowed).

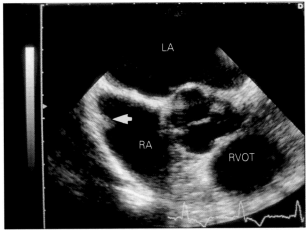

Fig. 3.32 Transoesophageal echocardiographic image obtained at a slightly higher level than *Fig. 3.31*. The thin oval fossa is readily distinguished from the thickened 'septum' or interatrial fold.

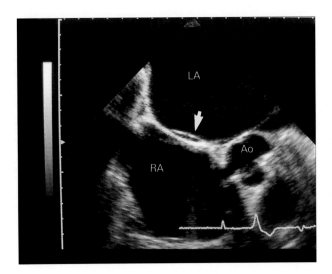

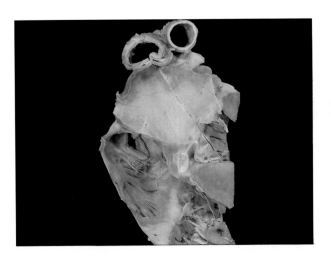

Fig. 3.33 High section through the right atrium showing the terminal crest on its lateral wall (arrowed). The left coronary leaflet of the aortic valve is traversed tangentially, and appears as a round mass in the left ventricular outflow tract.

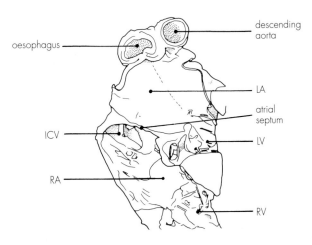

Fig. 3.31 Low oesophageal transverse section through the inferior limit of the atrial septum and through the mitral and tricuspid orifices. The interatrial fold is seen most clearly between the atria posteriorly (*).

entire dimensions of a patent foramen in a single transverse plane (30). The communication usually runs from inferior to the rim of the fossa (the limbus) on the right side of the septum, superiorly through the defect, rather than from anterior to posterior, and the average patent foramen measures only 5mm in size (31). In normal subjects, a small fluid-filled space is sometimes seen between the flap valve of the fossa (the primary septum) and the rim around the edge of the oval fossa (part of the overlying secondary septum) (Fig. 3.30), but this may be a normal variant as it is not always associated with a persistent defect or potential shunt. If the primary septum overlying the rims of the fossa is redundant and more mobile than normal, with an excursion towards either atrium during each heart

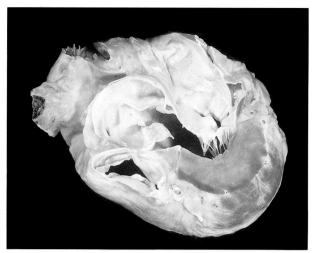

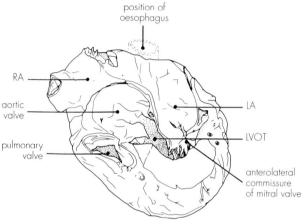

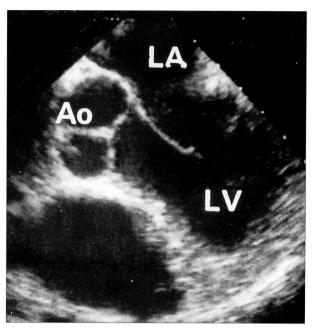

Fig. 3.35 Echocardiographic image of the left ventricular outflow tract. The mitral leaflet, the mitral curtain, and the left ventricular surface of the ventricular septum, are shown with considerable clarity.

Fig. 3.34 Transverse section through the left ventricular outflow tract, and the mitral leaflets near the anterolateral commissure.

beat of more than 1.5cm, then by definition, there is an aneurysm of the atrial septum (32). This, too, may be a normal variant representing one end of the spectrum of mobility of the septum (33).

The posterior rim enclosing the atrial septum is much more accessible to detailed imaging from the oesophagus than from standard precordial and subcostal planes. It is also possible to observe that the superior rim of the fossa (the so-called secondary septum) is, in reality, the infolded atrial wall (Fig. 3.31). Thus, in transoesophageal echocardiographic images of the atria, the presumed septum often looks very thickened, especially posteriorly (Fig. 3.32). This is a normal finding, and the appearances are due to the presence of fat in the groove between the atrial walls. Surgeons have

recognized for many years that there is a plane of potential cleavage between the atria superiorly and posteriorly (Waterston's groove). This groove extends down to the border of the true interatrial septum that is relatively small (34) and is not thickened. The true septum between the atrial cavities is the flap valve of the oval fossa. The fat seen in the interatrial groove on transoesophageal echocardiography thus lies outside the heart.

The terminal crest within the right atrium can be identified on the lateral wall as a smooth rounded protuberance (Fig. 3.33), marking the junction of the smooth-walled atrium with the pectinate muscles within the appendage (see *Figs. 3.28* and *3.38*). This crest should not be confused with localized thrombus or tumour.

The left ventricular outflow tract

If the probe is held at the same depth from which the four-chamber views are obtained, and if the tip is subsequently flexed upwards, an image of the left ventricular outflow tract is obtained in a true anatomical transverse plane (Figs. 3.34 and 3.35). Structures here can

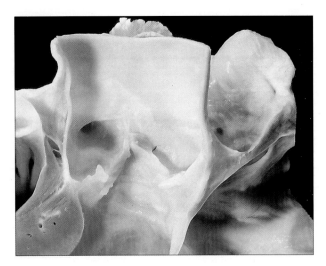

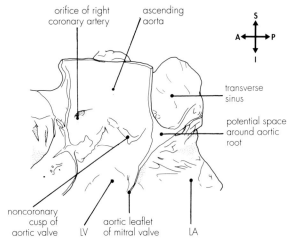

orifice of right coronary artery

ascending aorta

transverse sinus

potential space around aortic root

noncoronary cusp of aortic valve

LV

aortic leaflet of mitral valve

LA

S
A — P
I

Fig. 3.36 Sagittal section through the base of the aortic root. The orifice of the right coronary artery is visible. Posteriorly, the pericardial reflection in the floor of the transverse sinus is seen to enclose a triangular space between the posterior wall of the aortic root and the roof of the left atrium.

be identified in great detail because of their relative proximity to the transducer. The outflow tract is well aligned for colour flow mapping, but not well enough aligned for accurate pulsed Doppler interrogation. Minor modulations of the position and orientation of the probe can be used to scan between the anterior (aortic) leaflet of the mitral valve and the aortic root via the mitral curtain. Around the base of the aortic root, and outside the heart, is a potential circular space that is bounded by adjacent structures, including the left atrium posteriorly and the right ventricle anteriorly. It is triangular in cross section, and it is roofed over by the reflections of the epicardium (Fig. 3.36). This potential space is usually small and contains only some epicardial fat. It is, however, the most common site of para-aortic abscesses, and so it should be examined carefully during the transoesophageal study in any patient

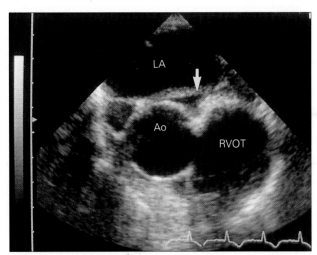

Fig. 3.37 Transverse echocardiographic image of the proximal ascending aorta. The transverse pericardial sinus is seen (arrowed), and should not be confused with the left coronary artery.

with suspected infective endocarditis (see *Chapter 9*). Above the epicardial reflection, the transverse sinus of the pericardial cavity is easily identified between the anterior and superior aspects of the left atrium and the posterior or inner aspect of the ascending aorta (Fig. 3.37).

The right ventricle and outflow tract

Transverse imaging planes traverse the right ventricular cavity and the outflow tract approximately at right angles to the direction of flow, and these structures are the most distant of any cardiac structures when imaged from the oesophagus (Fig. 3.38). For both reasons, therefore, they are not particularly well demonstrated on either imaging (see *Fig. 3.33*) or colour flow mapping. In particular, it is difficult to assess abnormalities in the outflow tract when these can only be shown in a stacked series of successive images seen in the transverse plane.

BASAL TRANSVERSE-AXIS IMAGES

When the probe is pulled back by 1 or 2cm from the middle of the left atrium, it is possible to obtain a large number of short-axis images at the base of the heart which are unique to transoesophageal echocardiography (Fig. 3.39). Access for these images is limited only when the probe is pulled back above the level of bifurcation of the trachea and air within it prevents further imaging. With mild clockwise and anticlockwise rota-

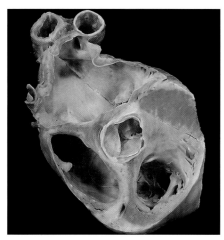

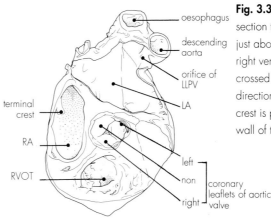

Fig. 3.38 Transverse anatomical section through the proximal aorta, just above the aortic leaflets. The right ventricular outflow tract is crossed at right angles to the direction of flow. The terminal crest is prominent at the lateral wall of the right atrium.

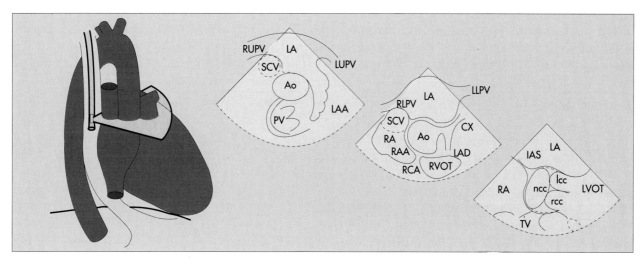

Fig. 3.39 Diagram demonstrating the position of the probe from which basal transverse-axis images are obtained.

tion of the probe, and minor adjustments to the depth and angulation of the transducer, the great arterial trunks can be followed over their central segments. It is usually unnecessary to flex or extend the tip of the probe to any great degree, except to ensure that it is kept in contact with the oesophageal mucosa.

The aortic valve

Scanning up from the left ventricular outflow tract brings the aortic valve into view in an oblique section through the sinuses of Valsalva (see *Fig. 3.38*) (Fig. 3.40). The right coronary and noncoronary leaflets are most clearly identified. The left coronary leaflet is seen initially in a transverse section through its middle, which appears as a circular structure in the left ventricular outflow tract (see *Fig. 3.33*). This is a normal appearance that should not be confused with a prolapsing

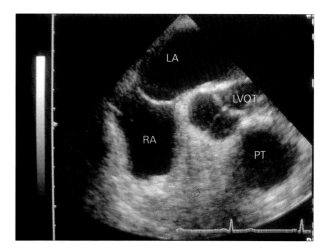

Fig. 3.40 In this image of the aortic valve, which was obtained in a true anatomical transverse plane, the noncoronary and right coronary leaflets of the valve are traversed tangentially. The commissure between these leaflets is shown well, but the left coronary leaflet is not demonstrated so clearly.

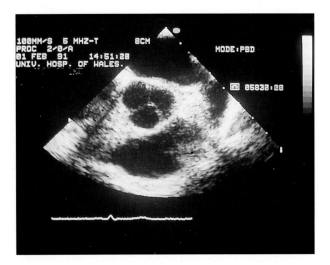

Fig. 3.41 Some tilt of the probe produces an image of the aortic valve in which the leaflets are shown in a short-axis scan. In this example, three leaflets are seen to meet symmetrically during diastole.

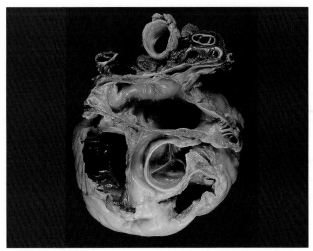

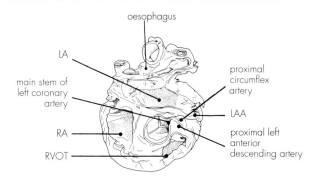

Fig. 3.42 Transverse anatomical section through the main stem of the left coronary artery.

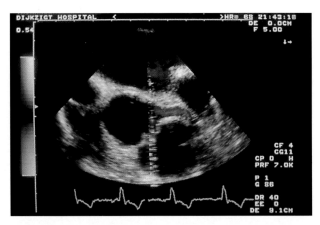

Fig. 3.43 Imaging shows a wide origin of the main stem of the left coronary artery, and the colour flow map demonstrates that flow is laminar. Compare with *Fig. 3.42*.

vegetation. If the leaflets are to be seen in true cross section (Fig. 3.41), some lateral tilt of the probe is required, because the aorta ascends initially along a line corresponding to the long axis of the heart (from below and to the right, to above and to the left). Coaptation of the leaflets can usually be seen clearly. The commissures may be identified, and colour flow mapping can be performed, but the aorta is not well aligned for a pulsed Doppler examination.

The coronary arteries

The origins and proximal portions of the coronary arteries can be identified by scanning up from the leaflets of the aortic valve towards their orifices at the level of the sinutubular ridge. The left coronary artery is located in the middle of the left sinus of Valsalva, and its main stem lies approximately at right angles to the interrogating ultrasound beam (Fig. 3.42). This relationship is ideal for accurate imaging of the vessel, unless the wall is calcified when there may be considerable masking of more distant structures (35). Colour flow mapping is possible (Fig. 3.43) but pulsed Doppler interrogation is difficult and unreliable. Movement of the heart makes it difficult to position the sample volume to obtain signals during both inspiration and expiration and throughout the cardiac cycle. Beyond the bifurcation of the left coronary artery, the proximal segment of the circumflex artery can be followed laterally for several centimetres between the left ventricle and the left atrial appendage until it turns posteriorly. The proximal portion of the left anterior descending artery

can also be seen, and is better aligned for pulsed Doppler studies (see *Chapter 11*). The right coronary artery is often more difficult to image than the left since considerable tilt of the probe is required to follow the vessel as it runs downwards and to the right. The origin of the right coronary artery can usually be identified, but it is unusual to see more than the proximal

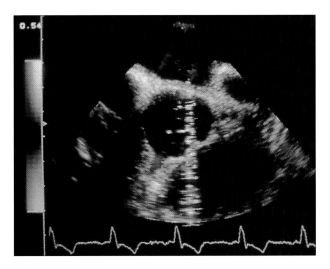

Fig. 3.44 Laminar flow is demonstrated within the proximal part of the right coronary artery. There is a considerable midline artefact on this colour map.

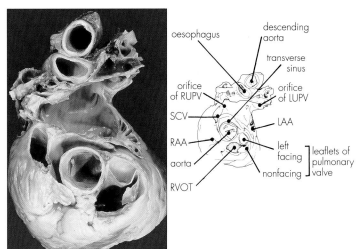

Fig. 3.45 Transverse section through the upper right ventricular outflow tract and the pulmonary valve. The leaflets that are shown are the nonfacing and left-facing ones.

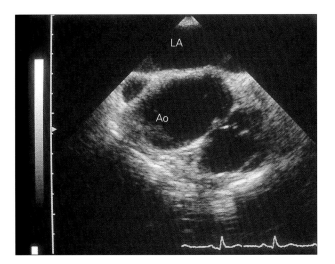

Fig. 3.46 Only two pulmonary leaflets, the nonfacing and left-facing ones, are seen in this echocardiographic image that was obtained in an anatomical transverse plane. Compare with *Fig. 3.45*.

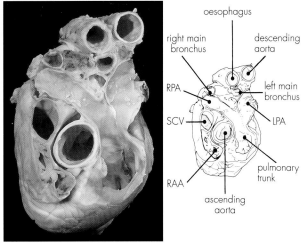

Fig. 3.47 Transverse section through the pulmonary trunk, also showing the proximal parts of the right and left pulmonary arteries. The relationship between the oesophagus and the descending thoracic aorta is well shown.

part of the vessel. Nevertheless, it is usually possible with colour flow mapping to identify that proximal flow is laminar (Fig. 3.44).

The pulmonary valve and pulmonary trunk

The pulmonary valve is seen in the same imaging planes as the aortic valve, lying anteriorly and to the left (Fig. 3.45). It, too, is not sectioned in its true short axis, and so it is usually impossible to see all three of its leaflets simultaneously (Fig. 3.46). Above the pulmonary valve, the pulmonary trunk is usually

demonstrated well in basal imaging planes, and it can be followed from the valve to the bifurcation (Figs. 3.47 and 3.48a). This portion of the vessel is very well aligned for both colour flow mapping (Fig. 3.48b) and pulsed Doppler interrogation. Beyond the bifurcation, only a short segment of the left pulmonary artery may be seen since the left main bronchus is interposed between it and the oesophagus (Fig. 3.49). It can, however, be seen again near the hilum in images in the longitudinal axis. Echocardiographic access to the right pulmonary artery is usually unrestricted, and it can be followed from the bifurcation towards its division into the major lobar branches.

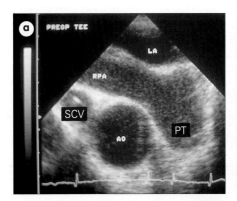

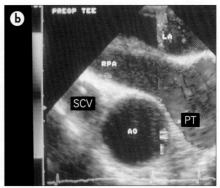

Fig. 3.48 Image (a) and colour flow map (b) of the pulmonary trunk, obtained in a patient with a large left atrium. The imaging plane is well aligned for Doppler studies, and normal laminar flow is displayed. There is a catheter in the superior caval vein. Compare with *Fig. 3.47*.

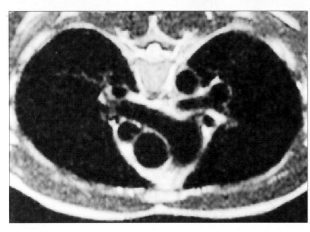

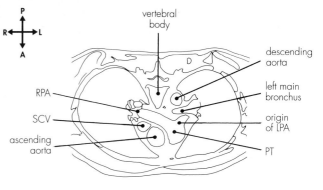

Fig. 3.49 Magnetic-resonance image of the pulmonary trunk. The left main bronchus is interposed between the oesophagus and the origin of the left pulmonary artery.

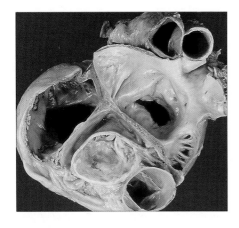

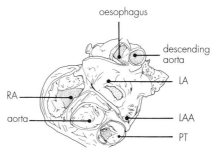

Fig. 3.50 Transverse anatomical section at the level of the atrial appendages. The prominent pectinate muscles within the left appendage, and the smoother and blunter right appendage, are demonstrated. The aortic valve in this heart is heavily calcified and stenosed.

The superior caval vein

The distal superior caval vein cannot be imaged from the precordium but it is readily demonstrated in its short axis on transoesophageal imaging (see *Fig. 3.48a*). It lies anterior to the right pulmonary artery and lateral to the ascending aorta (see *Fig. 3.47*). It is located by scanning upwards in successive transverse planes from the right atrium. It is poorly aligned for Doppler studies, so these are still best performed from the right supraclavicular fossa.

The atrial appendages

The atrial appendages are inaccessible from the precordium but are clearly seen on transoesophageal echocardiography (Fig. 3.50), making this the ideal technique for establishing atrial arrangement (situs) and for searching for thrombus in patients with atrial arrhythmias or systemic embolism.

The left appendage (Fig. 3.51) is located by pulling the probe back for a very short distance above the level of the anterolateral commissure of the mitral valve, and

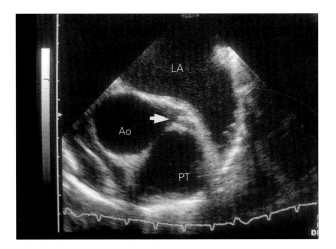

Fig. 3.51 Image of a normal left atrial appendage. The origin of the left coronary artery is also visible (arrowed).

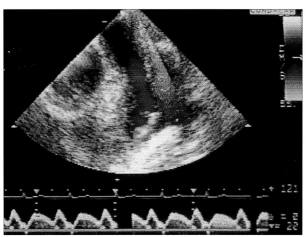

Fig. 3.52 This colour flow map shows normal flow (blue) filling the left atrial appendage, and also normal drainage of blood from the left upper pulmonary vein into the left atrium (red).

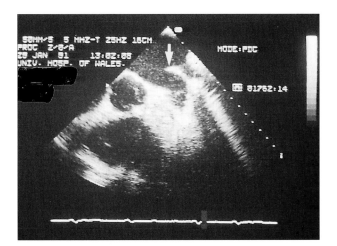

Fig. 3.53 There is a bulbous fold (arrowed) between the orifice of the left upper pulmonary vein and the left atrial appendage. In some views, this might be confused with a left atrial mass such as a thrombus.

then rotating it slightly in an anticlockwise direction. The orifice and body of the appendage may not lie in the same horizontal plane so that minor adjustments of the orientation of the probe may be required to show the entire appendage in one image. The normal left atrial appendage is described as being 'ear' shaped, and has a pointed tip and a narrow junction with the smooth-walled component of the atrium. The endocardial surface within the appendage is often quite irregular, and folds of the wall of the appendage that are identified on transoesophageal echocardiography should not be confused with a small thrombus. Routine assessment of the atrial appendages should include an assessment of function (Fig. 3.52) (36), as discussed more fully in *Chapter 4*.

The right appendage is seen by scanning up from the atrial septum above the level of the tricuspid valve and lateral to the distal right ventricular outflow tract. It has a much broader junction with the venous component of the atrium than does the left atrial appendage. It also has a blunted tip that lies anterior and to the right of the proximal ascending aorta (see *Chapter 15*).

The pulmonary veins

All four pulmonary veins can be identified on transoesophageal echocardiography since their junctions with the left atrium are readily located. The upper pulmonary veins are often imaged over several centimetres, so it is usually possible to obtain pulsed Doppler recordings from their extracardiac portions. The left upper pulmonary vein is the most easy to locate (see *Fig. 3.52*). Its junction with the left atrium lies just posterior to the orifice of the left atrial appendage and in the same transverse plane. It runs just lateral to the lateral wall of the appendage, between it and the descending thoracic aorta. The fold in the atrial wall between the orifice of the left upper pulmonary vein and the left atrial appendage may appear to be quite thick or even bulbous (Fig. 3.53), but this is a normal variant (Fig. 3.54) that should not be confused with an atrial mass. The right upper pulmonary vein enters the left atrium at approximately the same level as the left upper pulmonary vein, and it can be located by rotating the probe in a clockwise direction until the superior caval vein is seen, and then by using colour flow mapping to identify its orifice. The inferior pulmonary veins enter the left atrium while running in an almost

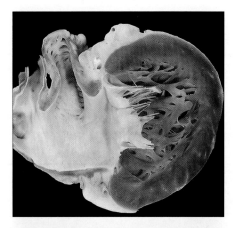

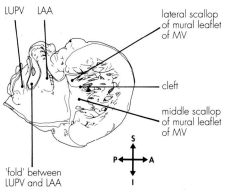

LUPV   LAA

lateral scallop
of mural leaflet
of MV

cleft

middle scallop
of mural leaflet
of MV

'fold' between
LUPV and LAA

Fig. 3.54 A longitudinal anatomical section through the lateral left atrium and left ventricle, imaged from the right side. Between the left atrial appendage and the left upper pulmonary vein, the fold in the atrial wall has been sectioned tangentially.

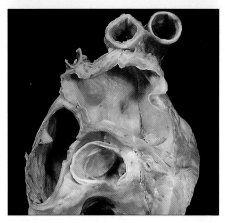

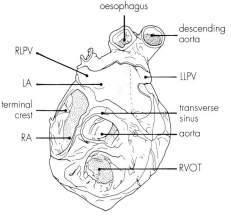

oesophagus

descending
aorta

RLPV

LA

terminal
crest

RA

LLPV

transverse
sinus

aorta

RVOT

Fig. 3.55 Basal transverse section that shows the proximity of the orifices of the lower pulmonary veins to the oesophagus. In this section, the transverse sinus of the pericardium is also clearly seen.

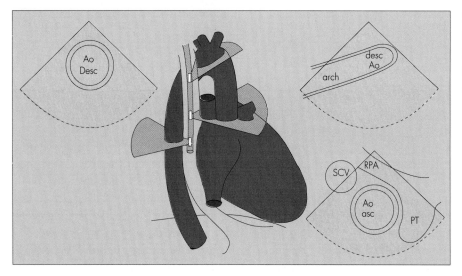

Ao
Desc

desc
Ao

arch

SCV   RPA

Ao
asc

PT

Fig. 3.56 Diagram demonstrating the positions of the probe and transducer from which the various transoesophageal views of the aorta and the arch are obtained.

true coronal plane (Fig. 3.55), some 1–2cm inferior (see *Figs. 3.22* and *3.28*) and slightly posterior to the origins of the ipsilateral upper pulmonary veins. Further information about pulmonary venous anatomy is provided in *Chapter 5*.

THE AORTA

Very little of the aorta can be seen on precordial imaging, but transoesophageal echocardiography produces excellent images of most of its intrathoracic course (Fig. 3.56). The only limitation is that it is impossible to obtain images of the upper half of the ascending aorta and the proximal third of the aortic arch because of the interposition of the trachea between these structures and the oesophagus (Fig. 3.57).

The ascending aorta is identified in basal transverse scans above the aortic valve, and it is then followed superiorly by slowly withdrawing the probe until images are lost once the transducer is above the level of the carina. In patients with annuloaortic ectasia or a tortuous

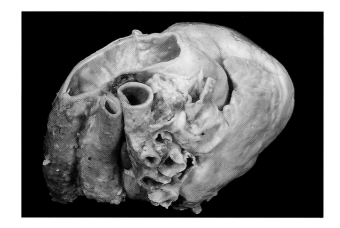

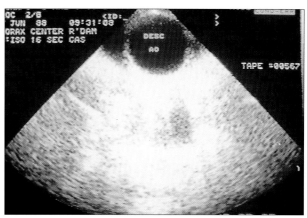

Fig. 3.58 The descending thoracic aorta (Desc Ao) is identified as a large artery that lies posterior to the oesophagus. Unless the vessel is very tortuous, it is seen almost in a circular cross section.

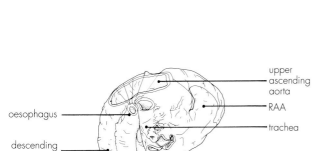

Fig. 3.57 The same specimen as shown in *Fig. 3.5*, which has been re-photographed from above, to demonstrate the interposition of the trachea between the oesophagus and the proximal part of the aortic arch. As indicated, a considerable part of the arch cannot be imaged.

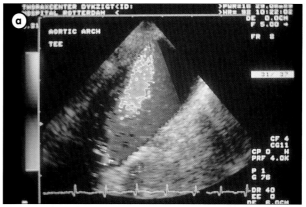

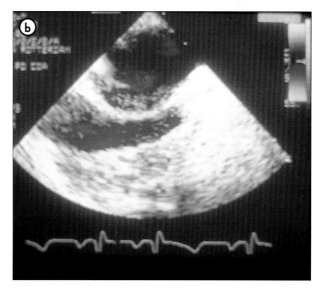

proximal aortic root, the initially more horizontal and rightward course of the aorta than normal allows the proximal portion of the ascending aorta to be seen, together with the aortic valve, in a standard basal view, with some added flexion of the tip of the probe.

The descending thoracic aorta and the oesophagus are closely related (see *Fig. 3.57*). The upper descending aorta is lateral to the oesophagus (see, for example, *Fig. 3.47*) but the two structures coil around each other so that the aorta lies more posterior to the oesophagus at the level of the diaphragm. It is very easy to scan the whole course of the descending thoracic aorta if it is first identified by rotating the probe in an anticlockwise direction from a position high in the stomach (Fig. 3.58). The aorta can be imaged for a short distance below the diaphragm, and then kept in view by slowly rotating the probe as it is withdrawn. Once the upper descending thoracic aorta is reached (at approximately 25cm from the teeth), the lumen of the aorta broadens out into the distal part of the transverse aortic arch (Fig. 3.59a). In order to image as much of the arch as

Fig. 3.59 (a) Image of the distal half of the aortic arch obtained with the transverse planar transducer and some retroflexion of the tip of the probe. There is normal laminar flow around the arch. (b) Image of the thoracic aorta at the junction between the distal arch and the upper descending thoracic aorta. Anterior to the aorta, the left brachiocephalic vein is shown with laminar flow in it, away from the transducer.

possible, the tip of the probe should then be extended and rotated in a clockwise direction. Occasionally, the brachiocephalic vein can be identified in front of the aorta (Fig. 3.59b). The demonstration of continuous laminar flow at low velocity, confirms that this structure is a vein rather than, for example, a false lumen in a patient with aortic dissection.

LONGITUDINAL PLANE IMAGING

The ability of transoesophageal imaging to demonstrate details of intracardiac anatomy, as well as provide images of the great vessels, has been considerably enhanced by the development of transoesophageal probes that have two phased-array transducers (37). The additional transducer is mounted 1cm proximal to the other one, at the tip, in order to image in longitudinal planes that are perpendicular to the traditional ones (Fig. 3.60). At present, some biplane probes incorporate a reduced number of separate elements into each transducer, and so the definition of the images is reduced, compared with usual. In many circumstances, nonetheless, the additional anatomical information that can be obtained (38–40) outweighs this disadvantage.

When switching from the transverse to the longitudinal transducer, some modification of the position of the probe is often required to optimize the quality of the image. Good ultrasonic contact with the mucosa may not be achieved for both transducers simultaneously. Once good contact is obtained between the longitudinal transducer and the ventricles from the fundus of the stomach, or between it and the posterior wall of the left atrium from within the oesophagus, the depth of the probe should not be altered significantly while imaging in the longitudinal axis. Successive imaging planes are produced by rotating the probe in a clockwise or an anticlockwise direction while scanning through the heart and great vessels from one hilum to the other (Fig. 3.61). From the oesophagus, part of the left atrium is always visible at the top of the image. Starting from the right side, gradual anticlockwise rotation progressively demonstrates the right atrium and increasing amounts of the right ventricle, and then increasing amounts of the left atrium and the left ventricle.

Longitudinal images are displayed on the echocardiographic monitoring screen with the head of the patient to the right, and the posterior surface of the heart at the top, as if the patient was lying prone with the examiner looking from his or her right side. It is not possible to display these images in a more conventional orientation, with the ultrasonic source depicted on the left or the right side of the screen, since the controls of the machine only allow the source to be shown at the top of the screen (as is usual), or at 180° to this. The 'head-to-the-right' configuration is the same as that

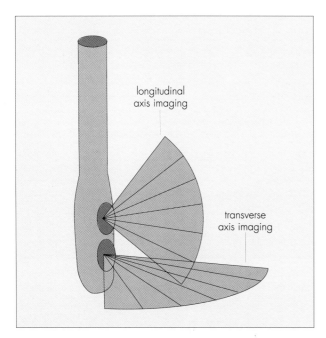

Fig. 3.60 Diagram of the tip of a biplane probe showing the orientation of the imaging planes obtained when using the two transducers.

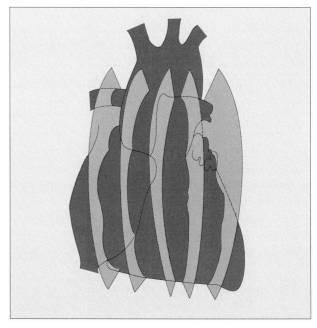

Fig. 3.61 Schematic representation of the orientation of longitudinal-axis transoesophageal imaging planes to the heart.

which is used when displaying precordial long-axis images, although in these, the anterior surface of the heart is shown at the top of the screen. Although echocardiographic cross sections in the longitudinal plane are displayed in this way, the anatomical sections are most easily understood if they are displayed in their true orientation, with the head to the top of each section; they are also shown as a series of slices viewed from the right side of the heart. This means that, in the following account, corresponding anatomical and echocardiographic images are displayed differently, with the echocardiographic cross sections rotated to the right (that is, in a clockwise direction) through 90°.

Transgastric longitudinal plane imaging

Once the standard short-axis cross section of the left ventricle has been obtained in the transverse plane, switching to the longitudinal transducer produces a long-axis image through the anterior and inferior walls of the left ventricle. This cross section includes the apex of the left ventricle (Fig. 3.62). If the longitudinal image includes the papillary muscles (and both are seen in the same image), then foreshortening may occur since the longitudinal imaging plane is directed towards the distal lateral free wall of the ventricle above the true apex. If the probe is withdrawn slightly and its tip is flexed while using the longitudinal transducer, the imaging plane is directed away from the apex and towards the base of the heart, and it becomes possible to display the left ventricular outflow tract and the proximal ascending aorta, as well as the

anterior and basal posterior walls of the left ventricle. This unconventional transoesophageal echocardiographic view corresponds closely to a conventional parasternal long-axis image but viewed from the opposite side of the heart. Its only advantage as part of a transoesophageal study is that it is the view that best allows Doppler interrogation of the left ventricular outflow tract and the aortic valve.

If the image of the ventricles in the transverse plane is adjusted so that the right ventricular cavity is present in the middle of the screen, switching to the longitudinal transducer will provide a longitudinal image through the middle of the right ventricle. This image is similar to that which can be obtained unusually with a transverse transducer (see *Fig. 3.12*), as it shows the anterosuperior and inferior (mural) leaflets of the tricuspid valve. When transgastric imaging of the liver in the transverse plane demonstrates the hepatic veins draining posteriorly towards the hepatic portal, and the inferior caval vein in cross section, then switching to longitudinal planar imaging shows a considerable length of the inferior caval vein in its own long axis (Fig. 3.63). Maintaining this image and transducer orientation as the tip of the probe is withdrawn through the cardia allows examination of the junction of the inferior caval vein with the floor of the right atrium.

Oesophageal longitudinal plane imaging

Directing the ultrasonic beam towards the right side of the heart produces a long-axis cross section through the superior caval vein as it enters the right atrium

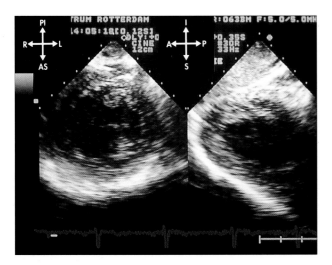

Fig. 3.62 Transverse (on the left) and longitudinal (on the right) transgastric images of the left ventricle. The longitudinal section includes the apex and parts of the inferior and anterosuperior walls of the ventricle.

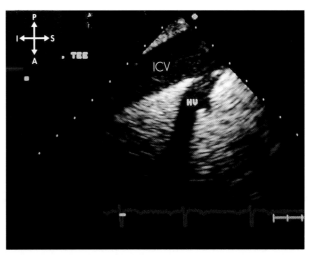

Fig. 3.63 Longitudinal image of the inferior caval vein showing its junction with the hepatic vein.

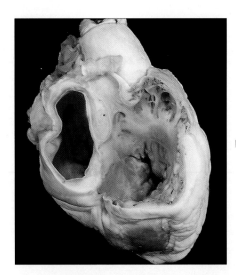

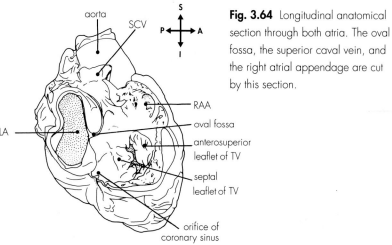

Fig. 3.64 Longitudinal anatomical section through both atria. The oval fossa, the superior caval vein, and the right atrial appendage are cut by this section.

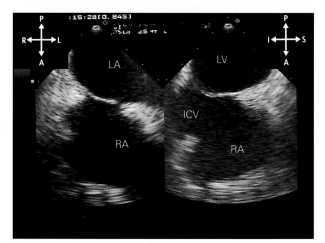

Fig. 3.65 Longitudinal image obtained by directing the transducer towards the right side of the heart in a patient with mitral stenosis, and an enlarged left atrium that contains spontaneous echo contrast. There is a catheter (arrowed) in the right atrium. Both caval veins are shown in longitudinal section, and the right atrial appendage is demonstrated at the bottom right of the image. Compare with *Fig. 3.64*.

Fig. 3.66 Transverse (on the left side) and longitudinal (on the right side) images through a normal, intact atrial septum. On the longitudinal image, the orifice of the inferior caval vein is also shown.

(Figs. 3.64 and 3.65). Posteriorly, the right pulmonary artery is cut in cross section, and anteriorly, an oval section through the right lateral aspect of the ascending aorta may be seen if the aorta is enlarged or tortuous. With some anticlockwise rotation, the right atrial appendage is demonstrated. In all of these images, the plane traverses the atrial septum, and so biplane imaging may prove to be the best method of studying the whole septum (Fig. 3.66) while searching for small defects or a patent foramen, or of measuring the size of a defect. While still scanning to the right side of the heart, but after some anticlockwise rotation, longitudinal imaging demonstrates the anterosuperior and inferior (mural) leaflets of the tricuspid valve (Fig. 3.67). The aortic root and the leaflets of the aortic valve are demonstrated clearly, wedged in the centre of the heart. The origin of the right coronary artery is shown (Fig. 3.68), and indeed, imaging of the anterior aortic root in the longitudinal axis may be the most reliable means of identifying this. When the transducer is withdrawn so that it occupies a position in the oesophagus just distal to the carina, and if the tip of the probe is flexed slightly, a long segment of the ascending aorta is seen (Fig. 3.69). In most adults, this segment measures 6–7cm in length, and so most of the upper ascending aorta can be imaged with this technique.

Longitudinal imaging directly forwards from the oesophagus in a sagittal plane not only depicts the aorta, but also a portion of the left ventricular outflow tract (Fig. 3.70). Angulation of the tip of the probe towards the right side of the patient opens up the whole

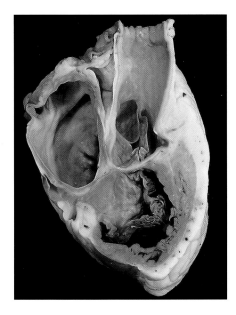

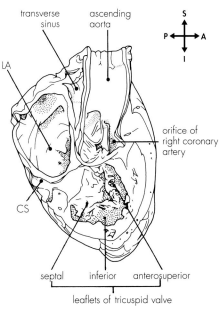

Fig. 3.67 More medial anatomical section than *Fig. 3.64*, still in the longitudinal axis. The anterosuperior and inferior leaflets of the tricuspid valve have been cut. Within the aortic root, only the base of the noncoronary leaflet has been sectioned, and the origin of the right coronary artery is demonstrated. This plane also shows the transverse sinus of the pericardium and the distal part of the coronary sinus.

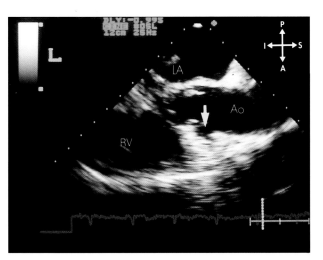

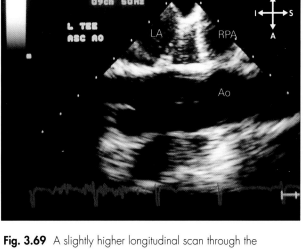

Fig. 3.68 Longitudinal transoesophageal image through the aortic root showing the origin of the right coronary artery (arrowed). Compare with *Fig. 3.67*.

Fig. 3.69 A slightly higher longitudinal scan through the ascending aorta, which is seen clearly over a length of 7cm. The right pulmonary artery is shown in cross section.

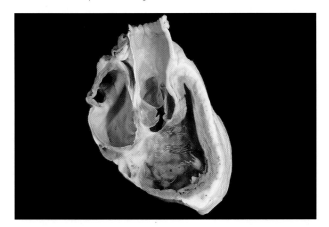

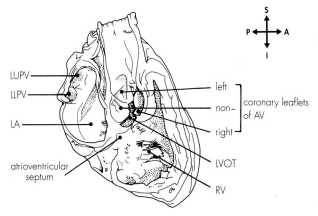

Fig. 3.70 Anatomical section obtained in the sagittal plane that passes directly forward from the oesophagus. This plane is medial to the anterosuperior and inferior leaflets of the tricuspid valve, and to the atrial septum. In the centre of the heart, the section passes near to the atrioventricular septum and it crosses the left ventricular outflow tract and the noncoronary and right coronary leaflets of the aortic valve.

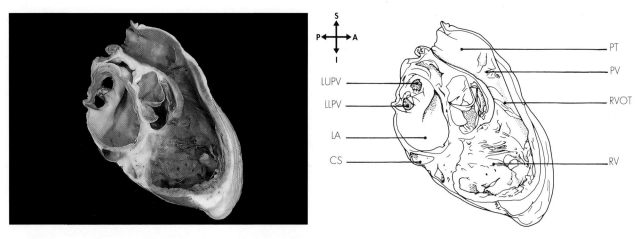

Fig. 3.71 Angulation of the probe from the position in which an image corresponding to *Fig. 3.70* is produced, results in this section in which the whole of the right ventricle is demonstrated, together with the pulmonary valve and the proximal pulmonary trunk.

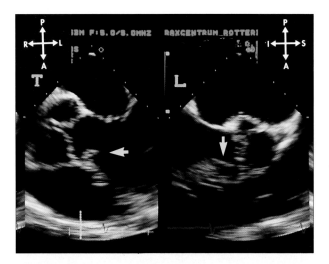

Fig. 3.72 Transverse (on the left) and longitudinal (on the right) echocardiographic sections. The transverse image shows the left ventricular outflow tract with a shelf (arrowed) attached to the upper ventricular septum. On switching to the longitudinal transducer, the pulmonary valve is demonstrated, and the shelf (arrowed) can be seen as a structure running along the upper ventricular septum.

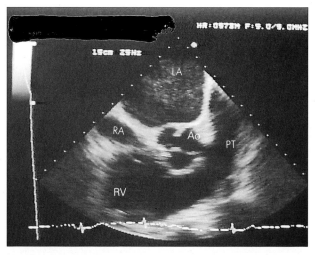

Fig. 3.73 Echocardiographic image corresponding to the anatomical section shown in *Fig. 3.71*.

outflow tract of the right ventricle, which is seen together with the tricuspid valve, the pulmonary valve, and the proximal part of the pulmonary trunk (Fig. 3.71). Thus, when the left ventricular outflow tract is shown by the transverse image, switching to the longitudinal transducer and flexing the tip of the probe slightly, produce a clear image of the right ventricular infundibulum and the pulmonary valve (Fig. 3.72). In some of these views, both atria together with the anterosuperior and inferior tricuspid leaflets are seen (Fig. 3.73). These views are unique to transoesophageal echocardiographic imaging in the longitudinal plane,

and probably represent one of its main contributions for the assessment of intracardiac morphology in congenital heart disease. The right ventricular outflow tract, however, runs almost at right angles to the ultrasonic beam, so neither colour flow mapping nor pulsed Doppler studies can be performed satisfactorily. From a higher position of the transducer, the longitudinal image shows the pulmonary trunk and its bifurcation (Fig. 3.74).

If the orientation of the tip of the probe is restored to an anatomical sagittal plane, further longitudinal images that are produced as the probe is turned towards the left side of the patient, show the leaflets of the mitral valve near the posteromedial commissure, and the left ventricle (Fig. 3.75). The medial portions of the mitral leaflets are not well demonstrated in the transverse plane on transoesophageal echocardiography, but the

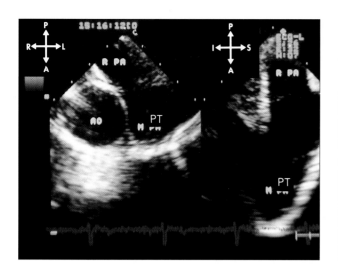

Fig. 3.74 Biplane images of the pulmonary trunk; the transverse-axis image is on the left and the longitudinal image on the right.

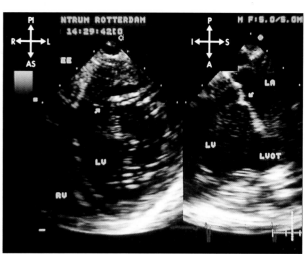

Fig. 3.76 Transverse (on the left) and longitudinal (on the right) images of the mitral valve near the posteromedial commissure (arrowed). Compare with *Fig. 3.75* and *3.77*.

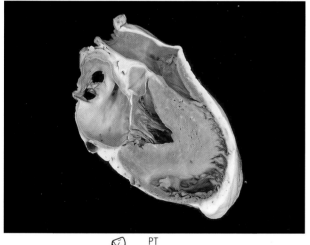

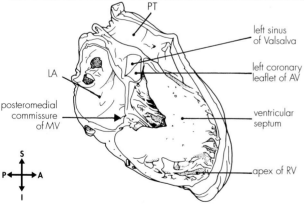

Fig. 3.75 Anatomical section that cuts the ventricular septum and the medial parts of the mitral leaflets. Only a small part of the aortic root is included in this section, near the base of the left coronary leaflet of the aortic valve.

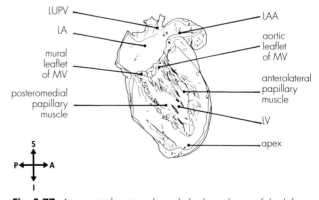

Fig. 3.77 Anatomical section through the lateral part of the left ventricle. Both papillary muscles are seen, and the orifices of the left atrial appendage and the left upper pulmonary veins are identified.

longitudinal axis approach shows the closure line of the valve clearly (Fig. 3.76). The ventricular septum is crossed very tangentially by longitudinal imaging planes, and so it is not demonstrated very clearly. In the more lateral images through the left ventricle (Fig. 3.77), its anterior and inferior walls are seen, although the apex is not demonstrated as readily as it is from the transgastric longitudinal approach. The left atrial appendage and the left upper pulmonary vein are demonstrated arising from the high lateral wall of the left atrium. Finally, the left pulmonary artery and the pulmonary veins can be followed in cross section towards the left hilum.

It seems likely that one of the major applications of longitudinal transoesophageal imaging in adults will be the study of aortic disease. The main benefit of the second transducer is that it provides additional views of the complex pathology found in patients with aortic dissection or aneurysm. Longitudinal planar images of the descending aorta show the vessel in its long axis (Fig. 3.78), while at the arch they give short-axis cross-sectional images, and sometimes show the origins of the brachiocephalic vessels.

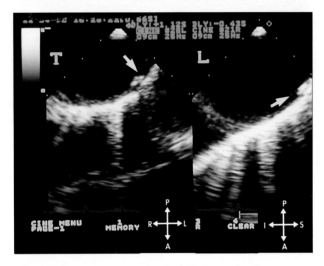

Fig. 3.78 Transverse image (on the left) obtained at the junction of the upper descending component of the thoracic aorta with the distal aortic arch; this explains why the cross section is ellipsoid rather than circular. The longitudinal section shows a considerable length of the outer wall of the descending aorta. There is an atheromatous plaque (arrowed).

THE ORGANIZATION OF A TRANSOESOPHAGEAL ECHOCARDIOGRAPHIC STUDY

Unlike transthoracic echocardiography, a 'second look' is much more difficult to accomplish if an initial transoesophageal echocardiographic study is, for technical reasons, incomplete or nondiagnostic. At the same time, a desire to perform a careful and comprehensive, but also time-consuming, study has to be set against the discomfort to the patient if the procedure is prolonged unnecessarily. Thus, the investigation should be performed logically and efficiently, integrating the use of the different imaging and Doppler modalities.

In patients who are ill, attention should first be directed towards answering the specific clinical questions that prompted the examination. In those who are well, and who tolerate the procedure well, the transverse planar images can be obtained in sequence from the gastric fundus to the aorta. To save time, we suggest that

Sequence of Imaging Planes During Normal Transoesophageal Echocardiographic Investigation		
Standard examination	**Additional studies Longitudinal axis**	**Additional studies Acquired disease**
Transgastric planes		
LV and RV, short axis	apex, anterior and inferior walls of LV	RV inlet, TV
MV subvalvar apparatus and orifice	subvalvar apparatus	
Transoesophageal planes lower oesophagus		
coronary sinus	inferior caval vein	floor of LA (in patients with prosthetic MV)
tricuspid valve	biplane views of commissures	
four-chamber view		
midoesophagus		
mitral valve	posteromedial commissure of MV	pulsed Doppler studies
atrial septum	biplane views of atrial septum	contrast study/Valsalva
pulmonary veins		pulsed Doppler studies
LV outflow tract		
upper oesophagus/basal views		
aortic valve		
coronary arteries	RCA origin	
atrial appendages		flow in LA appendage
ascending aorta	ascending aorta in long axis	
superior caval vein	SCV in long axis	
pulmonary trunk		
thoracic aorta		
descending aorta	longitudinal views	
aortic arch	longitudinal views	

Fig. 3.79 Summary of the sequence of imaging planes that should be used, and the structures that are seen, during a normal transoesophageal echocardiographic investigation.

colour flow mapping should be performed after each new set of imaging planes has been studied from the standard positions of the probe, rather than attempting a second examination of the same planes for colour flow mapping alone. This approach also avoids unnecessary manipulation of the probe. When complex abnormalities of colour flow are found, their interpretation is greatly aided by the use of colour M-mode recordings, which can be analysed for the exact timing and location of flow events much more quickly than can be achieved by recording and playing back cine loops.

The transverse plane and longitudinal plane images have been described separately in this chapter since the vast majority of transoesophageal echocardiographic studies are performed with a probe having only a single plane (transverse). When a biplane probe is used, however, it is more efficient to integrate the use of the transverse and longitudinal planar transducers throughout the study. One sequence of performing a complete investigation with such a probe is given in Fig. 3.79. In future, it is likely that multiplane probes will also be available. In such circumstances, the type of probe to be used in any particular patient may be selected on the basis of whether very high-quality imaging of a single structure is required, or if it is more important to analyse complex anatomy or pathology in multiple planes. To achieve either of these goals, it is axiomatic that cardiologists need to extend their knowledge and three-dimensional understanding of, cardiac anatomy.

REFERENCES

1. Schlüter M, Hinrichs A, Thier W *et al.* Transesophageal two-dimensional echocardiography comparison of ultrasonic and anatomic sections. *Am J Cardiol* 1984;**53**:1173–8.

2. Mitchell MM, Sutherland GR, Gussenhoven EJ *et al.* Transesophageal echocardiography. *J Am Soc Echo* 1988;**1**:362–77.

3. Seward JB, Khanderia BK, Oh JK *et al.* Transesophageal echocardiography: technique, anatomic correlations, implementation, and clinical applications. *Mayo Clin Proc* 1988;**63**:649–80.

4. Weller IVD, Williams CB, Jeffries DJ *et al.* Cleaning and disinfection of equipment for gastrointestinal flexible endoscopy: interim recommendations of a Working Party of the British Society of Gastroenterology. *Gut* 1988;**29**:1134–51.

5. Spire B, Barre–Sinoussi F, Montagnier L, Chermann JC. Inactivation of lymphadenopathy-associated virus by chemical disinfectants. *Lancet* 1984;**i**:899–901.

6. Clausen TG, Wolff J, Hansen PB *et al.* Pharmacokinetics of midazolam and α-hydroxy-midazolam following rectal and intravenous administration. *Br J Clin Pharmacol* 1988;**25**:457–63.

7. Bell GD, Morden A, Coady T *et al.* A comparison of diazepam and midazolam as endoscopy premedication assessing changes in ventilation and oxygen saturation. *Br J Clin Pharmacol* 1988;**26**:595–600.

8. Hamdy NAT, Kennedy HJ, Nicholl J, Triger DR. Sedation for gastroscopy: comparative study of midazolam and diazemuls in patients with and without cirrhosis. *Br J Clin Pharmacol* 1986;**22**:644–7.

9. Raza SM, Masters RW, Zsigmond EK. Comparison of the hemodynamic effects of midazolam and diazepam in patients with coronary occlusion. *Int J Clin Pharmacol Ther Toxicol* 1989;**27**:1–6.

10. Engberding R, Hasfeld I, Chiladakis I *et al.* [Transesophageal echocardiography: increased risk by rise in arterial blood pressure and cardiac arrhythmias?] *Herz Kreisl* 1988;**20**:233–6.

11. Taylor WJR, Llewellyn–Thomas E, Sellers EA. A comparative evaluation of intramuscular atropine, dicyclomine, and glycopyrrolate using healthy medical students as volunteer subjects. *Int J Clin Pharmacol* 1970;**3**:358–64.

12. Gilman AG, Goodman LS, Gilman A. *Goodman and Gilman's The Pharmacological Basis of Therapeutics, 6th Edition.* New York: MacMillan, 1980.

13. Cormier B, Starkman C, Kulas A *et al.* L'echographie par voie oesophagienne. Interêt de la technique à propos d'une expérience préliminaire concernant 320 patients (385 examens). *Ann Med Interne (Paris)* 1989;**140**:561–5.

14. Shovron PJ, Eykyn SJ, Cotton PB. Gastrointestinal instrumentation, bacteremia and endocarditis. *Gut* 1983;**24**:1078–93.

15. Dennig K, Sedlmayr V, Seling B, Rudolph W. Bacteremia with transesophageal echocardiography [Abstract]. *Circulation* 1989;**80**:II-473.

16. Görge G, Erbel R, Henrichs J *et al.* Positive blood cultures during transesophageal echocardiography [Abstract]. *J Am Coll Cardiol* 1990;**15**:62a.

17. Delaye J, Etienne J, Feruglio GA *et al.* Prophylaxis of infective endocarditis for dental procedures. Report of a Working Party of the European Society of Cardiology. *Eur Heart J* 1985;**6**:826–8.

18. Sreeram N, Sutherland GR, Fraser AG *et al.* The evolution of transesophageal echocardiography: Indications from clinical

experience of 1,000 patients [Abstract]. *J Am Coll Cardiol* 1990;**15**:62A.

19. Daniel WG, Angermann C, Curtius J *et al.* Safety of transesophageal echocardiography — A European multicenter study. *Eur Heart J* 1989;**10** (Abstract Supplement):206.

20. Khanderia B, Seward J, Oh J *et al.* Safety of transesophageal echocardiography in awake patients: experience with 400 procedures [Abstract]. *J Am Coll Cardiol* 1989;**13**:225a.

21. Geibel A, Kasper W, Behroz A *et al.* Risk of transesophageal echocardiography in awake patients with cardiac diseases. *Am J Cardiol* 1988;**62**:337–9.

22. Urbanowicz JH, Kernoff RS, Oppenheim G *et al.* Transesophageal echocardiography and its potential for esophageal damage. *Anesthesiology* 1990;**72**:40–3.

23. Taams MA, Gusssenhoven EJ, Cahalan MK *et al.* Transesophageal Doppler color flow imaging in the detection of native and Björk–Shiley mitral valve regurgitation. *J Am Coll Cardiol* 1989;**13**:95–9.

24. Wittlich N, Erbel R, Drexler M *et al.* Color-Doppler flow mapping of the heart in normal subjects. *Echocardiography* 1988;**5**:157–72.

25. Nimura Y, Miyatake K, Izumi S. Physiological regurgitation identified by Doppler techniques. *Echocardiography* 1989;**5**:385–92.

26. Klein AL, Burstow DJ, Tajik AJ *et al.* Age-related prevalence of valvular regurgitation in normal subjects: a comprehensive color flow examination of 118 volunteers. *J Am Soc Echocardiogr* 1990;**3**:54–63.

27. Levine RA, Triulzi MO, Harrigan P, Weyman AE. The relationship of mitral annular shape to the diagnosis of mitral valve prolapse. *Circulation* 1987;75:756–67.

28. Zenker G, Erbel R, Kramer G *et al.* Transesophageal two-dimensional echocardiography in young patients with cerebral ischemic events. *Stroke* 1988;**19**:345–8.

29. Gueret P, Lacroix P, Bensaid J. Assessment of mitral valve prolapse by transesophageal echocardiography [Abstract]. *J Am Coll Cardiol* 1990;**15**:94a.

30. Mugge A, Daniel WG, Klopper JW, Lichtlen PR. Visualization of patent foramen ovale by transesophageal color-coded Doppler echocardiography. *Am J Cardiol* 1988;**62**:837–8.

31. Hagen PT, Scholz DG, Edwards WD. Incidence and size of patent foramen ovale during the first 10 decades of life: an autopsy study of 965 normal hearts. *Mayo Clin Proc* 1984;**59**:17–20.

32. Schreiner G, Erbel R, Mohr–Kahaly S *et al.* [Detection of aneurysms of the atrial septum using transesophageal echocardiography.] *Z Kardiol* 1985;**74**:440–4.

33. Silver MD, Dorsey JS. Aneurysms of the septum primum in adults. *Arch Pathol Lab Med* 1978;**102**:62–5.

34. Sweeney LJ, Rosenquist GC. The normal anatomy of the atrial septum in the human heart. *Am Heart J* 1979;**98**:194–9.

35. Taams MA, Gussenhoven EJ, Cornel JG *et al.* Detection of left coronary artery stenosis by transesophageal echocardiography. *Eur Heart J* 1988;**9**:1162–6.

36. Suetsugu M, Matsuzaki M, Toma Y *et al.* [Detection of mural thrombi and analysis of blood flow velocities in the left atrial appendage using transesophageal two-dimensional echocardiography and pulsed Doppler flowmetry.] *J Cardiol* 1988;**18**:385–94.

37. Omoto R, Kyo S, Matsumura M *et al.* Biplane color transesophageal Doppler echocardiography (color TEE): its advantages and limitations. *Int J Card Imaging* 1989;**4**:57–8.

38. Stümper OFW, Fraser AG, Ho SY *et al.* Transoesophageal imaging in the longitudinal axis: a correlative echocardiographic–anatomic study and its clinical implications. *Brit Heart J* 1990;**64**:282–8.

39. Seward JB, Khanderia BK, Edwards WD *et al.* Biplanar transesophageal echocardiography: anatomic correlations, image orientation, and clinical applications. *Mayo Clin Proc* 1990;**65**:1193–213.

40. Bansal RC, Shakudo M, Shah PM, Shah PM. Biplane transesophageal echocardiography: technique, image orientation, and preliminary experience in 131 patients. *J Am Soc Echo* 1990;**3**: 348–66.

4

Atrial lesions

Massimo Pozzoli
John H Smyllie
Jos R T C Roelandt

INTRODUCTION

One of the most important areas in which transoesophageal echocardiography has added substantial new insight to clinical knowledge, is the study of the atria and their related structures. As previously indicated, much of the new information available from the use of the transoesophageal technique is purely related to the close proximity of the lower oesophagus to the left atrium. Thus, by a series of manipulations of the transoesophageal probe, multiple cross-sectional images of the left and right atria can be obtained. The structures that can be scanned include the left and right atrial appendages, the interatrial septum, the pulmonary and systemic venous connexions, and the right and left atrioventricular junctions. As it is inappropriate to discuss abnormalities of all these structures in one chapter, the transoesophageal evaluation of specific abnormalities are described elsewhere. Congenital lesions, such as atrial septal defects, unroofed coronary sinus, anomalous pulmonary venous drainage, and obstruction or leakage of interatrial baffles, are described in detail in *Chapter 14*. The complexities involved in the recording and analysis of pulmonary venous flow are outlined in *Chapter 5*, and acquired abnormalities of the mitral and tricuspid valves are discussed in *Chapter 6*. This chapter focuses on the current status and future prospects for the use of transoesophageal echocardiography in the diagnosis of atrial lesions. In particular, it concentrates on the complex role of the atria as sites of both systemic and pulmonary emboli.

CARDIAC SOURCES OF SYSTEMIC EMBOLIZATION

Embolization from within the heart may account for many cases of cerebral ischaemia. Unfortunately, the diagnosis of cerebral embolism from the heart is often difficult, and previous studies have shown that cross-sectional precordial echocardiography yields little additional information when the clinical cardiac findings are normal (1,2). In approximately one-third of patients with a cerebral ischaemic event, the cause remains undefined despite considerable diagnostic effort (2). It has been suggested that many of these episodes may be secondary to occult cardiac sources (3). Transoesophageal echocardiography has recently been welcomed as an effective method for the detection of intracardiac sources of emboli in patients with peripheral embolization and, more particularly, with cerebral ischaemic events. Several reports from different centres concordantly indicate that transoesophageal echocardiography can detect potential causes of embolism, many of which were missed by the precordial approach in 30–60% of patients (4–7). The cardiac conditions that produce an increased risk for systemic embolization are summarized in Fig. 4.1, which also indicates our impression at the Thoraxcentre of the respective diagnostic values of the transoesophageal and precordial techniques.

Transoesophageal echocardiography may give additional information in patients with cardiac disease that is known to provide a risk for embolization, such as rheumatic valvar disease or valvar prosthesis. It may also reveal intra-atrial thrombi and/or spontaneous echocardiographic contrast, which are normally missed by precordial echocardiography. When thrombotic material is visualized, a transoesophageal study can be repeated to assess the results of therapeutic interventions. In patients with cryptogenic stroke, this technique can be used to detect occult cardiac abnormalities such as a patent oval foramen or an atrial septal aneurysm, which may represent the source of embolization.

In our experience, compliance for a transoesophageal study is excellent in patients with mild neurologic involvement. Pop and associates were able to carry out an investigation in all 72 patients with transient ischaemic attacks who were included in their prospective study, without the need to administer sedatives (4). Patients with a major stroke can also be investigated with a high success rate and without complications (6). Patients during evolution of a stroke, however, and those incapable of collaborating because of severe cognitive (advanced receptive aphasia) or psychological problems, should be excluded from the investigation. Hemiparesis involving the cranial nerves does not usually hamper the examination. When involuntary movements, apraxia, or

major disturbances of swallowing are present, we prefer to induce adequate sedation with benzodiazepines. The probe can then be inserted directly into the oesophagus, without requiring the patient to collaborate in swallowing. Attempts to swallow the probe in these patients can induce a feeling of frustration that may result in a refusal to continue the procedure.

LEFT ATRIAL THROMBI AND SPONTANEOUS ECHO CONTRAST

Left atrial thrombus is a well-recognized cause of systemic embolization (8,9). Known predisposing factors for the formation of atrial thrombi include mitral valvar disease (in particular, rheumatic), atrial fibrillation, and left atrial enlargement. Due to the limited sensitivity of the diagnostic methods that were previously available, little information exists on the prevalence, the pathophysiologic mechanism, and the natural history of left atrial thrombi, particularly when associated with conditions other than mitral stenosis. For the same reason, the indications for anticoagulant therapy are still determined empirically, and the efficacy of the treatment is not sufficiently proven.

Thrombi can occur at any site within the left atrial cavity, although the left atrial appendage is most often involved. The morphology of these thrombi can vary greatly from ball-like masses to flattened, plaque-like mural structures, and their size can range from a huge accumulation of thrombotic material occupying a large part of the atrial cavity (Fig. 4.2) to a small pedunculated structure detectable on the atrial side of either the native or the prosthetic mitral valve (Fig. 4.3).

It has been shown in several studies that precordial echocardiography has low sensitivity for the detection of left atrial thrombi (10,11). This is partly due to the fact that half of the thrombi lie within the left atrial appendage, which is almost inaccessible from the precordium. In addition, the masking effect of either thickened rheumatic mitral valves or valvar prostheses, reduces the ability of precordial cross-sectional echocardiography to image thrombi placed within the main left atrial cavity (Fig. 4.4).

In contrast, transoesophageal studies give an unimpaired view of the left atrium and permit exploration of the left atrial appendage (12). The technique of scanning the left atrium through multiple basal short-axis and four-chamber cross sections has already been discussed. The atrial walls can be thoroughly explored, and atrial soft tissues such as thrombi can be visualized, both within the main part of the left atrium and the appendage (Figs. 4.5 and 4.6). On the transoesophageal

Cardiac Sources of Systemic Emboli — Transoesophageal versus Precordial Echocardiography		
Cardiac lesions	Transoesophageal	Precordial
Masses		
left atrial thrombus	+++	+
left atrial appendage thrombus	+++	−
left atrial myxoma	+++	++
mitral valve/prosthesis vegetations	++	+
aortic valve/prosthesis vegetations	+	+
left ventricular thrombus	+	++
Other conditions		
left atrial spontaneous echocardiographic contrast	+++	+
atrial septal defect (paradoxical embolism)	+++	+
patent oval foramen (paradoxical embolism)	+++	+
prolapse of mitral valve	+*	++
atrial septal aneurysm	+++	+
− = insufficient + = sufficient ++ = good +++ = excellent * = with biplane transoesophageal imaging, +++		

Fig. 4.1 Cardiac sources of systemic emboli — the relative values of transoesophageal versus precordial echocardiography.

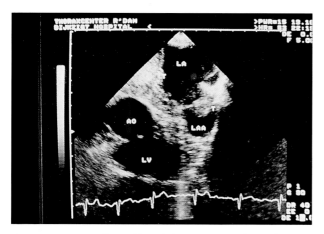

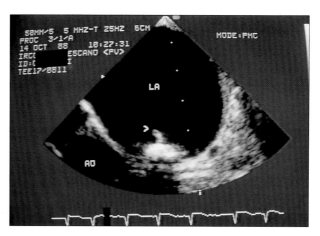

Fig. 4.2 Transoesophageal basal short-axis scan of the left atrium in a patient with mitral stenosis. A large part of the main atrial cavity and the appendage is occupied by thrombus (T).

Fig. 4.3 Transoesophageal transverse-axis image in a patient with mitral valvar prosthesis. A pedunculated, mobile thrombus (arrowed) is attached to the atrial side of the valve.

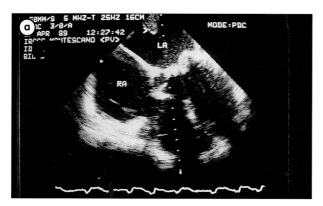

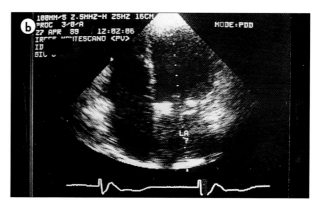

Fig. 4.4 Transoesophageal and precordial four-chamber views in a patient with a mitral bio-prosthesis. (a) From the transoesophageal approach, thrombus (arrowed) attached to the posterior wall of the left atrium and protruding into the atrial cavity, is clearly visible. (b) On the precordial image, no definite structure could be visualized in the corresponding site despite a high setting of the gain control.

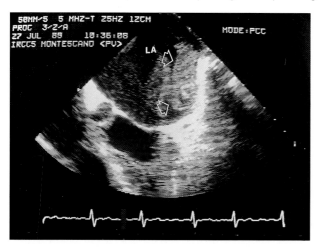

Fig. 4.5 Transoesophageal transverse view in a patient with mitral stenosis. An example of a large thrombus attached to the lateral wall of the left atrium is shown (arrowed). The transoesophageal image allows the differentiation of thrombus from the underlying myocardium and from a cloud of spontaneous echocardiographic contrast surrounding the mass.

images, the characteristic echocardiographic 'texture' of thrombus is easy to differentiate from the underlying myocardium, and the contours facing the atrial cavity are clearly delineated. Thus, left atrial thrombus can be readily differentiated from myocardial structures and spontaneous echocardiographic effects (see *Fig. 4.5*).

If little diagnostic doubt exists in the case of large atrial thrombi, small lesions within the appendage may be difficult to differentiate from the crenellated configuration of the appendage produced by the pectinate muscles. Furthermore, as previously mentioned in *Chapter 3*, the bulbous appearance of the wall that separates the appendage from the left upper pulmonary vein must not be misinterpreted as thrombus. Doppler investigation of flow within the left appendage can provide valuable additional information to differentiate small thrombi from wall structures. Indeed, the detection of an abnormally low flow in a patient with a sus-

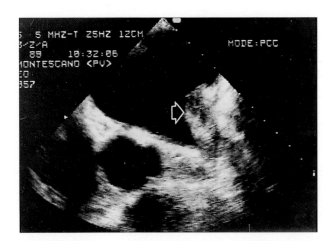

Fig. 4.6 Transoesophageal basal short-axis of the left atrium at the level of the appendage in a patient with mitral stenosis and recent stroke. The cavity of the appendage appears almost completely filled by mural thrombus (arrowed).

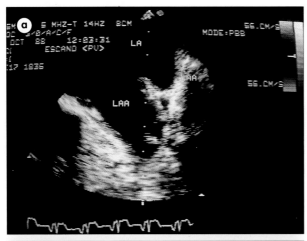

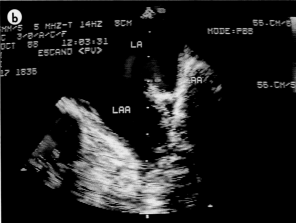

Fig. 4.7 Transoesophageal short-axis scan of the left atrial appendage in a patient with stroke. (a) A small echogenic structure, more protruding and mobile than the usual appearance of pectinate muscles, is seen at the apex of the appendage. (b) Colour flow mapping shows absence of significant flow velocity within the appendage. This finding would support the diagnosis of thrombus formation secondary to very low velocity flow.

pected mass should reinforce the presumptive diagnosis of thrombus (Fig. 4.7).

In patients with either native mitral valvar disease or a mitral prosthesis, emboli can also arise from the valvar leaflets or from the sewing ring (see *Fig. 4.3*). Transoesophageal echocardiography can identify such lesions with remarkable consistency when they are large and mobile, but difficulties arise in the distinction of small thrombi, vegetations, calcified areas, and suture material (Fig. 4.8).

Apart from allowing the diagnosis of left atrial thrombus, transoesophageal echocardiography provides new insight into some unresolved questions related to its pathogenesis and natural history. Once the diagnosis of thrombus has been made, serial examinations can be used to assess the effect of therapy. Mugge and associates, who investigated a group of patients with left atrial thrombus, were able to demonstrate the rapid resolution of thrombi in 14 of 16 patients (13). On the basis of this encouraging observation, the transoesophageal technique may be employed to follow up patients found to have intra-atrial thrombus and, for this reason, undergoing anticoagulation. In cases where anticoagulants have proved ineffective, other alternative treatments, such as fibrinolytic agents or inhibitors of platelet function, can be assessed in the same manner. In this respect, we believe that transoesophageal echocardiography may also have a relevant application whenever anticoagulants are administered in a patient in atrial fibrillation prior to cardioversion.

Since cardiac transplantation was introduced as an accepted treatment for patients with end-stage cardiac failure, a new category of patients is at risk of developing atrial thrombus and peripheral embolism. Angermann and associates used the transoesophageal approach to visualize the anastomoses between the atria of donors and recipients (14). The occurrence of spontaneous contrast and mural thrombi was observed in proximity to the suture line. Furthermore, pseudoaneurysms of the reconstructed atrial septum were detected by the transoesophageal approach. Thus, this investigation should be considered in recipients of transplanted hearts subsequent to cerebral ischaemic episodes. The findings obtained might be useful in explaining some of the neurologic events that occur occasionally after a heart transplantation (15).

The spontaneous contrast effect is an echocardiographic phenomenon attributed to an increased echo reflection which occurs when the red cells 'clump' together. This appearance is often associated with mural thrombi, and is commonly seen where there is low flow within a cardiac chamber. Spontaneous echocardiographic contrast appears as swirling clouds of echoes,

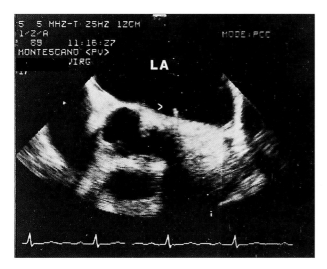

Fig. 4.8 Transoesophageal short-axis cross section of the left atrium at the level of the appendage in a patient with mitral prosthesis. The small, fixed, echo-dense structure (arrowed), visible just above the insertion of the prosthesis, is probably due to suture material.

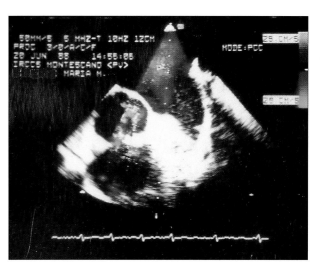

Fig. 4.10 Transoesophageal colour flow mapping of the left atrium and appendage in a patient with 'lone' atrial fibrillation. The appendage appears colour free while spontaneous echocardiographic contrast is present in its cavity. These two findings concordantly indicate the presence of blood stasis within the appendage.

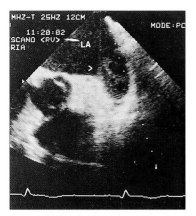

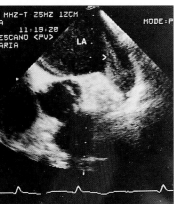

Fig. 4.9 Transoesophageal short-axis images of the left atrial appendage in a patient with atrial fibrillation. A thick cloud of spontaneous contrast is visible within the appendage. These two different frames give the impression of the characteristic swirling movement of the spontaneous contrast which is most apparent in real time.

neous contrast (16). If its detection within the left atrium by precordial cross-sectional echocardiography is exceptional, it would have been visualized with the transoesophageal approach in two-thirds of patients with mitral valvar stenosis and in over one-third of patients with mitral valvar replacement (16). Moreover, in these conditions, the presence of spontaneous contrast is associated with an increased risk of thromboembolism. Spontaneous echocardiographic contrast can also be seen in patients with atrial fibrillation without mitral valvar disease (Fig. 4.10), and subsequent to cardiac transplantation.

BLOOD FLOW WITHIN THE LEFT ATRIAL APPENDAGE

In patients in sinus rhythm, the left atrial appendage appears as a vigorously contracting structure. Correspondingly, both pulsed and colour flow Doppler identify significant velocities of flow into and out of its cavity. Normal flow has a biphasic configuration. The positive velocities indicate blood flow towards the transducer and represent ejection coinciding with left atrial contraction and the electrocardiographic P wave. The negative velocities indicate flow in the opposite direction and represent filling of the appendage in ventricular systole. This pattern differs significantly from normal flow in the left upper pulmonary vein (Fig. 4.11). Therefore, although both the left atrial appendage and the left upper pulmonary vein are in close proximity

either occupying the main left atrial cavity or localized to the appendage (Fig. 4.9). Due to its characteristic motion and indistinct contours it can readily be differentiated from both signal 'noise' and atrial thrombus. It must be remembered, nonetheless, that an appropriate high-gain setting is required to detect mild forms of sponta-

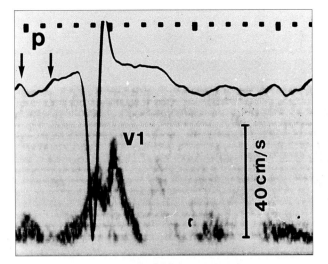

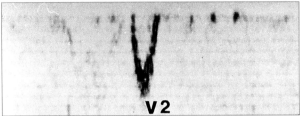

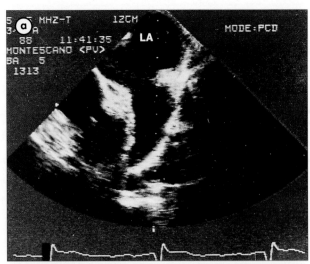

Fig. 4.11 Pulsed wave Doppler of the flow within the left atrial appendage in a subject in sinus rhythm. The normal biphasic to-and-fro pattern is shown. This waveform follows the electrocardiographic P wave. The positive (V1) and negative (V2) components represent ejection from and filling of, the appendage, respectively.

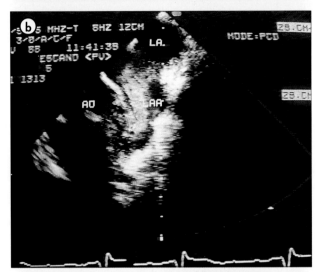

(Fig. 4.11), there should be no confusion as to which cavity is being interrogated by the pulsed Doppler modality. Doppler studies using colour flow confirm the biphasic pattern of ejection from left atrial appendage and filling, by demonstrating the rapid sequence of changes of colour (blue and red) (Fig. 4.12); since this change is rapid, the colour M mode may be more helpful for the precise timing of these events.

Patterns of flow in patients with atrial arrhythmias

In patients with atrial flutter, the same biphasic pattern of flow in the left atrial appendage follows each electrocardiographic 'flutter' wave, resulting in a 'saw-tooth' profile on the pulsed Doppler trace (Fig. 4.13). The peak velocities of both the positive and negative components are smaller than those seen in normals. Patients with atrial fibrillation, either in isolation or in association with other pathologies, can be subdivided

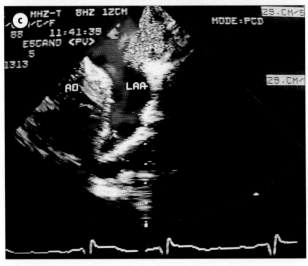

Fig. 4.12 Transoesophageal echocardiogram of the left atrial appendage. (a) The normal appearance of the appendage as imaged by a transoesophageal basal short-axis section. (b and c) Colour flow maps obtained in the same patient. The appendage is opacified by red (ejection phase) and subsequently by blue (filling phase). Note the close proximity of the flow coming from the left upper pulmonary vein into the atrium.

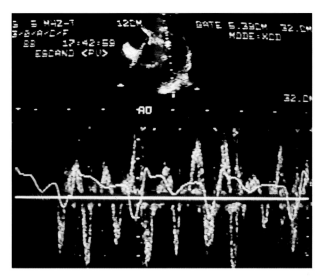

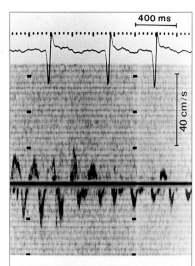

Fig. 4.14 Velocity of flow within the left atrial appendage recorded by transoesophageal pulsed wave Doppler in a patient in atrial fibrillation. In this patient, a significant velocity of flow with a multiphasic irregular pattern is seen.

Fig. 4.13 Transoesophageal pulsed Doppler recording of the flow within the left atrial appendage in a patient in atrial flutter with 2:1 block. This shows a saw-tooth pattern with two biphasic waveforms corresponding with each R–R electrocardiographic interval.

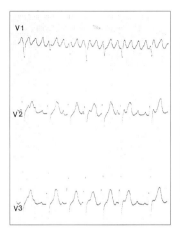

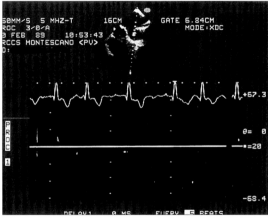

Fig. 4.15 Pulsed wave Doppler of the left atrial appendage in a patient with mitral stenosis and atrial flutter with variable block. No significant flow could be detected by Doppler.

Echocardiographic Variables			
	Thrombus and/or spontaneous echo contrast	No thrombus or spontaneous echo contrast	P value
	10 patients	32 patients	
V1 (cm/s)	3.5±5.6	45±26	<0.001
V2 (cm/s)	2.5±4.2	44±19	<0.001
LAA diameter (mm)	25±10	17±6	<0.005
LA diameter (mm)	53±10	40±9	<0.002
V1=peak positive flow velocity within the left atrial appendage V2=peak negative flow velocity within the left atrial appendage			

Fig. 4.16 Echocardiographic variables in patients with and without thrombi and/or spontaneous echocardiographic contrast within the left atrial appendage. For an illustration of V1 and V2, see *Fig. 4.11*.

on the basis of flow patterns detected by transoesophageal pulsed Doppler. The first group has a 'multiphasic' pattern of flow in which the time intervals between each waveform, as well as the peak velocities, are irregular (Fig. 4.14). The second group has no significant flow detectable by either pulsed Doppler or colour flow mapping (Fig. 4.15). The latter technique shows that the left atrial appendage is free of colour throughout the whole cardiac cycle (see *Fig. 4.9*). This subset of patients has a high incidence of either the appearance of a spontaneous echocardiographic contrast effect or mural thrombus localized within the left atrial appendage (17,18). In our recent experience, the presence of thrombus and/or spontaneous echocardiographic contrast was closely associated with reduced velocity of flow within the appendage (Fig. 4.16). Thus, these patients would be expected to be at higher risk for systemic embolization. Interestingly, we have ob-

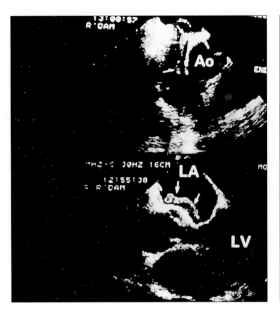

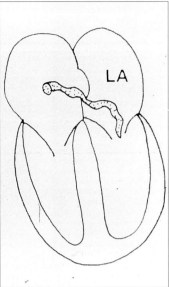

Fig. 4.17 Transoesophageal echocardiograms in a patient with both pulmonary and systemic embolization. A worm-like thrombus (arrows) within the right and left atria and across the septum is clearly visible. This transoesophageal study led to the demonstration of paradoxical embolization in a patient with a patent oval foramen.

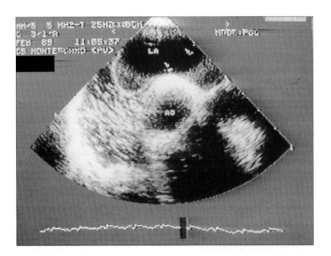

Fig. 4.18 Transoesophageal short-axis image of the atria during the peripheral injection of agitated saline as a contrast medium. The right atrium is completely opacified. A few bubbles become visible (arrowed) in the left atrium, immediately after a Valsalva manoeuvre. This is a reliable sign of patency of the oval foramen. (By courtesy of Dr R Tramarin, Centro Medico Montescano, Pavia).

served an absence of significant flow within the appendage in three patients with sinus rhythm and a history of recent stroke. In these patients, the isolated standstill of the appendage was associated with the presence of mural thrombus and/or spontaneous echo contrast within the appendage. The clinical potential of Doppler interrogation of the left atrial appendage requires further evaluation. Our experience would indicate that the absence of flow within the appendage might represent a predisposing factor for systemic em-

bolism. Moreover, because of the close association between the absence of significant flow and the detection of thrombi, the assessment of this pattern may represent a useful confirmatory sign for differentiating small thrombi from pectinate muscles. Thus, when echogenic masses are seen within the appendage, and flow cannot be detected by Doppler, the presence of thrombus should be strongly suspected (see *Fig. 4.7*).

PARADOXICAL EMBOLIZATION AND PATENT OVAL FORAMEN

Paradoxical embolization from the systemic venous circulation and the right heart is a recognized complication of an atrial septal defect. Recent interest has focused on the role of the patency of the oval foramen in the pathogenesis of paradoxical emboli (Fig. 4.17) (3). In normal circumstances, the oval foramen becomes functionally closed within a few days of birth, and anatomical closure usually occurs within the first year of birth (19). A patent foramen, however, can persist in the normal population with an incidence that progressively declines with increasing age. Overall, as judged in a large autopsy study, persisting patency is observed in approximately one-quarter of normal hearts (20).

Since the size of the foramen is usually very small, precordial cross-sectional imaging cannot detect its presence within an otherwise normal interatrial septum. The investigation of the oval fossa purely by means of cross-sectional images does not allow any reliable diagnosis of a patent foramen, even with the transoesophageal approach. Therefore, when its presence needs to be confirmed, it is necessary to rely on contrast or colour Doppler echocardiography in order to detect a minor right-to-left shunt across the interatrial septum. The transient elevation of the right atrial pressure produced by coughing or other Valsalva-like manoeuvres, causes an inversion of the normal pressure gradient between right and left atria. When a patent foramen is present, these manoeuvres produce a small right-to-left shunt that can be detected using a peripheral injection of venous contrast, during either precordial or transoesophageal echocardiographic monitoring. This method involves the injection of 10–20ml of agitated saline into an antecubital vein, while the patient performs a Valsalva manoeuvre. When the right atrium becomes opacified, the patient is invited to release the respiratory effort; at this moment, the presence of a patent foramen can be recognized by the immediate appearance of microbubbles within the cavities of the left heart (Fig. 4.18). To increase the sensitivity of this procedure, we have used three repeated injections. Using precordial echocardiography in conjunction with a peripheral injection of venous contrast, Lechat and associates were able to demonstrate a patent foramen in 40% of patients with an ischaemic stroke, and in only 10% of a control group (3). This study shows, convincingly, that patency of the foramen may be implicated in the genesis of an embolic stroke. Since the reported prevalence of this abnormality is less than that found at autopsy, however, the sensitivity of precordial contrast echocardiography is probably low. The transoesophageal technique, providing a fine delineation of the oval fossa and excellent visualization of the echocardiographic contrast within the cardiac chambers should be the most sensitive method. A patent foramen can be found by contrast transoesophageal echocardiography in approximately one-third of patients with a recent stroke (6,21). The prevalence of this finding in patients with ischaemic stroke and normal extracranial carotid arteries, however, may be as high as 54%, although it is only 24% in patients with significant lesions of the carotid arteries (6).

Alternatively, colour flow mapping can be used to detect a right-to-left shunt through a patent foramen during Valsalva or Valsalva-like manoeuvres. Since the resulting colour jet is usually small and nonturbulent, the echocardiographic section must precisely transect the fossa. Such imaging is best performed with a biplane probe in the longitudinal axis, but even then, it can be difficult during a Valsalva manoeuvre because of the movements of the heart induced by the forced respiration. The advantage of the contrast method is that the appearance of microbubbles in the left heart cavities, immediately after the opacification of the right atrium, is easily detectable without requiring the direct visualization of the fossa. In addition, other intra-atrial flows, such as those which come from the right upper pulmonary vein, may simulate transseptal flow, and the diagnosis by colour flow Doppler is made more difficult. For these reasons, we consider the method that uses contrast to be far better for the diagnosis of patency of the oval foramen. This investigation may be important in those patients with cerebral ischaemic events of suspected embolic origin and should be performed whenever a precordial echo (inclusive of contrast study) has failed to detect any potential source of systemic emboli. In addition, this examination may have important implications in normal subjects who practice underwater diving, since patency of the oval foramen is probably implicated as a risk factor for the development of decompression sickness due to gas embolism (22).

OTHER CARDIAC SOURCES OF SYSTEMIC EMBOLI

Atrial septal aneurysm

Atrial septal aneurysm is an infrequent anatomic condition that has been related to atrial arrhythmias, a midsystolic click, prolapse of the mitral valve, and pulmonary and systemic embolization (23–26). It is a membranous mobile structure that can involve the entire atrial septum, and it may co-exist with either an atrial septal defect or patency of the oval foramen. Its noninvasive diagnosis became possible with the advent of cross-sectional echocardiography. The prevalence of this finding during precordial studies was significantly less than that found at autopsy. This would suggest that many septal aneurysms, because of their thin laminar structure and the poor orientation of the interrogating ultrasound beams, were missed by precordial ultrasound. In contrast, atrial septal aneurysm can be easily diagnosed by transoesophageal echocardiography due to the higher resolution of the images and the better orientation of the echocardiographic plane to the interatrial septum. In addition, the movements of the aneurysmal septum, which reflect the variation of the interatrial pressure gradient, can be followed during normal or forced respiration, the latter produced, for example, by coughing or a Valsalva manoeuvre. Contrast echocardiography allows the detection of co-existing patency of the foramen, or an atrial septal defect (Fig. 4.19). The transoesophageal technique should, thus, be a very useful technique for clarifying

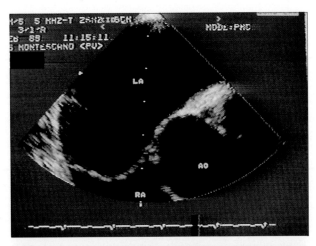

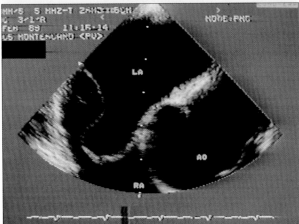

Fig. 4.19 Transoesophageal images of an atrial septal aneurysm. The membranous appearance of the aneurysm that separates the atria is seen. The two frames demonstrate the movement of the septum related to different respiratory phases. In this patient, the aneurysm involves the whole atrial septum and is associated with patency of the oval foramen (see *Fig. 4.18*). (By courtesy of Dr R Tramarin, Centro Medico Montescano, Pavia).

the role of septal patency in the genesis of systemic embolism. Whether an atrial septal aneurysm facilitates the formation of thrombus (which is only rarely seen at autopsy) or is only indirectly related to systemic embolism associated with other factors such as a patent oval foramen, prolapse of the mitral valve or atrial arrhythmias still needs to be determined.

Prolapse of the mitral valve

The association between prolapse of the mitral valve and stroke has been convincingly established in patients less than 45 years old (27), and the embolic nature of these episodes is demonstrated by cerebral angiography. The fact that valvar thrombi represent the

cause, however, is purely conjectural, and other alternative mechanisms such as atrial arrhythmias and bacterial endocarditis, can be involved. The diagnosis of a prolapse can usually be made from precordial echocardiography, although some authors have found the transoesophageal approach more sensitive (28). In young patients with cerebral ischaemia, a prolapse of the leaflets can be found by this method in up to 60% of cases, perhaps confirming the data previously obtained with precordial echocardiography. In studies that also include older patients, the prevalence of prolapse is much less, and its relation to the ischaemic episode is less clear (4,6).

If the transoesophageal approach can visualize the mitral valve with a superior quality of images, it should be remembered that, with standard probes, the valvar apparatus can be imaged in only one transverse plane. This plane is not optimal for the diagnosis of prolapse and this limitation, discussed in detail in *Chapter 6*, should be taken into account when the transoesophageal technique is used. In this respect, the limitations of the precordial four-chamber view in the diagnosis of mitral valvar disease should also be acknowledged for the transoesophageal approach.

Infective endocarditis, thoracic aortic disease, and aortic valvar disease are other important causes of systemic embolization and represent prime indications for a transoesophageal study. These subjects are discussed in their specific chapters.

Left ventricular thrombus, associated with either myocardial infarction or congestive cardiomyopathy, is recognized as an important cause of systemic embolization (29) but is more readily diagnosed by precordial than transoesophageal imaging. This is especially true of left ventricular thrombus occurring in the apical or anterior portion of the left ventricle. These areas are well-recognized blind spots for standard transoesophageal imaging. Recent experience suggests that biplane transducers that provide long-axis cross sections of the left ventricle, might overcome this limitation.

IMPLICATION FOR THE MANAGEMENT OF PATIENTS WITH SYSTEMIC EMBOLI

Before the advent of transoesophageal echocardiography, the diagnosis of a cardiac source of cerebral embolism was frequently uncertain. Precordial echocardiography was not considered a valuable technique for the investigation of these patients when a clinically detectable cardiac abnormality was not present. The role of precordial echocardiography was limited, even in patients with overt heart disease, due to the low sensitivity of the technique for detecting some of the intracardiac sources of emboli. The transoesophageal approach has overcome many of these limitations, so that it yields a large amount of important information.

As previously discussed, the sensitivity of this approach for the detection of the cardiac sources of emboli has been established. By combining the precordial and transoesophageal approaches, the clinician now has at his or her disposal, a powerful means of detecting these abnormalities. To establish the importance of this information in terms of clinical management, other factors should be considered. Firstly, the strength of the association between cardiac lesions and embolization should be taken into account. Some cardiac abnormalities, such as prolapse of the mitral valve and patency of the oval foramen, are very frequent in 'normal' populations and probably have a low risk for embolization. The diagnosis of these morphologic abnormalities, therefore, does not necessarily prove the embolic mechanism since it can be associated with other conditions that produce a risk of embolization, such as lesions of the carotid arteries. Secondly, the therapeutic impact of the diagnosis must be considered. The role of transoesophageal echocardiography (still a semi-invasive technique available only in a limited number of centres) in the diagnostic workup of patients with suspected emboli, therefore, should be evaluated by taking into consideration the clinical data and the information obtained from other techniques such as cerebral computed tomography, high-resolution ultrasound imaging, Doppler, and angiography of cerebral arteries.

At present, transoesophageal echocardiography has two main roles in the assessment of patients with cerebral ischaemic events of suspected embolic origin. Firstly, it can be performed in patients with overt cardiac disease who are at risk of left atrial thrombus if they have or have not suffered a cerebral ischaemic event; this would be particularly relevant when the indication for anticoagulant therapy is not clearcut (30). This could occur, for example, in a patient with lone atrial fibrillation, or in a patient with a mitral bio-prosthesis in sinus rhythm. The direct demonstration of thrombotic material, spontaneous echocardiographic contrast, or reduced flow within the left atrial appendage would, in these cases, reinforce the decision to give prophylactic anticoagulation. Serial examinations can then be performed to assess the effect of therapy.

Secondly, in patients with stroke and normal or inconclusive standard echocardiography, a transoesophageal study should be considered since it may demonstrate a cause for embolization in many patients studied. When a patent oval foramen is detected, some have advocated that deep venous phlebography should be performed, and those with detectable thrombus should be given anticoagulants. The management of a patent oval foramen with peripheral emboli may be more difficult since the origin and the type of paradoxical emboli may not be discovered. Use of antiplatelet inhibitors has been proposed for those with prolapse of the leaflets of the mitral valve.

The yield of transoesophageal studies will be more relevant in patients less than 45 years old. In older patients, other important causes of cerebral ischaemia, such as ulcerated carotid atheromas, are likely to be present and can sometimes co-exist with cardiac abnormalities (6). For this reason, the indication for transoesophageal echocardiography in this subset should probably be restricted to those patients in whom an ultrasonic study of the cerebral arteries and/or angiography has shown normal vessels, or when the side of the vascular abnormality is not concordant with the cerebral lesion.

RIGHT ATRIAL THROMBUS, SPONTANEOUS ECHO CONTRAST, AND PULMONARY EMBOLI

Spontaneous contrast and formation of thrombus would appear to be much less common in the right than in the left atrium, even though right atrial dysfunction frequently accompanies left atrial pathology and dysfunction. We have frequently observed patients in atrial fibrillation with bi-atrial enlargement, by transoesophageal echocardiography, who have spontaneous contrast and thrombus in the left atrium, and yet the right atrium is clear. The most likely explanation for this is that right atrial dysfunction is usually secondary to high right-heart pressures that are nearly always associated with varying degrees of tricuspid regurgitation. This results in abnormal, yet increased, flows of blood within the right atrium, thus preventing the formation of spontaneous echo contrast and thrombus.

In several cases, however, the visualization of mobile thrombus within the right atrium has been described, using precordial echocardiography in patients with overt or suspected pulmonary embolization (31–33). There is growing evidence that these mobile masses originate from deep venous thrombosis. Their echocardiographic appearance consists of elongated worm-like masses floating within the right atrium, and often through the tricuspid valve, with no apparent site of attachment. The diagnosis of these masses in most cases can be made by routine echocardiography. We believe that the transoesophageal approach should be considered whenever the diagnosis is difficult from the pre-

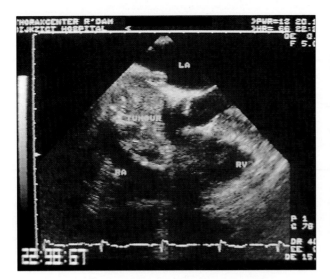

Fig. 4.20 Transoesophageal scan of right atrial myxoma. Note how well the site of attachment on the atrial septum is visualized from the transoesophageal approach. The transoesophageal study was also able to demonstrate the extension of the tumour across the atrial septum and its protrusion into the left atrium. This information prompted the surgeon to perform a wide excision of the septum.

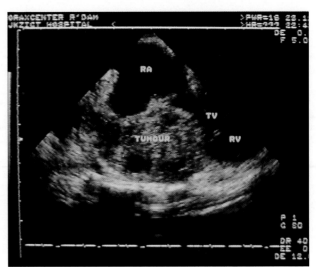

Fig. 4.21 Transoesophageal image of a large tumour involving the right atrium and partially obstructing the tricuspid orifice. The structure of the tumour is not homogeneous, and small cystic structures are visible within the mass. The biopsy of the tumour, performed under transoesophageal echocardiographic control, led to a diagnosis of angiosarcoma.

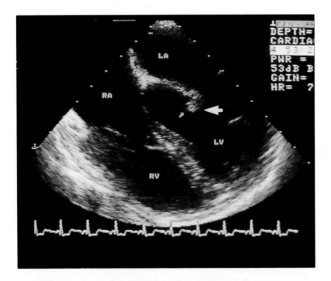

Fig. 4.22 Transoesophageal four-chamber view showing a small mass attached to the aortic leaflet of the mitral valve (arrowed). The diagnosis of a fibroelastoma of the mitral valve was confirmed at operation.

cordium because of images of nonoptimal quality. In these cases, other causes of mobile right atrial masses, including primary or secondary tumours, vegetations, a prominent Chiari network, or an Eustachian valve, must be excluded. Important diagnostic elements can be better differentiated by the transoesophageal examination; for example, myxomas can be recognized from the more homogeneous acoustic pattern and from the

site of their attachment (Fig. 4.20). Vegetations will usually be attached to the tricuspid valve.

CARDIAC TUMOURS

Atrial myxoma

A myxoma represents the single most frequent tumour occurring in the heart. It is more frequently localized within the left atrium, from which it often causes systemic emboli. Either a left or right atrial myxoma can be easily diagnosed by precordial echo, but the transoesophageal approach may provide new information about its morphology, acoustic structure, and site of attachment on the atrial septum. This information may be useful for the surgeon prior to the resection and it may be used after the operation to detect early recurrence of the tumour (Fig. 4.20).

Direct spread of a tumour up the inferior caval vein into the right atrium is a rare, but described, complication of renal carcinoma and Wilms tumour in children. The transoesophageal echo can be extremely useful for making this diagnosis, since the junction of the inferior caval vein and the right atrium can usually be well visualized. Moreover, as shown in Fig. 4.21, the extension and structure of a tumour, and its relation with the tricuspid valvar apparatus, can be assessed more precisely with transoesophageal imaging.

Angiosarcoma of the right atrium and ventricle has been seen in two patients in our institution. Both tumours were more clearly visualized by the transoesophageal approach and, in one patient, a biopsy of the tumour was carried out under transoesophageal echo-cardiographic control (Fig. 4.21). A mitral valvar fibro-elastoma was also diagnosed by the transoesophageal technique and differentiated from a vegetation or thrombus (Fig. 4.22).

REFERENCES

1. Knopman DS, Anderson DC, Asinger RW *et al.* Indications for echocardiography in patients with ischemic stroke. *Neurology* 1982;**32**:1005–11.

2. Hart RG, Miller VT. Cerebral infarction in young adults: a practical approach. *Stroke* 1983;**14**:110–4.

3. Lechat Ph, Mas JL, Lascault G *et al.* Prevalence of patent foramen ovale in patients with stroke. *N Eng J Med* 1988;**318**:1148–52.

4. Pop G, Sutherland GR, Koudstaal PJ *et al.* Transesophageal echocardiography in the detection of intracardiac emboli sources in patients with transient ischemic attacks. *Stroke* 1990;**21**:560–5.

5. Daniel WG, Engberding R, Erbel R *et al.* Transesophageal echocardiography in arterial embolism and central ischemic events — An European multicenter study in patients without pre-known cardiac disease [Abstract]. *Eur Heart J* 1989;**10** (suppl):204.

6. Tramarin R, Pozzoli M, Torbicki A *et al.* Integrated high resolution cardiovascular study of patients with ischemic stroke [Abstract]. *Eur Heart J* 1989;**10** (suppl):2001.

7. Stolberger C, Brainin M, Slany J. Transesophageal echocardiography in patients with embolic events [Abstract]. *Eur Heart J* 1989;**10** (suppl):204.

8. Wallach JB, Lukash L, Angrist AA. Interpretation of incidence of mural thrombi in left auricle and appendage with particular reference to mitral commissurotomy. *Am Heart J* 1953; **45**:252–4.

9. Askey JM, *Systemic Arterial Embolism.* New York: Grune Stratton, 1957.

10. Come PC, Riley MF, Markis JE, Malagold M. Limitations of echocardiographic techniques in evaluation of left atrial masses. *Am J Cardiol* 1981;**48**:947–53.

11. Shereshita NK, Moreno FL, Narcisso FV *et al.* Two-dimensional echocardiographic diagnosis of left atrial thrombus in rheumatic heart disease. A clinicopathologic study. *Circulation* 1983;**167**:341–7.

12. Ashemberg W, Shulter M, Kremer P *et al.* Transesophageal two-dimensional echocardiography for the detection of left atrial appendage thrombus. *J Am Coll Cardiol* 1986;**7**:163–6.

13. Mugge A, Daniel WG, Lichtlen PR. Left atrial appendage thrombi follow-up by transesophageal echocardiography [Abstract]. *Eur Heart J* 1989;**10** (suppl):207.

14. Angerman CE, Spes CH, Tammen AR *et al.* Transthoracic and transesophageal echocardiographic findings after orthotopic heart transplantation. In: Erbel R, Khandheria BK, Brennecke R, Meyer J, Seward J B, Tajik AJ, eds. *Transesophageal echocardiography: A new window to the heart.* Berlin:Springer–Verlag, 1989:330–8.

15. Sila CA. Spectrum of neurologic events following cardiac transplant. *Stroke* 1989;**20**:1586–9.

16. Daniel WG, Nellesen U, Shroeder E *et al.* Left atrial spontaneous echo contrast in mitral valve disease: an indicator for an increased thromboembolic risk. *J Am Coll Cardiol* 1988;**11**:1204–11.

17. Pozzoli M, Tramarin R, Torbicki A *et al.* Standstill of left atrial appendage: a new Doppler sign of thromboembolic risk? [Abstract]. *Eur Heart J* 1989;**10** (suppl):206.

18. Suetsogu M, Matsizaki M, Tomay *et al.* Detection of mural thrombi and analysis of blood flow velocities in the left atrial appendage using transesophageal two-dimensional echocardiography and pulsed Doppler flowmetry. *J Cardiol* 1988;**18**:385–94.

19. Patten BM. The closure of the foramen ovale. *Am J Anat* 1931;**48**:19–44.

20. Hagen PT, Scholz DG, Edwards WD. Incidence and size of patent foramen ovale during the first 10 decades of life: an autopsy study of 965 normal hearts. *Mayo Clin Proc* 1984;**58**:17–20.

21. Decoodt P, Kalenelenbogen R, Heuse D *et al.* Detection of patent foramen ovale in stroke by transesophageal contrast echocardiography [Abstract]. *Circulation* 1989;**II**(suppl):339.

22. Moon R E, Camporesi EM, Kisslo JA. Patent foramen ovale and decompression sickness in divers. *Lancet* 1989;**i**:513–4.

23. Hanley PG, Tajik AJ, Hynes JK *et al.* Diagnosis and classification of atrial septal aneurysm by two-dimensional echocardiography: Report of 80 consecutive cases. *J Am Coll Cardiol* 1985;**6**:13–82.

24. Iliceto S, Papa A, Sorino M, Rizzon P. Combined atrial septal aneurysm and mitral valve prolapse: detection by two-dimensional echocardiography. *Am J Cardiol* 1984; **54**:1151–3.

25. Silver MD, Dorsey JS, Aneurysm of the septum primum in adults. *Arch Pathol Lab Med* 1978;**73**:227–30.

26. Grosgogeat Y, Lhermitte F, Carpentier A *et al.* Aneurysme de la

cloison interauricolaire revele par une embolie cerebrale. *Arch Mal Coeur* 1973;**66**:169–77.

27. Barnett HJM, Bougner DR, Taylor DW *et al.* Further evidence relating mitral valve prolapse to cerebral ischemic events. *N Eng J Med* 1980;**307**:369–70.

28. Zenker G, Erbel R, Kramer G *et al.* Transesophageal two-dimensional echocardiography in young patients with cerebral ischemic events. *Stroke* 1988;**19**:345–8.

29. Cabin HS, Roberts WC. Left ventricular aneurysm, intraaneurysmal thrombus and systemic embolus in coronary heart disease. *Chest* 1980;**77**:463–9.

30. Lie JT. Atrial fibrillation and left atrial thrombus: an insufferable odd couple. *Am Heart J* 1988;**116**:1374–7.

31. Armstrong WF, Feigenbaum H, Dillon JC. Echocardiographic detection of right atrial thromboembolism. *Chest* 1985;**87**:801.

32. Bergman C, Monaghan M, Daly K, Jewitt DE. Right atrial embolus. Echocardiographic features. *Br Heart J* 1985;**53**:552.

33. Torbicki A, Pasierski T, Uchman B, Miskiewic Z. Right atrial mobile thrombi, two-dimensional echocardiographic diagnosis and clinical outcome. *Cor Vasa* 1987;**29**:293–303.

5

Pulmonary venous flow

Bernardino Tuccillo
Alan G Fraser

INTRODUCTION

Until transoesophageal echocardiography became available, it was extremely difficult to obtain accurate recordings of flow of pulmonary venous blood in adults. Now, however, it is possible to obtain excellent Doppler traces in almost all patients who are studied. As a result, interest in patterns of pulmonary venous flow, and their possible relevance for diagnosis and monitoring, is increasing rapidly. So far, pulmonary venous Doppler profiles remain a subject for research rather than proven clinical application, but initial expe-

rience suggests that they may be useful in certain circumstances. This chapter reviews some of the findings of early physiological studies of pulmonary venous blood flow, the normal patterns that have been described, and some potential applications during clinical transoesophageal echocardiographic examinations.

Precordial Doppler echocardiography has been used for some years in neonates and children to assess pulmonary venous flow, especially at the orifice of the right upper pulmonary vein (1,2); this is also occasionally possible in adults using an apical four-chamber approach (Fig. 5.1). On transoesophageal echocardiogra-

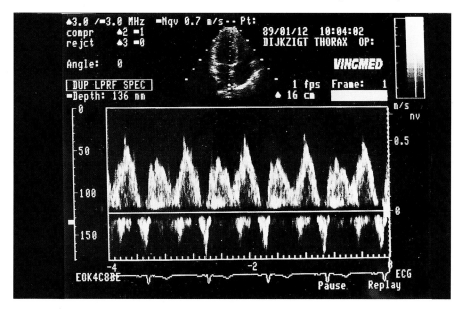

Fig. 5.1 Profile of flow at the orifice of the right upper pulmonary vein. This is obtained by using pulsed Doppler while imaging from the precordium in an apical four-chamber plane, as demonstrated in the small cross-sectional image. The pattern of flow is normal, and retrograde flow during atrial systole is demonstrated.

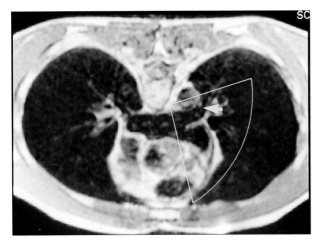

Fig. 5.2 MRI image of the heart obtained in an anatomic transverse section at the level of the upper pulmonary veins. They are seen to enter the left atrium while facing posteriorly but, for most of their extraparenchymal course, they are orientated more in a coronal plane. When the transoesophageal transducer is directed laterally, the veins are well aligned for pulsed Doppler interrogation. This is depicted for the left upper pulmonary vein (arrowed).

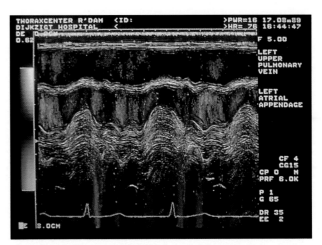

Fig. 5.3 Colour M-mode recording through the left upper pulmonary vein. This demonstrates cyclical changes in its diameter. In this patient with mitral regurgitation, there is retrograde flow into the pulmonary veins during ventricular systole, which is shown in blue, and this is associated with an increase in the size of the vein.

phy, however, the upper pulmonary veins appear to enter the left atrium facing posteriorly (Fig. 5.2), and so proper alignment from the precordium for accurate Doppler measurements of peak velocity is difficult. In addition, the pattern of flow at the orifice of a pulmonary vein may be influenced by turbulent jets within the atrium, which produce a profile that is different from that recorded within the vein itself. In contrast, it is usually easy to identify the orifices of the pulmonary veins when using transoesophageal echocardiography with colour flow mapping, and to sample flow from within their extraparenchymal portions.

In healthy subjects, the pulmonary veins are thin walled and compliant vessels. It has been reported that they can contain a sufficient volume of blood to fill the left ventricle with a normal stroke volume (3), making left ventricular filling relatively independent of beat-to-beat variations in right heart output. It has also been demonstrated that the pulmonary veins change dimension (and therefore, presumably, volume) during the cardiac cycle (3); there is, for example, an increase in size if there is retrograde pulmonary venous flow after atrial contraction. These observations have been confirmed during transoesophageal echocardiography (Fig. 5.3), but it is difficult to measure the dimensions of the pulmonary veins. Their walls are usually imaged, parallel with, rather than at right angles to, the direction of the ultrasonic beams, and so lateral resolution is poor. Furthermore, even if it were possible to measure the venous dimensions accurately, this could not be done for all four veins simultaneously and throughout

the cardiac cycle. It is evident, therefore, that transoesophageal echocardiographic techniques cannot measure pulmonary venous blood *flow*, but only *velocity profiles*. Why, then, is it anticipated that pulmonary venous velocity measurements may be of clinical value?

EXPERIMENTAL AND CLINICAL STUDIES OF PULMONARY VENOUS FLOW

The major controversy amongst physiologists who have studied flow within the pulmonary veins has been between those who have argued that flow within the pulmonary veins is 'driven' by systolic pressure waves transmitted from the right heart through the pulmonary capillary bed (4,5), and those who have reported that it is 'sucked' by pressure changes occurring within the left atrium and the left ventricle (6–10). It may be due in part to both mechanisms (11), but the argument now seems to have been resolved in favour of the latter hypothesis. Several studies have demonstrated that there is a close correlation between pulmonary venous flow and cyclical changes in left atrial pressure (1,9,12,13). Indeed, there is a constant and inverse relationship between pulmonary venous flow and the pressure in the left atrium, with venous peak velocities corresponding to troughs in left atrial pressure (Fig. 5.4). Clinical observations (13,14) also support the consensus that pulmonary venous flow is dependent on haemodynamic events within the left heart, since virtually normal patterns of venous flow have been recorded

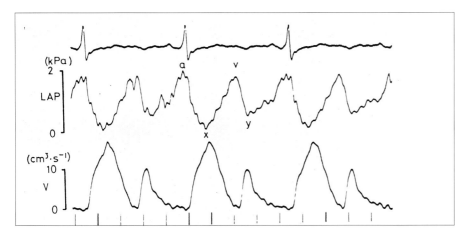

Fig. 5.4 Simultaneous recordings of pulmonary venous velocity (V) and left atrial pressure (LAP) obtained in a patient during cardiac catheterization. (Reproduced with permission of Rajagopalan B, Friend JA, Stallard T, Lee G de J. Blood flow in pulmonary veins: I. Studies in dog and man. *Cardiovasc Res* 1979; **13**:667–76).

in patients with a well-functioning Fontan circulation in which normal pulsatile pulmonary arterial flow is replaced by flow determined by right atrial contraction (1).

Since left atrial pressure is strongly influenced by left ventricular function, particularly during diastole when the mitral valve is open, it is possible that patterns of pulmonary venous flow may contain information about ventricular pressure and compliance, as well as left atrial function. An analogy can be drawn with patterns of systemic venous flow and right heart function. Many studies have demonstrated that Doppler velocity profiles recorded in the inferior and superior caval veins are altered when there is abnormal relaxation or decreased compliance of the right ventricle (15,16); for example, in patients with right ventricular hypertrophy secondary to pulmonary hypertension, abnormal relaxation of the ventricle may be reflected by diminished, or even absent forward flow within the distal caval veins in diastole, and by an increase in retrograde flow back up the caval veins during right atrial contraction.

Patients with decreased compliance of the right ventricle due to a restrictive cardiomyopathy, or other myocardial disease, have reduced ventricular filling during atrial systole (15) because the end-diastolic pressure is elevated. The most common findings on Doppler analysis of central venous flow are reduced or absent forward flow during systole, predominant forward flow during early diastole, and reversed flow during atrial contraction. In patients with more advanced disease, end-diastolic retrograde flow may occur before atrial contraction, due to a greatly elevated diastolic pressure. Thus, abnormal passive filling of the right ventricle can cause reversed flow in the central veins, as can abnormal atrial filling. Characteristic patterns of flow in the central veins are also observed in patients with pericardial constriction (17). During inspiration, there is an increase in forward flow, and on expiration there is reduced diastolic forward flow and a significant

increase in retrograde flow. In patients with tamponade, the right atrium is compressed throughout the cardiac cycle, and diastolic emptying is impeded (18,19). Systemic venous waveforms then show absence of any diastolic flow of blood into the right atrium.

Severe tricuspid regurgitation also causes typical alterations of flow from the central veins into the right atrium (20,21). If the regurgitant volume is large, or the right atrial pressure high, systolic retrograde flow occurs from the right ventricle through the right atrium and into the caval veins. The reversed flow on the Doppler velocity profile occurs at the same time as the v wave in the jugular vein. The velocity profile in the hepatic and caval veins is influenced by right atrial compliance, as well as by the degree of tricuspid regurgitation, but the finding of considerable reversed flow indicates severe tricuspid regurgitation. In such patients, forward flow into the right atrium occurs only during ventricular diastole.

Experimental studies of pulmonary venous flow, and extrapolations from more recent Doppler studies of systemic venous flow, all suggest that pulmonary venous Doppler traces may be able to provide information about the function of the left heart since abnormalities of left atrial or left ventricular function are reflected by changes in the pressure waveform of the left atrium. During ventricular systole, the pulmonary venous waveform may be influenced by changes in left atrial compliance or by mitral regurgitation. During ventricular diastole, the waveform may be affected by mitral stenosis and by left ventricular relaxation or compliance. During atrial systole, it may be influenced by conditions such as aortic incompetence, which cause a high left ventricular end-diastolic pressure.

Some of these relationships have already been documented in research studies performed in the operating room during cardiothoracic surgery, in which pulmonary venous flow was measured directly by placing electromagnetic flow probes around individual pulmonary veins (22). Clinical studies may confirm that pulmonary venous Doppler traces provide information about left heart function, without some of the problems and limitations associated with other noninvasive or semi-invasive techniques. Indeed, some properties, such as left atrial compliance, cannot at present be measured noninvasively by any other echocardiographic method.

TECHNICAL CONSIDERATIONS

The upper pulmonary veins are the most easy to locate. The left vein enters the left atrium just posterolateral to the orifice of the left atrial appendage (Fig. 5.5), and the right one can be found at the same level, entering from the right just behind the superior caval vein (Fig. 5.6). The lower pulmonary veins lie almost in a true coronal plane and enter the left atrium some 1–2cm below the orifices of the upper veins (Fig. 5.7). Unless an angle correction is used, velocities of flow recorded from within the lower veins are less than those obtained from the upper veins. For practical purposes, therefore, it is easier and quicker to record patterns of flow in the upper veins. Difficulty may be encountered only when the site of pulmonary venous drainage is anomalous or if the left atrium is very enlarged, for example, in patients with chronic mitral stenosis. In such patients, the orifices of the pulmonary veins may be displaced so far laterally by the expansion of the atrium

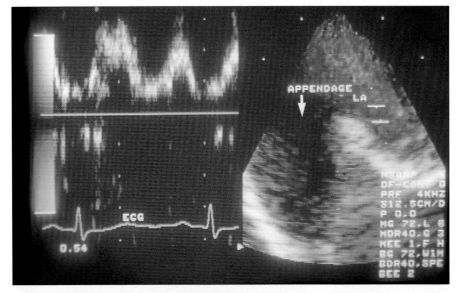

Fig. 5.5 Cross-sectional image of the left upper pulmonary vein. The superimposed colour flow map demonstrates laminar flow within the vein towards the posterior wall of the left atrium. The sample volume has been positioned approximately 1cm from the orifice of the vein, and the pulsed Doppler profile (left-hand panel) demonstrates normal biphasic flow.

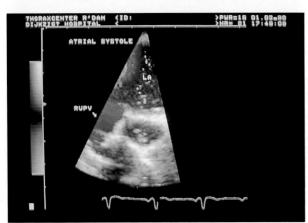

Fig. 5.6 Cross-sectional image of the right upper pulmonary vein. The vein enters the left atrium just lateral to the superior caval vein in a basal transverse plane. During atrial systole, the colour flow map shows normal laminar retrograde flow into the vein.

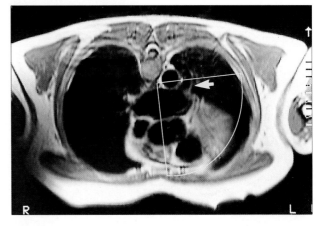

Fig. 5.7 MRI scan obtained in a transverse axis through the left atrium at the level of the lower pulmonary veins. When the transoesophageal transducer is directed towards their orifices as depicted for the left lower pulmonary vein (arrowed), the extraparenchymal portions of the lower pulmonary veins are not well aligned for recording peak velocities by Doppler techniques without angle correction.

that it is almost impossible, because of the extreme angle, to locate and interrogate them with Doppler. In these circumstances, the ultrasound beam may traverse extracardiac structures before it reaches the pulmonary veins, and so it is difficult to maintain images of good quality.

In the absence of pulmonary disease, flow profiles in the right and left upper pulmonary veins are the same, at least in patients who are supine (Fig. 5.8). They may be slightly different if patients are lying on one side, as is usually the case during an out-patient transoesophageal echocardiographic study in a conscious patient (Fig. 5.9). If traces are being documented for comparative purposes, the posture and the position of the sample volume should be recorded.

Since pressure differences between the left atrium and the pulmonary veins in healthy subjects are of the order of only 1–2mmHg, the normal peak velocities of pulmonary venous flow are 0.5m/s, or less. At such low velocities, however, it is inaccurate to apply the modified Bernoulli equation, and so inferences about pressure gradients between the pulmonary veins and the left atrium may be misleading. In order to measure the low-velocity waveforms accurately, high-quality traces should be recorded, using a low wall-filter setting and a small sample volume. The pattern of pulmonary venous flow may vary according to the sampling site, since colour flow mapping sometimes demonstrates simultaneous forward and reversed flows at opposite sides of the same vein (usually near the orifice) (Fig. 5.10). Care is required, therefore, to avoid placing the sample volume in the pulmonary vein at a site which may be unrepresentative; for example, the velocity profile may be difficult to discern because of turbulence, or it may be influenced in an unrepresentative manner, if the sample volume is placed adjacent to, or within, a localized retrograde jet. In our experience at the Thoraxcentre, the most clear signals are obtained if the

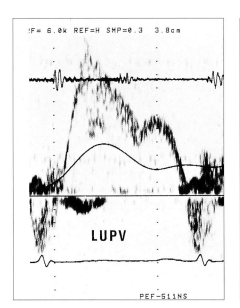

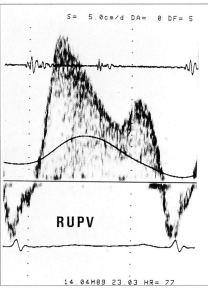

Fig. 5.8 Pulmonary venous velocity profiles. These were obtained consecutively at similar depths within the left (left-hand panel) and right (right-hand panel) upper veins in an anaesthetized and supine patient. The patterns of flow are virtually identical.

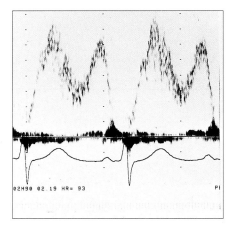

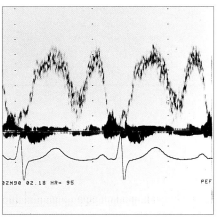

Fig. 5.9 Profiles obtained from within the left (left-hand panel) and right (right-hand panel) upper pulmonary veins during an out-patient transoesophageal echocardiographic study in a patient who is conscious and lying in a left lateral decubitus position. Although the patterns of flow are very similar, there is a difference between the veins in the peak velocities that have been recorded.

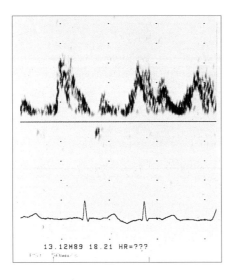
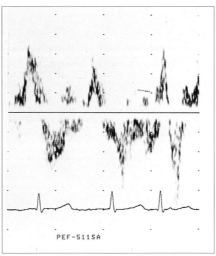

13.12M89 18.21 HR=???

PEF-511SA

Fig. 5.10 Pulsed Doppler profiles obtained during a single examination and at the same depth, from within the left upper pulmonary vein in a patient with constrictive pericarditis and very enlarged pulmonary veins. Sampling from the medial side of the vein demonstrated only antegrade flow (left-hand panel), while considerable retrograde flow was apparent when the sample volume was moved to the lateral side of the vein (right-hand panel).

sample volume is placed within the centre of the vein, between 1 and 2cm from the orifice (see *Fig. 5.5*). Signals recorded at the orifice may be unreliable, and those recorded from deeper within the pulmonary veins occasionally show different timing and velocity of individual components of the Doppler trace.

For careful analysis, traces should be recorded on paper at a fast speed, together with the electrocardiogram. A simultaneous phonocardiogram is helpful, but not essential, for reasons which are to be discussed. A pulsed Doppler recording of mitral valve inflow should be obtained for comparison during the same study.

THE NORMAL PULMONARY VENOUS FLOW PATTERN

Normal traces of pulmonary venous flow show biphasic or triphasic forward flow during ventricular systole and diastole, and transient retrograde flow during atrial systole (Fig. 5.11). A diagrammatic representation of a

typical trace is shown in Fig. 5.12, together with the names used to describe the different peaks and components of the waveforms.

The first phase of the pulmonary venous waveform occurs following atrial systole, and therefore coincides with atrial diastole and ventricular systole. It also includes the period of isovolumic relaxation, since the second phase of flow does not start until the mitral valve opens (Fig. 5.13); for this reason, it seems preferable to refer to 'systolic phase flow' rather than to 'systolic flow', within the pulmonary veins. The increase of velocity towards the first systolic peak coincides with the x descent of the left atrial pressure trace (see *Fig. 5.4*), and so, in the absence of mitral regurgitation, the slope of this part of the waveform relates to atrial relaxation, which is therefore a significant determinant of pulmonary venous flow. Contraction and descent of the atrioventricular junction also contribute to the reduction of left atrial pressure and, therefore, to pulmonary venous emptying. A second systolic peak may be observed on pulmonary venous waveforms, especially in

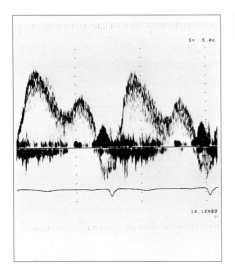

S= 5.0c

14.12M89

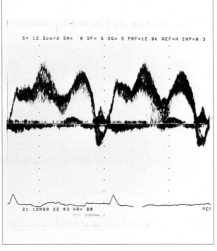

S= 12.5cm/d DA= 0 DF= 5 DG= 5 PRF=12.0k REF=H SMP=0.3

21.12M89 22.03 HR= 80

PEF

Fig. 5.11 Examples of normal pulmonary venous velocity profiles. These show biphasic (left-hand panel) and triphasic (right-hand panel) forward flow, with retrograde flow following atrial contraction. In both traces there are low velocity artefacts because the velocity range is low and the wall-filter setting is very low.

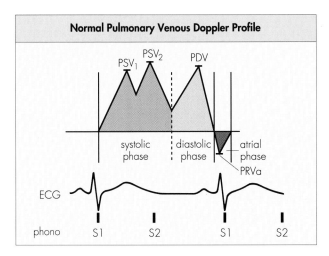

Fig. 5.12 Diagram of a normal pulmonary venous flow trace. This trace is annotated to show the separate components and their names. Abbreviations as in *Fig. 5.16.*

younger subjects. This peak seems to be related to motion of the junction during systole, and so it can be considered as a normal variant. Abnormalities of flow that occur in the systolic phase may reflect changes in left atrial compliance or pressure.

The second (diastolic) phase of pulmonary venous flow is characterized by a single antegrade wave that starts when the mitral valve opens (Fig. 5.13). It corresponds to the E wave of the Doppler trace and it coincides with the y descent of the left atrial pressure trace (see *Fig. 5.4*). Diastolic phase flow reaches its peak velocity after rapid filling, and then declines before the onset of atrial contraction. During early- and mid-diastole, the atrium acts as an open conduit, with blood flowing directly from the pulmonary veins to the left ventricle. Since the mitral valve is open, patterns of pulmonary venous flow at this time may reflect left ventricular relaxation and passive filling.

The third (atrial) phase of pulmonary venous flow occurs during atrial systole (Fig. 5.13) and coincides with the a wave of the left atrial pressure trace (see *Fig. 5.4*) and the A wave of the mitral Doppler profile. These events are not always manifest on the pulmonary venous Doppler profile, but usually there is transient and low-velocity retrograde flow into the pulmonary veins. Deviations from normal patterns during this phase are related mainly to changes of left ventricular compliance and end-diastolic pressure.

In order to establish the exact timing of the systolic and diastolic phases of pulmonary venous flow, it is necessary to record the venous Doppler profile simultaneously with electrocardiographic, phonocardiographic, and pulsed Doppler traces of flow across the mitral valve. This is impossible, partly because of the transoe-

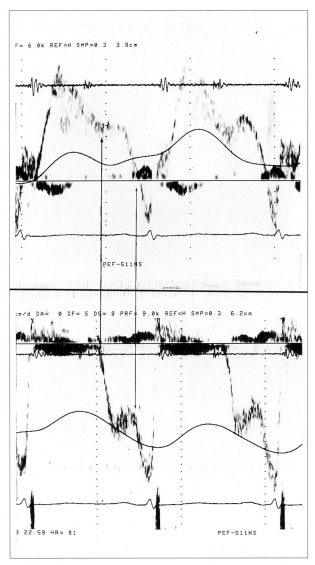

Fig. 5.13 Synchronized Doppler profiles. These are obtained from within the left upper pulmonary vein (upper panel) and at the orifice of the mitral valve (lower panel), produced by matching beats with similar R–R intervals. The onset of diastolic forward flow in the pulmonary vein corresponds to mitral valve opening, rather than aortic valve closure as shown by the second heart sound on the phonocardiogram. The atrial retrograde signal on the pulmonary venous profile coincides with the A wave of the mitral Doppler profile.

sophageal equipment that is currently available, and also because the orifice of the mitral valve and the pulmonary veins cannot be imaged simultaneously. Since the second heart sound on the phonocardiogram indicates the start of ventricular diastole but not the onset of flow across the mitral valve, it cannot be used to time the upstroke of the diastolic-phase signal on the pulmonary venous Doppler trace. As a compromise, therefore, a pulsed Doppler trace of flow across the mi-

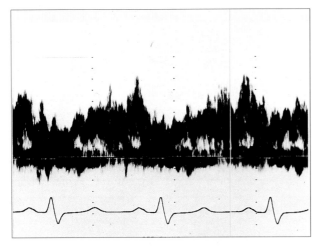

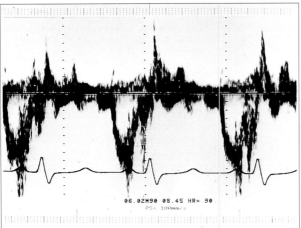

Fig. 5.14 Superimposed pulmonary venous (upper panel) and mitral (lower panel) Doppler profiles. These demonstrate the value of using the timing of the onset of mitral flow to determine the start of the diastolic phase of pulmonary venous flow (see the superimposed line). In this patient, the pulmonary venous trace appears to be of poor quality, but this is related to turbulence within the pulmonary vein caused by high flow due to a large left-to-right shunt through an oval fossa atrial septal defect.

Normal Values for Pulmonary Venous Flow			
	Dennig et al (n = 25)	Kreis et al (n = 17) young adults	Kreis et al (n = 20) adults
peak velocity of systolic flow (m/s)	0.43 ± 0.14	0.47 ± 0.09	0.60
second peak of systolic flow (m/s)	0.55 ± 0.17	0.60	0.62
peak velocity of diastolic flow (m/s)	0.38 ± 0.16	0.46 ± 0.11	0.50
time-velocity integral, systole (cm)	11 ± 5	14.4 ± 3.0	16.1
time-velocity integral, diastole (cm)	5 ± 3	7.7 ± 2.6	8.4
retrograde velocity, atrial systole (cm)	−0.3 ± 0.05	−0.22	−0.18
time-velocity integral, atrial retrograde flow (m/s)	0.3 ± 0.2	1.6	1.5

Fig. 5.15 Normal values for pulmonary venous flow recorded by transoesophageal echocardiography.

tral valve should be recorded, and beats of similar length superimposed in order to guide the interpretation and analysis of the pulmonary venous trace (Fig. 5.14).

It is difficult to acquire data about transoesophageal echocardiographic findings in normal subjects, but, nevertheless, several groups have now reported normal values of pulmonary venous Doppler measurements obtained from healthy patients and some volunteers (23,24). The available data are summarized in Fig. 5.15. The peak systolic velocity is usually slightly greater than the peak diastolic velocity, although they are quite similar. A scheme for digitising the velocity profiles is illustrated in Fig. 5.16. The time velocity integral of the systolic phase usually exceeds the diastolic integral, but

this does not necessarily mean that volumetric flow in the pulmonary veins is greater in systole.

The major difficulty encountered when analysing, or attempting to quantify, pulmonary venous Doppler traces, is that they can be extremely variable. In particular, the timing of the different components of the waveforms can vary between patients in their relation to the QRS complex. It might be easier to measure each component of the profile separately, but it is not always possible to identify them. It is necessary, therefore, to relate the waveform to the systolic and diastolic phases as defined by the Q wave and the onset of left ventricular filling through the mitral valve.

PHYSIOLOGICAL CHANGES IN PULMONARY VENOUS DOPPLER WAVEFORMS

The normal pattern of the pulmonary venous trace is influenced by age (25). There are usually two peaks of forward flow in systole in young subjects, while in older patients only one peak is observed. This pattern could be related to stiffness of the atrioventricular junction and reduced motion during ventricular systole. With increasing age, there is a decline in the velocities of diastolic pulmonary venous flow (Fig. 5.17), perhaps related to the changes of myocardial diastolic function that have been reported, such as increased stiffness and nonuniformity of relaxation (26). Reduced compliance of the left ventricle and higher diastolic pressures, also alter indices of diastolic function in older subjects, with lengthening of the isovolumic relaxation time and in-

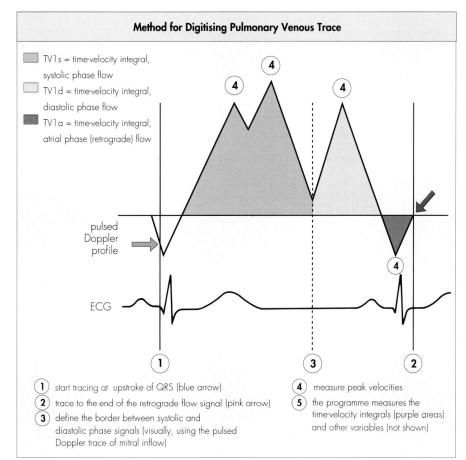

Method for Digitising Pulmonary Venous Trace

TV1s = time-velocity integral, systolic phase flow

TV1d = time-velocity integral, diastolic phase flow

TV1a = time-velocity integral, atrial phase (retrograde) flow

pulsed Doppler profile

ECG

(1) start tracing at upstroke of QRS (blue arrow)

(2) trace to the end of the retrograde flow signal (pink arrow)

(3) define the border between systolic and diastolic phase signals (visually, using the pulsed Doppler trace of mitral inflow)

(4) measure peak velocities

(5) the programme measures the time-velocity integrals (purple areas) and other variables (not shown)

Fig. 5.16 Method for digitising pulmonary venous Doppler profiles. PSV = (first) peak systolic velocity. PSV_2 = second peak systolic velocity. PDV = peak diastolic velocity. PRV_a = peak retrograde velocity during the atrial phase.

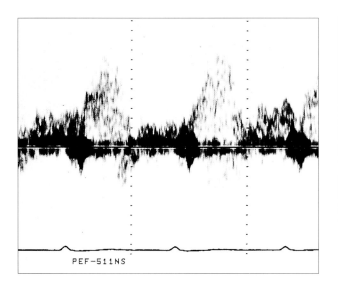

Fig. 5.17 Normal trace obtained in an 82-year-old man. There is reduced flow during ventricular diastole.

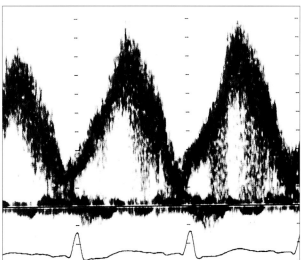

Fig. 5.18 Single forward flow wave in a patient with a heart rate of 118 beats per minute.

version on the pulsed Doppler mitral trace of the normal ratio between the early (E) and atrial (A) peak velocities.

Changes in heart rate also modify the pattern of pulmonary venous flow. As first shown in experimental studies (9), only one major pulse occurs when the heart rate is rapid (Fig. 5.18). Presumably, this represents coalescence of the normal systolic- and diastolic-phase signals.

Doppler flow profiles recorded from within the right heart usually show considerable variation with respiration. Pulmonary venous profiles, in contrast, appear to

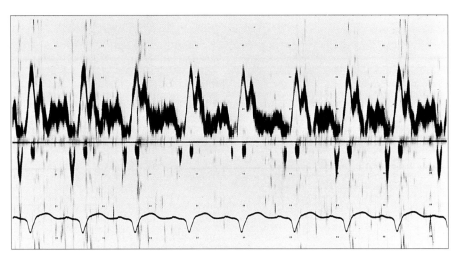

Fig. 5.19 Pulmonary venous profiles recorded during one respiratory cycle, starting with inspiration. The major variation to be seen is that, during expiration, there is a reduction in the velocity of atrial retrograde flow.

be influenced to a much lesser extent, perhaps because of the compliance of the pulmonary veins. Nevertheless, some variations do occur. On inspiration, there is a slight decrease in the velocities of antegrade flow and an increase in the velocity of atrial retrograde flow, (Fig. 5.19). The opposite effects are seen during expiration, with an increase in the velocities of antegrade flow. In clinical practice, these effects are so mild that they may be unimportant. The influence of respiratory disease and elevated intrathoracic pressures on pulmonary venous profiles recorded during a transoesophageal echocardiographic study has not yet been defined.

ARRHYTHMIAS

If there is retrograde conduction after a ventricular ectopic beat, atrial contraction occurs when the mitral valve is closed. This causes increased retrograde flow into the pulmonary veins (Fig. 5.20). The same phenomenon is observed in patients with atrioventricular dissociation, when the retrograde flow into the pulmonary veins coincides with cannon waves seen in the jugular venous pulse, and in patients with junctional rhythm and retrograde conduction (Fig. 5.21). Significant flow can be observed after each atrial contraction (27), and in some limited circumstances this may be helpful in diagnosing an arrhythmia.

Atrial flutter and atrial fibrillation are associated with reduced systolic emptying of the pulmonary veins (Fig. 5.22), probably because there is relatively little change in the volume of the left atrium, and the atrium is less compliant than normal. Most of the forward flow from the pulmonary veins appears to occur during ventricular diastole.

POTENTIAL CLINICAL APPLICATIONS

Mitral valvar disease

Pulmonary venous flow profiles may provide useful information about mitral valvar function (28–31). Changes in left atrial pressure due to mitral stenosis will influence pulmonary venous flow during diastole, and mitral regurgitation causes changes in pulmonary venous flow during ventricular systole. This may prove to be of value in grading the severity of mitral regurgitation, which is difficult even with Doppler colour flow mapping because of the myriad factors that influence the area of turbulence associated with a regurgitant jet. Pulmonary venous flow patterns, on the other hand, reflect changes in left atrial pressure, which are unrelated to patterns of turbulence in the left atrium.

Mitral regurgitation augments left atrial pressure, not only by increasing left atrial volume, but also by modifying the systolic phase of atrial filling. The atrial pressure is elevated, and normal emptying of the pulmonary veins during ventricular systole is reduced (Fig. 5.23a). In more severe degrees of regurgitation, there may be no forward flow from the pulmonary venous orifices into the left atrium during ventricular systole. Significant mitral regurgitation associated with a high v wave on the left atrial pressure trace causes retrograde pulmonary venous flow. This can vary from early, to late, or holosystolic retrograde flow (Fig. 5.23b, c and d), but in all instances the net time-velocity integral of forward flow during systole is reduced. Occasionally, the pulmonary venous Doppler trace may show turbulent flow during systole if the regurgitant jet is directed into the orifice of the pulmonary vein from which the recording is being obtained. If it can be obtained from an alternative position of the sample volume, a trace that is not affected by such turbulence will be more representative of the flow pattern in all the pulmonary veins. It has been suggested that the timing and duration of retrograde flow, which are more persistent in severe mitral regurgitation, can be useful indicators of the severity of incompetence (28). If the regurgitant jet is very eccentric, however, the timing of retrograde flow may vary slightly between opposite veins, and so this parameter is not always reliable.

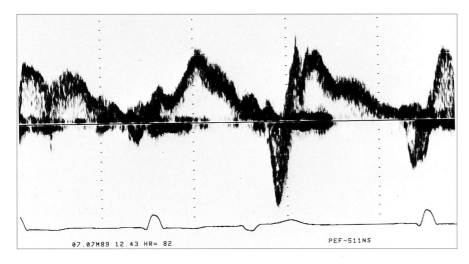

Fig. 5.20 Increased retrograde flow into the left upper pulmonary vein after a ventricular ectopic beat.

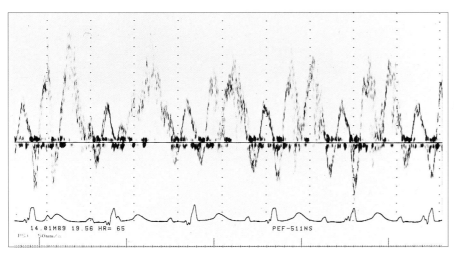

Fig. 5.21 Varying retrograde flow in a patient with atrioventricular dissociation, sinoatrial block, and a junctional escape rhythm. When atrial contraction is synchronous with ventricular contraction, there is a considerable increase in the velocity of retrograde flow (arrowed).

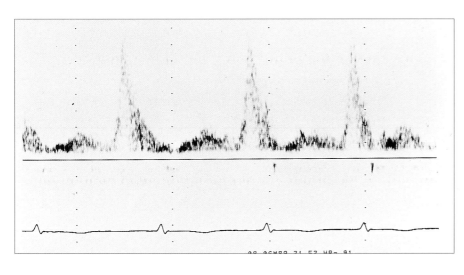

Fig. 5.22 Profile recorded within the left upper pulmonary vein in a patient who is in atrial fibrillation. There is a marked reduction in forward flow during systole.

In the operating room, transoesophageal echocardiography is sometimes used to assess valvar morphology and function in patients who are undergoing surgery of the mitral valve. Comparative studies using colour flow mapping may be difficult in such patients because, for example, the regurgitant jet is influenced by variations in the loading conditions of the left ventricle. Recordings of pulmonary venous flow before and after cardiopulmonary bypass offer another approach, since retrograde systolic phase flow disappears immediately after a successful repair (Fig. 5.24) (32,33). When a small residual leak causes a disproportionate amount of turbulence within the left atrium, the Doppler profile of pulmonary venous flow may help to distinguish significant, from trivial, persistent regurgitation. Used in conjunction with direct pressure recordings, which are often labile after cardiopulmonary bypass, this information may be helpful for making clinical decisions.

In patients with mitral stenosis, the left atrial pressure is elevated, particularly in late ventricular diastole. The left atrium may be very enlarged and the pulmonary veins also very dilated, so that velocities of pulmonary venous flow may be very low. If it is possible to obtain a pulmonary venous Doppler profile, however, it may show characteristic abnormalities (Fig. 5.25). In patients with co-existing atrial fibrillation, maximal forward flow occurs in early ventricular diastole. There may be retrograde flow during diastole, which starts before the time at which retrograde flow associated with atrial contraction would be seen. In patients in sinus rhythm, the duration of atrial retrograde flow is increased, and the peak negative velocity may be high (Fig. 5.26).

Diastolic function of the left heart

Pulsed Doppler recordings of flow across the mitral valve are a useful noninvasive index of changes in left ventricular function (34,35). The waveform depends on the temporal pattern of pressure gradients across the mitral valve, particularly the instantaneous gradient in early diastole, and it is determined by left ventricular compliance, the rate of relaxation, ventricular preload,

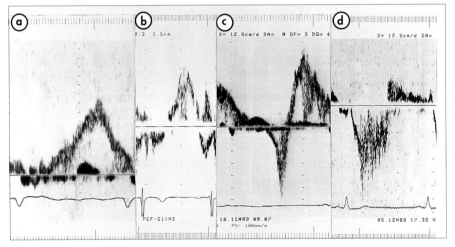

Fig. 5.23 Examples of pulmonary venous flow profiles obtained from the left upper pulmonary vein in four patients with mitral regurgitation. (a) Reduced velocity of forward flow during systole. (b) Early systolic retrograde flow. (c) Late systolic retrograde flow. (d) Holosystolic retrograde flow.

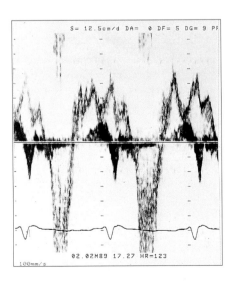
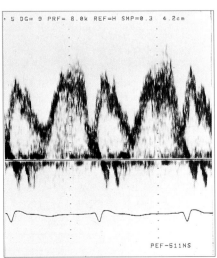

Fig. 5.24 Pre-bypass (left-hand panel) and post-bypass (right-hand panel) Doppler traces. These traces are from the left upper pulmonary vein in a patient with severe mitral regurgitation who underwent successful mitral valvar reconstruction. Before surgery, there is considerable retrograde flow into the pulmonary vein during systole, but the pattern is normal immediately after coming off cardiopulmonary bypass.

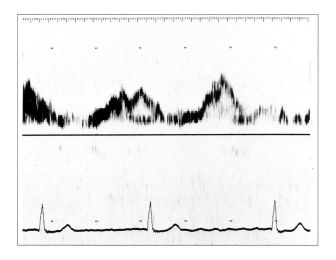

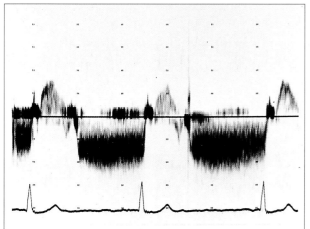

Fig. 5.25 Profile of flow in the left upper pulmonary vein (upper panel) in a patient with severe mitral stenosis and atrial fibrillation. There is almost no flow from the vein into the left atrium during ventricular systole, even though the patient had no mitral regurgitation. During diastole, indicated by the superimposed mitral Doppler trace (lower panel), the pulmonary venous velocity reaches its peak more slowly than normal, presumably due to a slower than normal early decline in pressure in the left atrium.

and other haemodynamic factors (16). As the left atrial pressure rises, the velocity of flow across the mitral valve during atrial systole increases. As the left ventricular end-diastolic pressure itself increases, however, the difference in pressure across the valve becomes less pronounced. This can result in apparent normalization of the mitral Doppler trace when both the ventricular and the atrial diastolic pressures are elevated. This process is called 'pseudonormalization', and it represents the major obstacle when using the mitral E/A ratio as an index of ventricular function (16). Pulmonary venous Doppler recordings may help in these circumstances to distinguish this pattern from a true normal one by showing an increase in pulmonary venous retrograde flow during atrial contraction when the left atrial pressure is elevated relative to that in the extracardiac pulmonary veins.

In patients with heart failure due to left ventricular dysfunction, there may be retrograde pulmonary venous flow that starts before the onset of the electrocardiographic P wave (Fig. 5.27). This abnormality on the Doppler venous trace almost certainly reflects a high left ventricular diastolic pressure. If further observations confirm that an elevated early diastolic pressure within the left ventricle causes reduced forward, or early retrograde, diastolic flow in the pulmonary veins, as well as increased retrograde flow during atrial systole, then these features of the Doppler profile may become useful as indicators of abnormal diastolic function. It may be possible to distinguish different patterns in patients with abnormal left ventricular compliance and ischaemic heart disease or an underlying dilated cardiomyopathy, from the patterns observed in patients with hypertrophic or restrictive cardiomyopathy; however, these applications for transoesophageal echocardiography remain speculative. At present, transthoracic

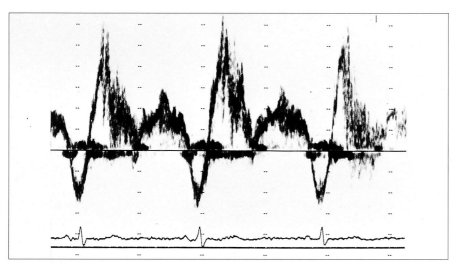

Fig. 5.26 Pulmonary venous Doppler profile from the left upper pulmonary vein in a patient with mitral stenosis and sinus rhythm. The velocity of forward flow during diastole is reduced when compared with normal, and there is an increase in the profile of retrograde flow during atrial systole.

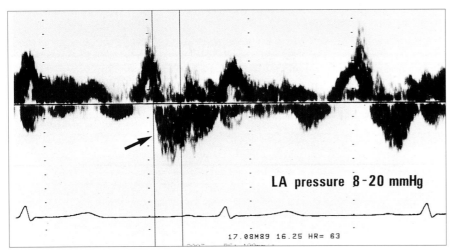

Fig. 5.27 Flow profile from the left upper pulmonary vein in a patient with congestive cardiac failure and a left atrial pressure of 8–20mmHg. There is retrograde flow into the vein which starts early in diastole (arrowed, first vertical line), before the onset of the P wave on the electrocardiogram (second vertical line).

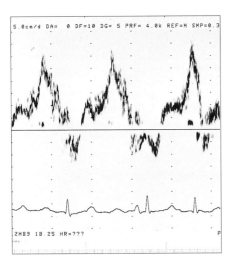

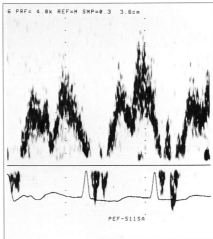

Fig. 5.28 Pulmonary venous profiles from a patient with constrictive pericarditis that extended around the left atrium and involved the orifices of the pulmonary veins. There is a reduced velocity of forward flow during ventricular systole (left-hand panel). After full excision of the pericardium and release of obstruction to the pulmonary veins, the pattern of flow is virtually normal (right-hand panel).

Doppler modalities remain the techniques of choice for the investigation of such problems.

It has recently been reported that there is a significant relationship between profiles of pulmonary venous flow and left atrial pressure (36). The percentage of total forward 'flow' from the pulmonary veins, which occurred during ventricular systole, was inversely related to mean left atrial pressure. This was true for the population that was studied while the chest was open during cardiac surgery, but it is not yet known whether or not the relationship is sufficiently close for it to be possible to use pulmonary venous traces to comment on the likely left atrial pressure in an individual patient. If this becomes possible, it may represent another application for transoesophageal echocardiographic monitoring during anaesthesia or in the intensive care unit.

Diastolic function of the heart is also abnormal in pericardial constriction. In such patients, reduced flow during ventricular systole may represent abnormal left atrial compliance, since we and others have observed

that this pattern is normalized immediately after pericardiectomy (Fig. 5.28) (37). The time-velocity integral of atrial retrograde flow is also increased in patients with constriction.

Aortic regurgitation

Patients with severe aortic regurgitation may show a rapid increase in early diastolic pressure in the left ventricle, with equalization of the left atrial and left ventricular pressures. If the regurgitant jet is directed towards the aortic (anterior) leaflet of the mitral valve, this generates a mild obstruction to inflow to the left ventricle. This in turn makes it difficult to analyse ventricular function from the pattern of flow. In severe aortic regurgitation, the pulmonary venous trace demonstrates an increase in the velocity and duration of retrograde flow during atrial contraction (Fig. 5.29a); this abnormality is exaggerated if there is a co-existing

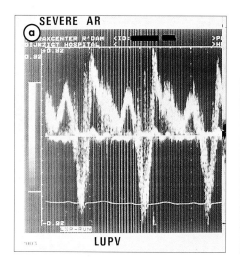

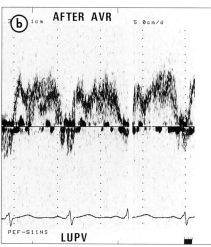

Fig. 5.29 (a) In this patient with severe aortic regurgitation caused by infective endocarditis, there is a considerable increase in the velocity of retrograde flow following atrial systole. (b) After aortic valvar replacement, the atrial retrograde flow wave has returned to normal.

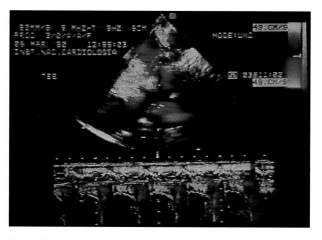

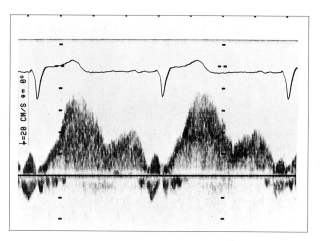

Fig. 5.30 Cross-sectional image and colour flow map from a patient with obstruction of the left upper pulmonary vein. The colour M-mode recording shows continuous turbulence near the orifice of the vein. Pulsed Doppler profiles obtained deep within the vein demonstrated a normal pattern of flow, while sampling within the turbulence demonstrated high velocities.

Fig. 5.31 Pulmonary venous flow profile recorded from the left upper pulmonary vein in a patient with severe aortic stenosis. Although the absolute velocity of flow during diastole is relatively normal (approximately 0.4m/s), the systolic velocity is much higher, and the ratio of systolic to diastolic peak velocities is considerably increased compared to normal.

reduction in left ventricular compliance. The pulmonary venous Doppler profile may return to normal immediately after successful surgical treatment (Fig. 5.29b).

Pulmonary venous obstruction

Transoesophageal echocardiography with colour flow mapping is an excellent technique for identifying obstruction of the pulmonary veins, caused, for example, by a mediastinal mass that constricts their extraparenchymal segments or narrows a pulmonary venous orifice, or by congenital heart disease (Fig. 5.30).

Aortic stenosis

In patients with severe aortic stenosis, left ventricular hypertrophy may impair diastolic filling, (38,39), and in patients who are decompensated, diastolic pressures may be elevated. These abnormalities are reflected in the pulmonary venous flow pattern by a reduction in the velocity of forward flow in diastole (Fig. 5.31). There may also be an increase in the velocity of retrograde flow during atrial systole. Similar changes may occur in patients with obstruction of the left ventricular outflow tract.

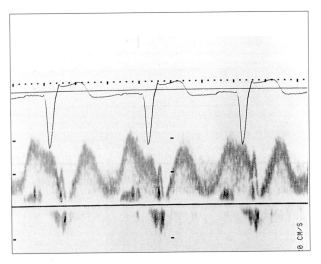

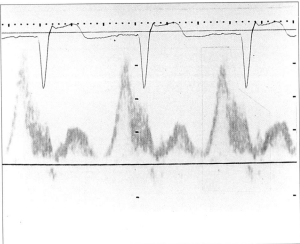

Fig. 5.32 Profiles recorded from the left upper (upper panel) and right upper (lower panel) pulmonary veins in a patient who has had a Mustard operation. The patient is supine, and the difference between the veins is presumably due to partial obstruction to emptying from the right upper vein during ventricular systole.

Congenital heart disease

Transoesophageal echocardiography is not performed as a routine investigation in babies or very young children with congenital heart disease, but it is emerging as a useful technique in the assessment of this disease in older patients, including patients who have had previous cardiac surgery and others who have poor precordial windows (40). Pulmonary venous traces can be obtained in children, as in adults, although analysis can be difficult because heart rates tend to be rapid.

Patients who have had a Mustard operation for complete transposition may develop obstruction of the pulmonary venous atrium or of an individual pulmonary vein (41). Transoesophageal echocardiography is an

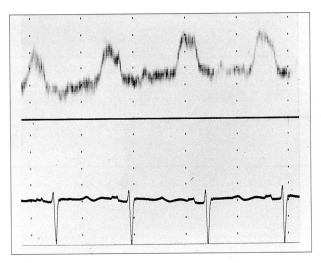

Fig. 5.33 Continuous flow recorded within the left upper pulmonary vein in a patient who had undergone a modified Blalock operation. Unfortunately, the graft from the left subclavian artery had been anastomosed directly to the pulmonary vein rather than to a branch of the left pulmonary artery.

excellent technique for analysing function of the atrial baffle and for assessing these complications (42). Obstruction of an individual pulmonary vein will be manifest on colour flow mapping and pulsed Doppler sampling as persistent turbulent inflow from the orifice of that vein. When pulsed Doppler profiles are recorded from within a nonobstructed pulmonary vein, they may give information about the severity of tricuspid regurgitation, just as information is available about mitral regurgitation when the circulation is anatomically normal. When there is no tricuspid regurgitation, impaired emptying of the pulmonary veins in systole may be caused by partial obstruction or by abnormal atrial compliance (Fig. 5.32) (43). Reduced velocities in diastole may be due to high filling pressures caused by abnormal systemic (right) ventricular function.

Characteristic patterns of flow occur in patients with anomalous pulmonary venous connexion or with systemic-to-pulmonary shunts. Increased flow through the pulmonary veins, for example, in patients with an atrial or a ventricular septal defect, may cause turbulent flow within the veins even in the absence of any obstruction. In congenital shunts, the pulmonary venous profile is altered by changes in atrial pressure such as those seen in large atrial septal defects. It is also altered in patients with obligatory unidirectional atrial shunting due to tricuspid or mitral atresia. If a modified Blalock shunt is accidentally connected to a pulmonary vein rather than to a branch of the pulmonary artery, this is obvious on the pulmonary venous profile (Fig. 5.33).

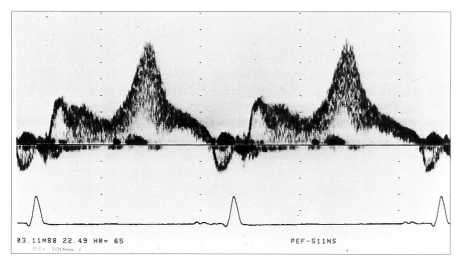

`03.11M88 22.49 HR= 65`　　　`PEF-511NS`

Fig. 5.34 Biphasic flow pattern recorded from the left upper pulmonary vein in a patient following a Fontan operation. Although the right heart circulation bypasses the right ventricle, there is a biphasic pattern of forward flow in the pulmonary veins, as normal.

Analysis of pulmonary venous flow can be helpful in patients with tricuspid or pulmonary atresia. It can identify differences in blood supply between the lungs and even between upper and lower pulmonary veins, such as those which may occur when this is determined by collateral vessels. In patients who have a surgically created Fontan circulation, study of pulmonary venous flow may be useful in analysing pathophysiologic changes (Fig. 5.34).

REFERENCES

1. Smallhorn JF, Freedom RM, Olley PM. Pulsed Doppler echocardiographic assessment of extraparenchymal pulmonary vein flow. *J Am Coll Cardiol* 1987;**9**:573–9.

2. Pickoff AS, Bennet V, Soler P, Ferrer PL. Detection of pulmonary venous flow by pulsed Doppler echocardiography in children. *Am Heart J* 1983;**105**:826–9.

3. Rajagopalan B, Bertram CD, Stallard T, Lee G de J. Blood flow in pulmonary veins: III. Simultaneous measurements of their dimensions, intravascular pressure and flow. *Cardiovasc Res* 1979;**13**:684–92.

4. Morkin E, Collins JA, Goldman HS, Fishman AP. Pattern of blood flow in the pulmonary veins of the dog. *J Appl Physiol* 1965;**20**:1118–28.

5. Szidon JP, Roland RH, Fishman AP. Origin of the pulmonary venous flow pulse. Am J Physiol 1968;**214**:10–4.

6. Morgan BC, Abel FL, Mullins GL, Guntheroth WG. Flow patterns in cavae, pulmonary artery, pulmonary vein and aorta in intact dogs. *Am J Physiol* 1966;**210**:903–9.

7. Dixon S, Nolan S, Morrow A. Pulmonary venous blood flow. The effects of alterations in left atrial pressure, pulmonary artery occlusion and mitral regurgitation in the dog. *Ann Surg* 1971;**174**:944–9.

8. Jenkins BS, Shiu MF, Webb–Peploe MM. Studies in pulmonary vein flow in man using an intravascular velocity probe and a twin lumen catheter. *Proc Physiol Soc* 1977;**271**:34–5P.

9. Rajagopalan B, Friend JA, Stallard T, Lee G de J. Blood flow in pulmonary veins: I. Studies in dog and man. *Cardiovasc Res* 1979; **13**: 667–76.

10. Rajagopalan B, Friend JA, Stallard T, Lee G de J. Blood flow in pulmonary veins: II. The influence of events transmitted from the right and left sides of the heart. *Cardiovasc Res* 1979;**13**:677–83.

11. Guntheroth WG, Gould R, Butler J, Kinnen E. Pulsatile flow in pulmonary artery, capillary, and vein in the dog. *Cardiovasc Res* 1974;**8**:330–7.

12. Friend JA, Lee GJ, Rajagopalan B, Stallard T. Measurement of by blood flow in the large pulmonary veins in the dog. *J Physiol* 1977;**269**:52–3P.

13. Keren G, Sherez J, Megidish R *et al*. Pulmonary venous flow pattern — its relationship to cardiac dynamics. A pulsed Doppler echocardiographic study. *Circulation* 1985;**6**:1105–12.

14. Keren G, Sonnenblick EH, LeJemtel TH. Mitral Anulus Motion. Relation to pulmonary venous and transmitral flows in normal subjects and in patients with dilated cardiomyopathy. *Circulation* 1988;**78**:621–9.

15. Appleton CP, Hatle LK, Popp RL. Demonstration of restrictive ventricular physiology by Doppler echocardiography. *J Am Coll Cardiol* 1988;**11**:757–68.

16. Nishimura RA, Abel MA, Hatle LK, Tajik AJ. Assessment of diastolic function of the heart:background and current applications of Doppler echocardiography. Part II. Clinical Studies. *Mayo Clin Proc* 1989;**64**:181–204.

17. Hatle LK, Appleton CP, Popp RL. Differentiation of constrictive pericarditis and restrictive cardiomyopathy by Doppler echocardiography. *Circulation* 1989;**79**:357–70.

18. Shabetai R, Fowler NO, Guntheroth WG. The hemodynamics of cardiac tamponade and constrictive pericarditis. *Am J Cardiol* 1970;**26**:480–9.

19. Appleton CP, Hatle LK, Popp RL. Cardiac tamponade and pericardial effusion:respiratory variation in transvalvular flow

velocities studied by Doppler echocardiography. *J Am Coll Cardiol* 1988;**11**:1020–30.

20. Sakai K, Nakamura K, Satomi G *et al.* Evaluation of tricuspid regurgitation by blood flow pattern in the hepatic vein using pulsed Doppler technique. *Am Heart J* 1984;**108**:516–22.

21. Pennestri F, Loperfido F, Salvatori MP *et al.* Assessment of tricuspid regurgitation by pulsed Doppler ultrasonography of the hepatic vein. *Am J Cardiol* 1984;**54**:363–8.

22. Skagseth E. Pulmonary vein flow pattern in man during thoracotomy. *Scand J Thorac Cardiovasc Surg* 1976;**10**:36–42.

23. Dennig K, Henneke KH, Rudolph W. Transesophageal Doppler echocardiographic evaluation of normal flow velocities within pulmonary veins. *Proceedings of Eighth International Symposium on Echocardiology*, Rotterdam 1989.

24. Kreis A, Lambertz H, Hanrath P. Pulmonary venous blood flow in normal subjects. Personal communication.

25. Klein A, Burstow DJ, Taliercio CP *et al.* Effect of age on pulmonary venous flow velocities in normal subjects [Abstract]. *J Am Coll Cardiol* 1989;**13**:50a.

26. Bonow RO, Vitale DF, Bacharach SL *et al.* Effect of aging on asynchronous left ventricular regional function and global ventricular filling in normal human subjects. *J Am Coll Cardiol* 1988;**11**:50–8.

27. Keren G, Bier A, Sherez J *et al.* Atrial contraction is an important determinant of pulmonary venous flow. *J Am Coll Cardiol* 1986;**7**:693–5.

28. Skagseth E. Pulmonary vein flow pattern in mitral incompetence, combined mitral stenosis/incompetence and after prosthetic valve replacement. *Scand J Thorac Cardiovasc Surg* 1976;**10**:43–52.

29. Skagseth E. Pulmonary vein flow pattern in mitral stenosis before and after commissurotomy. *Scand J Thorac Cardiovasc Surg* 1976;**10**:53–62.

30. Dennig K, Henneke KH, Dacian S, Rudolph W. Estimation of the severity of mitral regurgitation by parameters derived from the velocity profile of pulmonary venous flow using transesophageal Doppler technique [Abstract]. *J Am Coll Cardiol* 1990;**15**:91a.

31. Kreis A, Lambertz H, Gerich N, Hanrath P. Value of the transesophageal echocardiographic pulmonary venous flow in classification of mitral insufficiency [Abstract]. *Circulation* 1989;**80**:II-577.

32. Fraser AG, Tuccillo B, van der Borden S *et al.* Pulmonary venous flow in mitral regurgitation and after successful valve reconstruction [Abstract]. *J Am Coll Cardiol* 1990;**15**:74a.

33. Pearson AC, Castello R, Wallace PM, Labovitz AJ. Effect of mitral regurgitation on pulmonary venous velocities derived by transesophageal echocardiography [Abstract]. *Circulation* 1989;**80**:II-571.

34. Appleton C, Hatle L, Popp R. Relation of transmitral flow velocity patterns to left ventricular diastolic function: new insights from a combined hemodynamic and Doppler echocardiographic study. *J Am Coll Cardiol* 1988;**12**:426–40.

35. Danford DA, Huhta JC, Murphy DJ. Doppler echocardiographic approaches to ventricular diastolic function. *Echocardiography* 1986;**3**:30–40.

36. Kuecherer HF, Muhiudeen IA, Kusumoto F M *et al.* Estimation of mean left atrial pressure from transesophageal pulsed Doppler echocardiography of pulmonary venous flow. *Circulation* 1990;**82**:1127–39.

37. Schiavone WA, Calafiore PA, Currie PJ, Lytle BW. Doppler echocardiographic demonstration of pulmonary venous flow velocity in three patients with constrictive pericarditis before and after pericardiectomy. *Am J Cardiol* 1989;**63**:145–7.

38. Murakami T, Hess OM, Gage JE *et al.* Diastolic filling dynamics in patients with aortic stenosis. *Circulation* 1986;**73**:1162–74.

39. Maron BJ, Spirito P, Green KJ *et al.* Noninvasive assessment of left ventricular diastolic function by pulsed Doppler echocardiography in patients with hypertrophic cardiomyopathy. *J Am Coll Cardiol* 1987;**10**:733–42.

40. Stümper O, Elzenga NJ, Hess J, Sutherland GR. Transesophageal echocardiography in children with congenital heart disease — an initial experience. *J Am Coll Cardiol* 1990;**16**:433–41.

41. Vick GW, Murphy DJ, Ludomirsky A *et al.* Pulmonary venous and systemic ventricular inflow obstruction in patients with congenital heart disease: detection by combined two–dimensional and Doppler echocardiography. *J Am Coll Cardiol* 1987;**9**:580–7.

42. Kaulitz R, Stümper O F W, Geuskens R *et al.* Comparative values of the precordial and transesophageal approaches in the echocardiographic evaluation of atrial baffle function after an atrial correction procedure. *J Am Coll Cardiol* 1990;**16**:686–94.

43. Kaulitz R, Stümper O, Fraser AG *et al.* The potential value of transoesophageal evaluation of individual pulmonary vein flow after an atrial baffle procedure. *Int J Cardiol* 1990;**28**:299–308.

6

Diseases of the mitral and tricuspid valves

Alan G Fraser

INTRODUCTION

Transoesophageal echocardiography has some special advantages over precordial techniques when it is used to analyse the structure and function of the atrioventricular valves. Firstly, due to the proximity of the oesophagus to these structures, imaging demonstrates the valvar anatomy in considerably greater detail than is normally possible from either the apical or the parasternal approach. A higher frequency of ultrasound is used, giving better definition. Secondly, since transoesophageal echocardiographic planes approach the mitral and tricuspid valves from the atria, analysis of regurgitation is possible using colour flow mapping, even when there is considerable calcification in the valves or their annuluses, or when a prosthetic valve or annular ring has been inserted. In these circumstances, masking of the transmission of ultrasound from the precordial is overcome only by the oesophageal approach.

The increased information that is available when transoesophageal echocardiography is used to study the atrioventricular valves, has brought in its wake, an increased onus on the echocardiographer and cardiologist to produce more detailed and refined diagnoses. It is no longer adequate to report a crude diagnosis such as 'regurgitation due to prolapse', or 'stenosis', even when complementary precordial Doppler studies are performed to estimate their severity. Increasingly, and

particularly in emergencies or in severely ill patients, cardiac surgery may be performed for valvar disease without resorting to cardiac catheterization for confirmation of the diagnosis. In such patients, the transoesophageal study occasionally provides diagnostic information that cannot be corroborated by any other investigation, including catheterization. In addition, the increasing use of conservative techniques for the surgical repair of regurgitant valves (1,2), and the development of interventional procedures such as balloon valvotomy for stenotic valves (3,4), mean that more precise information is required in order to choose correctly, for each patient, from an increasing range of alternative treatments. For all of these reasons, a complete diagnosis based on a careful sequential analysis of both valvar structure and function is now required. The oesophageal approach helps to make this possible.

Transoesophageal echocardiography, nevertheless, does have some disadvantages compared with precordial techniques when it is used to analyse the atrioventricular valves. In particular, as discussed later, a transducer that only images in transverse planes is not sufficiently versatile to allow a complete study of the zone of coaptation of the mitral valve in all patients (5), nor can it always fully demonstrate the three leaflets of the tricuspid valve. From the oesophagus, colour Doppler mapping of flow at the mitral valve is usually technically excellent, but mapping of flow across the tricuspid valve may be less than ideal if either the right heart or the left atrium is very enlarged. Using pulsed Doppler from the oesophagus, it is possible to interrogate mitral or tricuspid inflow, but it can be difficult to place the sample volume between the tips of the leaflets without recording artefacts. In general, the quantification of mitral or tricuspid stenosis is performed better from the precordial approach (6,7). Most transoesophageal transducers do not yet incorporate the facility for continuous wave Doppler and so recording of the complete waveform of regurgitant jets, and analysis of pressure gradients in systole, are not possible. In the absence of calcification, grading of regurgitation through the atrioventricular valves using colour flow mapping is probably also performed best from the precordium, since it is possible to image the whole of the atrium while mapping the jet. Thus, the transoesophageal echocardiographic study should be viewed as only a part, albeit a very important one, of the full ultrasonic study of the atrioventricular valves. Precordial imaging, colour flow mapping, and continuous wave and pulsed Doppler studies, should also be performed, and should always form the foundations upon which a transoesophageal study is contemplated and planned.

IMAGING PLANES — MITRAL VALVE

The basic views of the mitral valve are obtained with the oesophageal transducer directed forwards or downwards from behind the left atrium, as discussed in *Chapter 3*. In addition, the valvar orifice may be seen in short axis as the tip of the probe is pulled back from the fundus of the stomach through the cardia. In order to understand the images of the valvar leaflets that are obtained in these views, it is necessary to appreciate the anatomical location and orientation of the leaflets, and their zone of coaptation, in relation to the imaging planes (Fig. 6.1). The junction between the aortic (anterior) and mural (posterior) leaflets, that is, the closure line along which the leaflets coapt, is called the commissure or the zone of coaptation. It extends from posteromedial to anterolateral extremes. The aortic leaflet has a similar surface area to the mural leaflet, although it arises from a much shorter segment of the atrioventricular junction (mitral annulus). The narrower, but longer, mural leaflet usually has three scallops, although it may have more, and can have none. The portions of the leaflets at their edges that are normally apposed to each other in systole have a slightly roughened appearance on visual inspection and are, therefore, referred to as the rough zone. The posteromedial end of the commissure of the valve is located close to

the ventricular septum, near its posterior border and opposite the orifice of the coronary sinus on the other side of the septum. From this site, the zone of coaptation curves upwards and towards the left. The anterolateral end of the commissure is adjacent to the high anterolateral free wall of the left ventricle, and only a few centimetres below the orifice of the left atrial appendage. Thus, the 'posterior' leaflet is attached to the

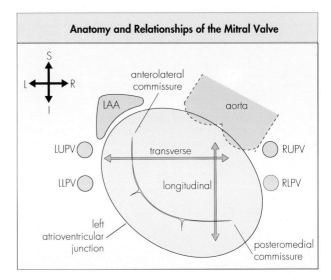

Fig. 6.1 Diagram of the leaflets and commissure of the mitral valve as seen from within the left atrium, demonstrating their relationships to adjacent structures. This view corresponds to that obtained by surgeons operating on the mitral valve, and also to the view obtained when looking anteriorly from the oesophagus. The horizontal and vertical lines illustrate the orientation of planes obtained with transducers that image in transverse and longitudinal planes, respectively.

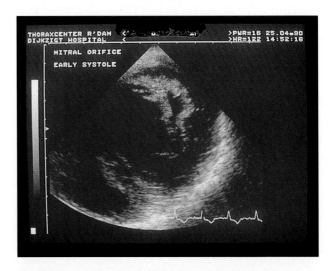

Fig. 6.2 Image of the leaflets of the mitral valve near the posteromedial end of the commissure, obtained with a transducer that images in the transverse plane, from a site in the distal oesophagus near the cardia.

lateral as well as to the posterior part of the atrioventricular junction, which explains why it is more accurately termed the mural leaflet. The aortic leaflet of the mitral valve is contiguous with the mitral curtain that extends upwards and merges with the posterior wall of the aortic root.

During a transoesophageal echocardiographic examination, withdrawal of the probe from the position

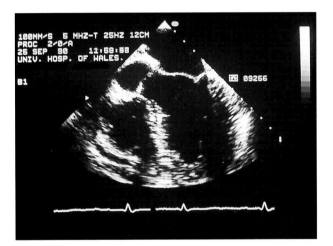

Fig. 6.3 The standard transverse transoesophageal image of the mitral valve in a four-chamber view. The zone of coaptation is shown in its middle third. This plane traverses a long segment of the aortic leaflet and a short portion of the mural leaflet.

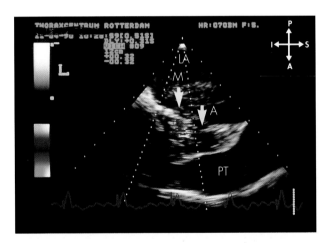

Fig. 6.4 Longitudinal image obtained near the posteromedial end of the commissure of the mitral valve. The aortic (A) and mural (M) leaflets are seen clearly in this systolic frame. Only a small portion of the left ventricle is displayed (the subaortic diverticulum), and between it and the right ventricle, the plane of imaging crosses portions of the membranous outlet and muscular ventricular septum. The systolic colour flow map shows that there is no mitral regurgitation at this site (in fact, there was fusion of the leaflets at the posteromedial end of the commissure). There is spontaneous echocardiographic contrast within the left atrium.

giving the low four-chamber view with the coronary sinus draining into the right atrium, and scanning towards the left ventricle, initially bring the mitral valve into view near the posteromedial end of the commissure (Fig. 6.2). The leaflets may be identified, but it is usually difficult with a transducer scanning only in the transverse plane to interrogate their edges near the posteromedial commissure and at right angles to the zone of coaptation, since the medial half of the zone of coaptation itself lies in a transverse plane (5). Occasionally, the edges of the leaflets near the posteromedial end of the commissure may be seen when the tip of the probe is tilted upwards, but it is difficult to perform this manoeuvre successfully. The images may also be confusing if there is prolapse of the aortic leaflet because the plane of imaging can incorporate the edges of the leaflets near the posteromedial end of the commissure and then, separately, their central portions towards the middle of the orifice of the valve. Most often, as the tip of the probe is withdrawn from the lower oesophagus towards the left atrium, the zone of coaptation is first demonstrated clearly only approximately half of the way from one end of the commissure to the other (Fig. 6.3). This standard transverse axial image crosses a large segment of the aortic leaflet and a small part of the mural leaflet, but it does not traverse either of these leaflets at right angles to the zone of coaptation. Clear images of the medial part of the zone of coaptation, in planes that are perpendicular to the edges of the leaflets, can be produced only by using a transducer that produces images in longitudinal planes (8). The longitudinal plane that crosses the mitral leaflets near the posteromedial end of the commissure also traverses the subaortic diverticulum of the left ventricle, and demonstrates the right ventricle anteriorly (Fig. 6.4).

The opposite holds true for studying the lateral third of the zone of coaptation, which runs almost in a true sagittal, or longitudinal, plane (see *Fig. 6.1*). Scanning in successive transverse planes as the probe is pulled backwards and rotated very slightly to the left (in an anticlockwise direction) demonstrates this part of the zone of coaptation very well (Fig. 6.5). In this region, the longitudinal transducer is not very useful and, indeed, it may be misleading if it is directed very laterally. What appears to be the zone of coaptation may, in fact, be the cleft between the lateral and middle scallops of the mural leaflet (see *Fig. 3.54*).

In the middle of the mitral valve, both transverse and longitudinal planes produce images that cross through substantial portions of both leaflets.

In systole, the atrioventricular junction that supports the leaflets of the valve does not lie in a single anatomical plane. Instead, it is curved as if it occupies the middle

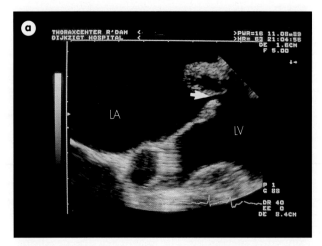
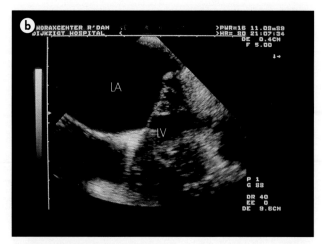

Fig. 6.5 (a) Cross-sectional image obtained with a transverse transducer positioned opposite the middle of the zone of coaptation. In systole (the timing of this frozen frame is indicated by the break in the green line displaying the electrocardiogram), there is prolapse of the mural leaflet, which balloons into the left atrium. The aortic leaflet appears more straight than normal, but this compensatory position is insufficient to maintain coaptation. A regurgitant orifice is clearly visible (arrowed). (b) In the same patient, an image in the transverse axis near the anterolateral end of the commissure shows mild prolapse of the mural leaflet, but at this site systolic coaptation is normal.

part of the surface of a hyperbolic paraboloid (Fig. 6.6) (9). The high points of the junction lie anteriorly (adjacent to the aortic root) and posteriorly, and so they are most easily viewed echocardiographically in the long-axis cross section obtained from a left parasternal approach. The low points of the atrioventricular junction are demonstrated from the precordium in an apical four-chamber view. In 15 normal subjects, the maximum distance between parallel planes passing through the low and high points of the junction was an average of 1.4cm (9). This shape accounts for the different prevalences of prolapse of the leaflets (10) which have been reported in studies of healthy individuals using different imaging planes but the same definition of prolapse — that is, the appearance of any part of the leaflet during systole above a line drawn between the edges of the atrioventricular junction in the same plane. The prevalence is higher when an apical four-chamber approach is used than when a parasternal long-axis plane is studied (10,11). The standard transoesophageal image through the middle of the mitral valve corresponds closely to an apical four-chamber view, except that it is approached from the opposite side of the heart. By extrapolating from precordial studies, therefore, it is likely that a high incidence of valvar prolapse will be found on transoesophageal echocardiography and that, in many subjects, this will be a false-positive diagnosis (12). Two recent studies have suggested that 'prolapse' (however it is defined) is indeed found more readily on transoesophageal

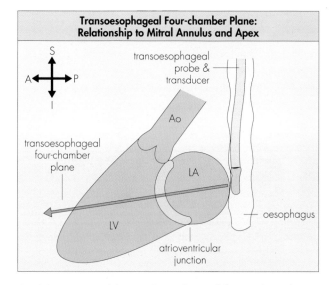

Fig. 6.6 Diagram of the nonplanar shape of the mitral annulus, related to the standard transverse transoesophageal plane of imaging. In the four-chamber views of the mitral valve, the plane of imaging (indicated by the arrow) passes through the low points of the atrioventricular junction.

echocardiography than on transthoracic echocardiography (13,14). The normal range of motion of the mitral leaflets when viewed from the oesophagus, however, has not been reported, and so exact criteria for the diagnosis of prolapse by transoesophageal echocardiography are not yet available. The diagnosis cannot be made safely on transoesophageal echocardiography alone if the degree of prolapse is very mild (for an

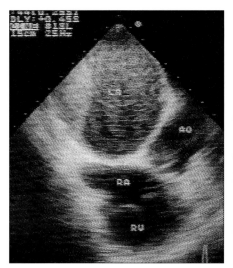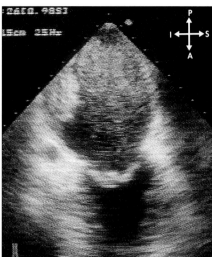

Fig. 6.7 Longitudinal images of the left atrium in a patient with mitral stenosis. No thrombus was observed on careful examination in transverse planes, but these views demonstrate that there is a laminar thrombus applied to the floor of the left atrium. There is spontaneous contrast within the left atrium. The right-hand image, through the left atrium and left ventricle, also shows the coronary sinus in the atrioventricular groove.

example, see *Fig. 3.27*), and if it is observed only in the four-chamber view.

The major implication of these anatomical considerations is that when transoesophageal echocardiography is performed with a single transducer that images in the transverse axis, it may fail to produce clear images of the valvar leaflets near the posteromedial end of the commissure, and it may miss pathology that is confined to this area or that extends there. Full analysis of the mitral valve can be performed with a biplane transoesophageal probe by using a transverse transoesophageal transducer in combination with transthoracic approaches, or with epicardial echocardiography in patients undergoing cardiac surgery (15).

MITRAL STENOSIS

In spite of its advantages, transoesophageal echocardiography is not the ideal technique for evaluating rheumatic mitral stenosis. Restricted motion, thickening and calcification of the leaflets, and involvement of the subvalvar apparatus, can usually be identified during a precordial study, while Doppler interrogation of flow across the mitral orifice is best performed from the apex (6). In severe mitral stenosis, particularly when the left atrium is very enlarged, the peak velocity of diastolic flow across the valve may exceed the limit at which it can be measured accurately (without aliasing) using pulsed Doppler techniques from the oesophagus. Use of continuous wave Doppler interrogation from the apex or the lateral precordium is then the best approach. Nevertheless, when a transoesophageal probe with integrated continuous wave and pulsed Doppler

modalities is available, estimates of the severity of mitral stenosis obtained with Doppler techniques from the oesophagus correlate closely with pressure gradients recorded at cardiac catheterization (16).

The role of transoesophageal echocardiography in patients with mitral stenosis is to supplement precordial studies, for example when operative treatment is being considered. It is the most accurate method of establishing whether or not there is thrombus in the left atrium, for example in patients who are being assessed for balloon valvotomy (17) and in those with atrial fibrillation who are being considered for cardioversion. Thrombus may be restricted to the left atrial appendage (18), or it may be laminar and closely applied to the wall of the left atrium so that it is only appreciated on detailed imaging in several planes (Fig. 6.7). In patients with mitral stenosis, transoesophageal echocardiography also demonstrates spontaneous contrast within the atria, much more often than transthoracic echocardiography does (19). This is a risk factor for embolism (20,21).

In special circumstances, transoesophageal echocardiography is helpful in analysing the morphology of a stenotic mitral valve. If the valve is not heavily calcified, the tendinous cords and the subvalvar apparatus may be imaged in more detail from the oesophagus than from the precordium. This makes it possible to deduce if there is cordal shortening or fusion, and to diagnose cordal rupture. It is usually impossible to image the cords along their entire length (from the tips of the leaflets to the papillary muscles) in a transverse plane; the longitudinal approach is better. Transoesophageal echocardiography can also determine if the leaflets are mobile or pliable. Fusion of the leaflets at the posteromedial end of the commissure (or its absence) can be identified by imaging in the longitudinal axis (Fig. 6.8), while imaging in transverse planes demonstrates fusion at the anterolateral end of the commissure. Knowledge of such details may be useful when selecting patients who are likely to benefit most from balloon valvotomy (22). One prospective study of transthoracic echocardiography demonstrated that patients with extensive subvalvar disease (such as thickening

or fusion) had a poor result (23). When the valve is heavily calcified, masking prevents imaging of the subvalvar structures from the oesophagus but, conversely, the oesophageal approach may be invaluable for making or excluding (as much as can ever be done by echocardiography) a diagnosis of infective endocarditis in a patient with a calcified mitral valve.

Colour flow mapping demonstrates well diastolic and systolic flow within the left atrium (Fig. 6.9). The zones of flow converging at the mitral valve, which are caused by aliasing as velocity increases when blood accelerates into the narrowed funnel of the restricted orifice, can be used to assess the severity of stenosis. Assuming that the pattern of flow into a valve is symmetrical (that is, that the isovelocity contours are hemispherical), then measuring the width of the zone of convergence (determined by the Nyquist limit in operation) and using the continuity equation allow the size of the orifice to be calculated. This method is independent of both the angle of incidence of the Doppler beam to the jet, and of the level of gain, and it is best performed with a low-pulse repetition frequency. The zone of convergence should be measured from the first colour alias to the centre of the valvar orifice. This may be easier to achieve when using the colour M-mode display (Fig. 6.10). It has not yet been reported whether or not these techniques give more information about mitral stenosis than is available from transthoracic Doppler studies. They are useful, therefore, in diagnosing the severity of mitral stenosis only in patients in

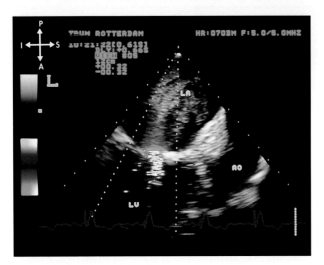

Fig. 6.8 Longitudinal image through the mitral valve in the medial third of the zone of coaptation in a patient with mitral stenosis. Colour flow mapping shows turbulent flow through the stenotic orifice. There is also considerable spontaneous contrast within the left atrium. The same patient as in *Fig. 6.4* is demonstrated here in a plane that is more to the left and nearer to the midpoint of the zone of coaptation.

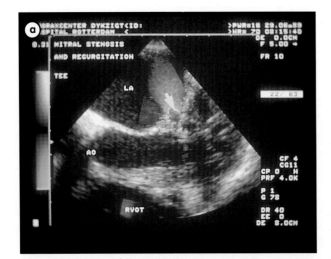
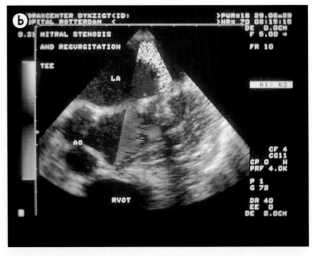

Fig. 6.9 (a) Diastolic and (b) systolic frames obtained in the transverse plane in a patient with mitral stenosis and regurgitation. The zone of flow converging into the mitral orifice in diastole is shown well (arrowed), but thickening and calcification of the leaflets mean that no flow is displayed within the left ventricle. In systole, the mitral regurgitant jet is clearly demonstrated.

whom adequate information cannot be obtained from the precordium, or in circumstances when Doppler estimates of pressure half-time may be unreliable (24).

Transoesophageal echocardiography can be used to guide and monitor mitral valvotomy at cardiac catheterization (25,26) if the procedure is performed under general anaesthesia. It is most useful for assessing the degree of mitral regurgitation before and after the intervention (Fig. 6.11a), especially if problems are encountered. It also depicts the site and size of the atrial septal defect caused by the transseptal puncture (Fig. 6.11b). It is less useful for guiding the transseptal puncture or the placement of the balloon across the orifice of the valve (Fig. 6.12). Both the needle and the catheter cast linear shadows on the echocardiogram,

making it difficult when imaging in only two dimensions to distinguish between a view along the length of the catheter and a view that incorporates a linear echo caused by the beam of ultrasound crossing the catheter at right angles to its short axis. Furthermore, when the balloon is inflated, any gas within it causes masking. If the mitral orifice is obstructed, there is then a rapid and marked increase in spontaneous echocardiographic contrast within the left atrium. It has not yet been demonstrated by randomized trials that the advantages of transoesophageal echocardiography during interventional catheterization outweigh the disadvantages of general anaesthesia, but the technique may have a role in reducing the high incidence in some series of tamponade related to transseptal puncture (27). Both

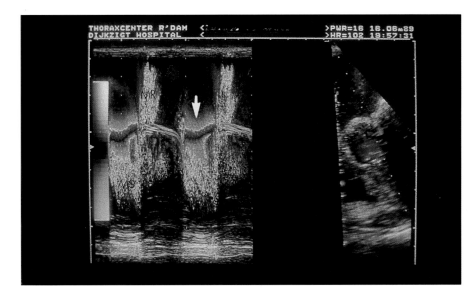

Fig. 6.10 The cursor for colour M-mode sampling has been placed across the mitral orifice (right-hand panel). The M-mode display increases the temporal and spatial resolution of flow events. The width of the zone of convergence in diastole (arrowed) is seen very clearly, as well as turbulence within the diastolic jet once it reaches the left ventricle. This patient has a central systolic jet of regurgitation (MR) of relatively short duration. MS = mitral stenosis.

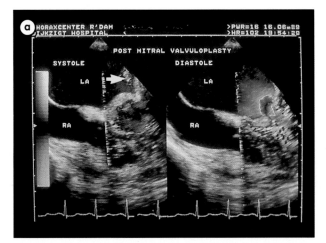

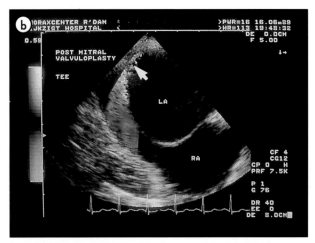

Fig. 6.11 (a) Systolic and diastolic frames obtained immediately after balloon dilatation of the mitral valve. There is only trivial mitral regurgitation (arrowed). (b) The patient has an enlarged left atrium, and the septum is displaced towards the right. There is a very posterior atrial septal defect (arrowed) following transseptal puncture, with a residual left-to-right shunt.

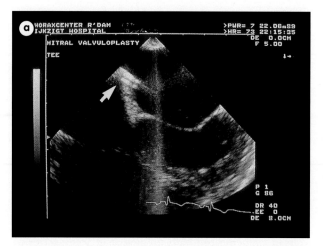 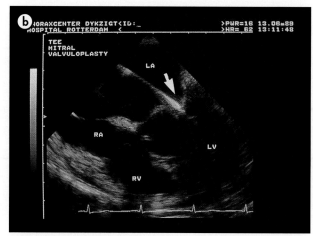

Fig. 6.12 (a) In this patient, transoesophageal echocardiography during cardiac catheterization confirms that the transseptal puncture is through the central portion of the atrial septum (arrowed). (b) In this four-chamber view that was obtained before the balloon was inflated, the echocardiogram suggests that it is correctly positioned across the orifice of the valve (arrowed).

transoesophageal and transthoracic echocardiography demonstrate residual left-to-right shunting (28,29).

MITRAL REGURGITATION

When using echocardiography to assess a patient with mitral regurgitation, the cardiologist should aim to identify the anatomical site of regurgitation, and to define the nature of the underlying structural problem. The first step in this process (Fig. 6.13) is to study the pattern of closure of the edges of the leaflets along the whole zone of coaptation, in order to identify if and where they fail to coapt. Only then is it appropriate to search for evidence of causes such as rupture, elongation or retraction of cords, infarction or rupture of a papillary muscle, perforation of a leaflet, and dilatation of the atrioventricular junction. The pattern of motion of the bodies of the leaflets should also be studied, but it is less important to diagnose abnormalities such as prolapse than it is to determine the relationship between the edges of the leaflets. Finally, the significance of the resulting regurgitation should be assessed using different methods. Together with the clinical assessment, this will indicate if treatment is required. When reconstructive surgery is considered, the echocardiographic analysis tells the cardiac surgeon where normal coaptation must be restored, and suggests how this might be achieved.

Scheme for Echocardiographic Analysis of Regurgitant Mitral Valves

Analyse the pattern of closure of the edges of the leaflets, between the posteromedial and anterolateral commissures
(1) is coaptation normal ?
(2) is apposition normal ?

Assess the size of the atrioventricular junction (mitral annulus)
(3) is the atrioventricular junction enlarged ?

Consider unusual causes or sites of regurgitation
(4) is there perforation of a leaflet ?
(5) congenital disease (such as an isolated cleft of the aortic leaflet, or insertion into the aortic leaflet of a shelf obstructing the left ventricular outflow tract)
(6) calcification of the atrioventricular junction

Study the subvalvar apparatus for associated abnormalities
(7) regional wall-motion abnormalities of the left ventricle ?
(8) papillary muscular infarction or rupture ?
(9) cordal elongation or rupture ?
(10) cordal fusion or retraction ?

Assess motion of the bodies of the leaflets
(11) prolapse ?
(12) retraction ?
(13) restriction ?

Assess the type and severity of the mitral regurgitation jet
(14) direction and nature of the jet (free standing or along the atrial wall)
(15) colour flow mapping (maximal area of turbulence, related to the area of left atrium in the same plane, or the length of the jet)
(16) timing and duration of regurgitation (colour M-mode recording)
(17) Doppler studies of flow across the mitral orifice (continuous wave if available; pulsed Doppler for timing of mitral inflow)
(18) pulmonary venous Doppler (influence of regurgitation reduced antegrade velocities, or retrograde flow, during systole)

Fig. 6.13 This scheme attempts to provide a logical framework for studying regurgitant mitral valves during transoesophageal echocardiography, but with minor modifications it is applicable to other echocardiographic approaches. In routine practice, it is rarely necessary to analyse all these aspects of structure and function in an individual patient.

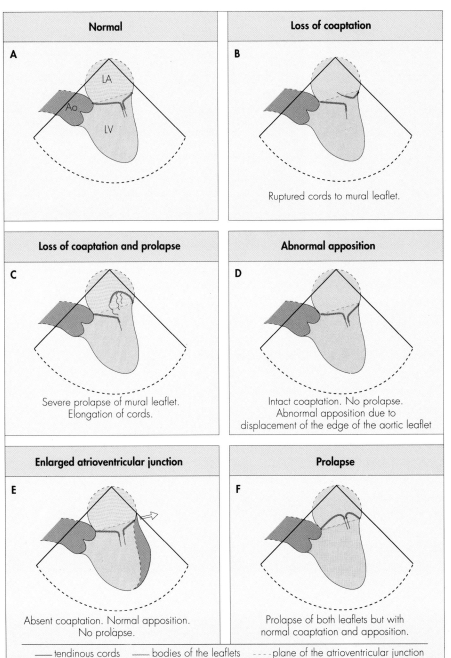

Fig. 6.14 Diagrammatic representation of common abnormalities found when studying patients with mitral regurgitation. These diagrams represent the patterns of closure found when imaging the midportions of the mitral leaflets in a transverse plane. In practice, the limitations of this imaging plane mean that it is not always possible to demonstrate these abnormalities so clearly. The pattern illustrated in F may be found in valves that are competent.

Normal

A

LA

Ao

LV

Loss of coaptation

B

Ruptured cords to mural leaflet.

Loss of coaptation and prolapse

C

Severe prolapse of mural leaflet.
Elongation of cords.

Abnormal apposition

D

Intact coaptation. No prolapse.
Abnormal apposition due to
displacement of the edge of the aortic leaflet

Enlarged atrioventricular junction

E

Absent coaptation. Normal apposition.
No prolapse.

Prolapse

F

Prolapse of both leaflets but with
normal coaptation and apposition.

—— tendinous cords   —— bodies of the leaflets   ----plane of the atrioventricular junction

Analysis of the morphology of regurgitant valves

A full transoesophageal study of the mitral valve, including its subvalvar components, starts during transgastric imaging of the left ventricle. Regional wall-motion abnormalities caused by myocardial infarction should be noted, along with any associated loss of function of the papillary muscles. As the tip of the probe is pulled back towards the cardia of the stomach and the atrioventricular groove, the papillary muscles and the cords are traced upwards until they merge with the leaflets. Infarction of a papillary muscle causes fibrosis and scarring, which may result in more dense or bright echoes, and it can cause calcification within the papillary muscles. It is difficult on transoesophageal echocardiography using a transverse transducer to appreciate elongation or retraction of cords since they cannot be imaged along their entire length in a single transverse plane. The presence of these abnormalities can be deduced from the thickness and mobility of the cords, and by excessive or restricted motion of the associated leaflet.

The zone of coaptation of the mitral valve is examined best when a biplane probe is used and the transducers are positioned opposite the left atrium. When the leaflets coapt normally, their edges remain in contact throughout systole and the rough zones are symmetrically aligned opposite each other (Fig. 6.14).

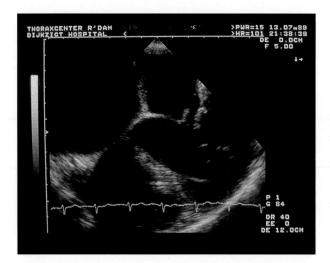

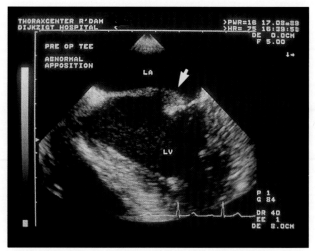

Fig. 6.15 Four-chamber view demonstrating loss of coaptation of the mitral valve due to rupture of cords to the aortic leaflet. There is no prolapse of the body of either leaflet, but there is a large regurgitant orifice in the middle of the zone of coaptation because of 'prolapse' of the edge of the leaflet.

Fig. 6.16 Abnormal apposition of the mitral leaflets demonstrated in a transverse image. The aortic leaflet reaches to the atrioventricular junction, although in this patient, conventional parasternal imaging in the long-axis plane did not demonstrate any of the criteria for the diagnosis of prolapse from the precordium. The edge of the aortic leaflet overlaps the mural leaflet at the site of coaptation and protrudes towards the left atrium (arrowed). This was associated with a regurgitant jet that was directed posterolaterally.

When the atrioventricular junction is enlarged, for example in a patient with a dilated left ventricle, coaptation is lost in the middle of the commissure, but the rough zones remain aligned opposite each other. Most commonly, coaptation is lost when there is abnormal motion of the edge of one leaflet. The relationship of the edges of the leaflets in systole is then obviously asymmetrical. An example is cordal rupture, which produces loss of coaptation when the edge of the affected leaflet prolapses (Fig. 6.15).

Occasionally, no echocardiographic abnormality is found in a patient with mitral regurgitation apart from mild asymmetry of the leaflets at their line of closure (30). One leaflet protrudes over the edge of the other towards the left atrium (Fig. 6.16). This subtle abnormality is called abnormal apposition. It is rarely appreciated on transthoracic imaging, but is frequently seen on transoesophageal imaging. Regurgitation is probably due to overlap of the free edge of one leaflet above the limit of the normally positioned rough zone of the opposite leaflet. Anatomical studies suggest that regurgitation can occur if this overlap is as little as 3 or 4mm (31). The regurgitant jet is eccentric and directed away from the protruding leaflet onto the atrial surface of the overlapped leaflet. If transoesophageal imaging fails to demonstrate a morphological basis for regurgitation in an individual patient, then this pattern on colour flow mapping suggests that the cause may be abnormal apposition. This can be the mechanism of mitral regurgitation in patients who fulfil the classical criteria for mitral valvar prolapse, as well as in those who do not, which is another reason why the pattern of closure of the edges of the leaflets should be assessed separately from motion of the bodies of the leaflets.

Rupture of a papillary muscle is always obvious. It is usually diagnosed on precordial echocardiography (32), but an emergency transoesophageal study may be required to make the diagnosis in a ventilated patient who has life-threatening pulmonary oedema (33). A ruptured papillary muscle is flail, and its torn head prolapses into the left atrium during systole (34). It is associated with torrential mitral regurgitation, often into a relatively small left atrium. In contrast, rupture of tendinous cords is much less likely to cause sudden clinical deterioration since it is often superimposed on chronic regurgitation in a patient with a dilated left atrium. The affected portion of the leaflet prolapses (35), and from its edge, the fine strands of ruptured cords may be seen trailing into the left atrium and fluttering in the regurgitant jet (Fig. 6.17) (36). This pattern is usually appreciated only on frame-by-frame analysis. Occasionally, primary cords rupture flush at the site of their insertions into the edge of a leaflet, so the absence of trailing strands of tissue does not reliably exclude cordal rupture. It is rarely important to make this precise diagnosis. In patients who are selected for

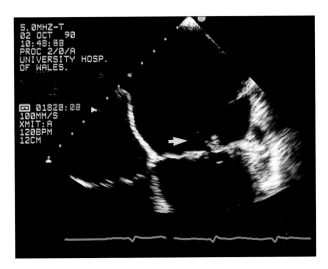

Fig. 6.17 Image obtained from a frozen video frame, demonstrating the fine strands of ruptured cords (arrowed) trailing from the prolapsed free edge of the mural leaflet of the mitral valve.

reconstructive surgery, ruptured cords are seen on inspection, and the segment of the leaflet that has lost its cordal tethering is usually excised as part of the repair. It is more important on echocardiography to define the extent of any resulting loss of coaptation.

If coaptation and apposition are entirely normal, and if the atrioventricular junction is not enlarged, then alternative explanations for regurgitation must be sought. Perforation of a leaflet may be demonstrated directly or, if it is small, inferred from the location and direction of the associated regurgitant jet (for an example, see *Fig. 13.8b*) (37). The most common cause of perforation is infective endocarditis, as discussed in *Chapter 9*, and so there may be associated vegetations or abscesses, or a communication between the left ventricular outflow tract and the left atrium (38). Congenital causes of mitral regurgitation should also be considered. Incompetence of the valve may be a consequence of tethering of the aortic leaflet by attachments of a subaortic fibrotic shelf, as discussed in *Chapter 7*, or it may be secondary to obstruction of the left ventricular outflow tract in hypertrophic cardiomyopathy (39). A true cleft of the aortic leaflet (not associated with any abnormality of the atrioventricular septum) may be detected, but its orientation towards the aortic root is most readily demonstrated in a parasternal short-axis view (40,41). It is difficult to reproduce this imaging plane on transoesophageal echocardiography, at least

when using a transverse transducer, although it is possible when imaging from the fundus of the stomach. Regurgitation across the left atrioventricular valve associated with atrioventricular septal defects is discussed in *Chapter 12.*

In this account of morphological changes revealed by transoesophageal echocardiography in patients with mitral regurgitation, abnormal motion of the bodies of the leaflets is deliberately discussed last. Traditionally, prolapse is the most reported abnormality of the leaflets in patients with mitral regurgitation of degenerative or other nonrheumatic aetiology. Indeed, it has often been deemed adequate on its own as an explanation of the cause or mechanism of regurgitation. The term 'prolapse', however, is used ambiguously (cardiologists and cardiac surgeons have different definitions), and its incidence depends on the plane in which the valve is imaged. Prolapse is usually used to refer to protrusion of the *body of a leaflet* into the left atrium, above a notional line drawn between the limits of the atrioventricular junction in the same plane, but it is abnormal apposition or asymmetrical prolapse of the *edge of a leaflet* that causes loss of coaptation, and regurgitation. Indeed, there may be marked prolapse of the bodies of both leaflets but no regurgitation in a valve in which the edges of the leaflets and the rough zone are neither abnormal nor displaced. The alternative term, 'billowing', has been proposed for this condition (42). Even when there is unambiguous prolapse of the edges of both leaflets, however, the valve may still be competent if the junction between the leaflets is symmetrical, and coaptation is maintained. Recognition of these difficulties has led to the elaboration of major and minor criteria that should be satisfied before making a clinical diagnosis of mitral valvar prolapse (43), and to the suggestion that prolapse should only be diagnosed on echocardiography if the point of coaptation, as well as the leaflets, are displaced towards the left atrium (44). Prolapse is seen well on a transoesophageal study, but reporting its presence without providing further details of coaptation or apposition, rarely describes all of the diagnostic information that can be obtained.

Other, less-common abnormalities of motion of the mitral leaflets may also be associated with regurgitation. In patients with rheumatic mitral disease, fusion or shortening of the cords may cause retraction of a leaflet so that it cannot move normally towards the atrioventricular junction in systole. The aortic leaflet is particularly affected, and when its motion is arrested during systole, the body of the leaflet appears angulated and normal coaptation becomes impossible (Fig. 6.18). Another uncommon pattern occurs in patients who have had a posterior or inferobasal myocardial infarction.

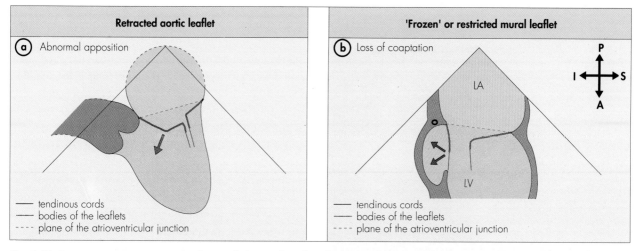

Fig. 6.18 Diagrammatic representation of unusual abnormalities found when performing echocardiography in patients with regurgitant mitral valves. (a) This transverse image demonstrates retraction of the aortic leaflet, resulting in abnormal apposition. (b) This diagram of a longitudinal planar image illustrates restricted motion of the mural leaflet caused by dilatation and systolic expansion of an infarcted basal segment of the left ventricular myocardium involving the posteromedial papillary muscle.

Expansion of the zone of infarction maintains tension on the posteromedial papillary muscle and on the cords to the posteromedial end of the commissure and the mural leaflet throughout the cardiac cycle. The mural leaflet becomes so restricted in its motion that it appears immobile on echocardiography. Both of these conditions (retraction or restriction of a leaflet) can be associated with abnormal apposition or loss of coaptation, and both can cause significant regurgitation. At present, only qualitative criteria are available for their diagnosis.

When imaging from the precordium, the size of the atrioventricular junction (mitral annulus) is usually measured in the parasternal long-axis plane (45). A similar approach is used by surgeons performing epicardial echocardiography (30). On transoesophageal echocardiography, however, it is difficult to reproduce these measurements because the standard plane corresponds to an apical four-chamber view. This approach has been used for some studies from the precordium (46) but criteria for the measurement of the atrioventricular junction from the oesophagus, and normal values, have not yet been reported. Better measurements for comparison with the long-axis approach may be possible using biplane probes. The morphology and function of the atrioventricular junction should also be assessed, since calcification within it is a common cause of regurgitation (47).

Assessment of regurgitation

The location and direction of the jet regurgitating through an incompetent valve are related to its mor-

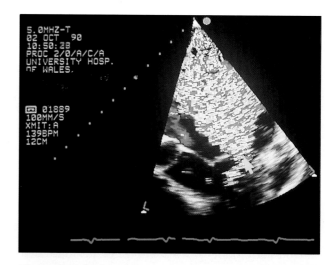

Fig. 6.19 Central regurgitant jet (arrowed) arising from the middle of the orifice of the mitral valve in a patient with a dilated atrioventricular junction. In this, the regurgitant orifice is not directly imaged.

phology. In patients with a dilated atrioventricular junction but no primary abnormality of the valve, and in those with rheumatic mitral regurgitation (48), the regurgitant jet usually arises from the centre of the zone of coaptation. It is directed into the middle of the left atrium as a free-standing jet (Fig. 6.19). In contrast, the regurgitant jet in a patient with loss of coaptation or abnormal apposition, is almost always eccentric. Mapping of the left atrium with pulsed Doppler to

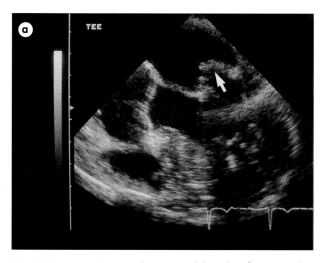

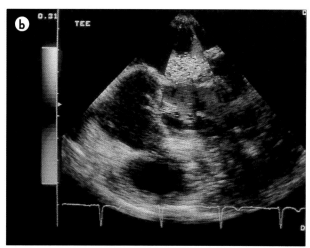

Fig. 6.20 (a) Cross-sectional image and (b) colour flow map obtained in a patient with prolapse of the mural leaflet (arrowed) and severe mitral regurgitation. There is a broad regurgitant jet that passes medially behind the aortic leaflet.

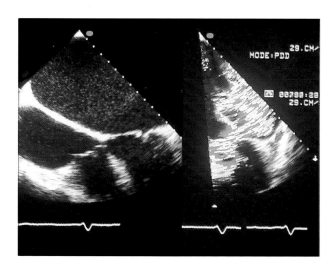

Fig. 6.21 Cross-sectional image (on the left) and colour flow map (on the right) in a patient with abnormal apposition of the aortic leaflet, resulting in a severe regurgitant jet directed posterolaterally around the left atrium.

detect regurgitation is much more sensitive from the oesophagus than from the precordium (49), but colour flow mapping is the best method. When the mural leaflet prolapses, the jet is directed anteromedially (Fig. 6.20) while in lesions of the aortic leaflet, it is directed posterolaterally (Fig. 6.21) (50). These eccentric jets initially hug the atrial surface of the opposite leaflet and then the atrial wall. They may track all the way around the posterior wall of the atrium and travel back towards the valve. If the morphology of the valve is unclear, then

the site and orientation of flow within the left ventricle accelerating into the regurgitant orifice, and the direction of the jet within the left atrium, are helpful in determining which leaflet is abnormal (51).

Echocardiographic grading of the severity of regurgitation is difficult from any approach (52), and the transoesophageal one is no exception. No absolute 'gold standard' exists against which new methods can be tested or compared since even angiographic criteria are influenced by many variables that are not directly related to the size of the regurgitant orifice. Similar factors influence the area of turbulence detected on colour flow mapping (53–55); these include heart rate, systemic blood pressure, left ventricular preload and afterload, left atrial pressure, and stroke volume. Thus, for example, the length of a jet is related to the drop in pressure across the orifice. In addition, the shape of a mitral regurgitant jet is influenced by its relationship to the walls of the left atrium. Central or free jets recruit blood cells from multiple lateral eddies around their high-velocity central core, and this amplifies the area of disturbed flow which is identified and displayed on the colour map as a region of 'turbulence'. Thus, a high-velocity central jet may cause a disproportionately large area of turbulence, even when the actual volume of regurgitant flow is relatively low. In contrast, the behaviour of jets that hug the wall of the atrium is altered since they can recruit blood cells into the regurgitant stream from one side only. This so-called Coanda effect causes jets which adhere to a surface to become flattened, and their width, as detected by colour flow mapping in planes at right angles to the interface between the fluid jet and the solid wall, does not increase (56). Thus, a high-volume mitral regurgitant jet that remains closely applied to the surface of a leaflet and then to the wall of the atrium, may appear to be relatively unimpressive on colour flow mapping (for an example, see *Fig. 13.8a*) (57). Not surprisingly, estimates of the severity of eccentric mitral regurgitant jets derived from colour flow mapping correlate poorly with angiographic grades (48).

It is easy to recognize mitral regurgitant jets using colour flow mapping from the oesophagus, especially if the area being interrogated is limited to the left atrium. Rapid sampling allows maps of excellent quality to be obtained. Even minor disturbances of flow are appreciated when the colour gain is high (Fig. 6.22). Regurgitation is detected in normal subjects (58), including a majority of those aged over 50 years (59). These qualities, however, may be a disadvantage when regurgitation is graded. There may be several separate regurgitant jets in a single patient (60) in addition to the four streams of pulmonary venous inflow. The patterns of turbulence caused by regurgitation may be quite irregular, making accurate and reproducible mapping of their areas difficult, especially if the rate of sampling of the colour map is slow. This is not an important consideration in patients with very severe regurgitation (Fig. 6.23), but it may be important in those with moderate regurgitation. It is also important to discriminate between turbulence within the left atrium caused by mitral regurgitation and that due to turbulent flow entering from the pulmonary veins. Using transoesophageal echocardiography, the whole of the left atrium and the entire course of a regurgitant jet are rarely demonstrated in a single plane or on a single image. In practice, most systems that are used for the clinical grading of regurgitation, rather than for research, employ simple methods that do not involve measuring the area of turbulence in relation to the area of the left atrium.

The most common approach has been to document the depth to which the regurgitant jet penetrates the left atrium; for example, the jet may be present only in the vicinity of the orifice, or it may reach a distance of less than one-third, less than two-thirds, or more than two-thirds, of the way from the atrioventricular junction towards the posterior left atrial wall. Such methods have been used mostly in precordial (61) and epicardial (62) echocardiographic studies, where they have been shown to correlate well with the results of left ventriculography, but they are also applicable to the transoesophageal approach (63). Timing the duration of a jet is also of some value since regurgitation associated with valvar prolapse may be restricted to late systole (60); that caused by obstruction of the left ventricular outflow tract may be midsystolic (39), and trivial regurgitation of a normal valve sometimes occurs only in early systole (64). It is difficult to assess this during real-time colour flow mapping, and recording and replaying cine loops is impractical during a transoesophageal study. The most useful, and also the quickest way of establishing the timing and duration of a regurgitant jet, is to study its colour M-mode display. The frequency of sampling of flow is much faster than on a cross-sectional image and so accurate information is obtained easily. Problems may arise when a jet is very

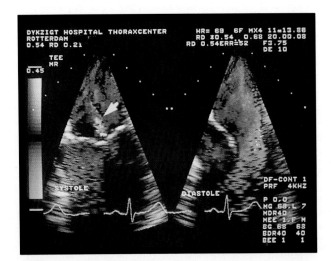

Fig. 6.22 Systolic (on the left) and diastolic (on the right) colour flow maps in a healthy subject. There is mild, and normal central regurgitation (arrowed). This occurred at the beginning of systole, and the jet did not reach the middle of the left atrium.

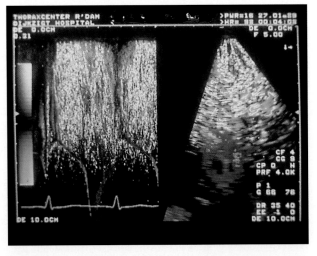

Fig. 6.23 Colour flow map and colour M-mode recording in a patient with very severe mitral regurgitation. It is impossible to discern the origin, direction, or limits of the jet that fills all of the atrium that is imaged.

eccentric if it is not appreciated that its timing may vary between different parts of the left atrium.

The severity of regurgitation can also be analysed by studying flow converging into the regurgitant orifice from the left ventricle in a manner which is analogous to the use of zones of convergence for studying the severity of mitral stenosis. The area of accelerating flow within the left ventricle correlates with the angiographic grade of regurgitation (51), especially when the regurgitant orifice is relatively small. It has been shown *in vitro* that a colour M-mode recording provides a clear display of the radius of 'first aliasing' over time, which can be integrated and used to calculate the regurgitant stroke volume (65).

Another indicator that can be considered when transoesophageal echocardiography is used to grade the severity of mitral regurgitation is the Doppler waveform of flow within the pulmonary veins. This is discussed in more detail in *Chapter 5*. In essence, significant mitral regurgitation is associated with prolonged retrograde flow into the pulmonary veins during ventricular systole, instead of the normal pattern of antegrade flow (or emptying) of blood from the veins into the left atrium (66,67). This feature is helpful in assessing the significance of mitral regurgitation when it is suspected that the colour flow map may be misleading. It is responsive to acute changes in the severity of regurgitation (68).

Simple methods of assessing regurgitation are adequate for most clinical purposes. It is easy to diagnose trivial or severe regurgitation. When more accurate quantification is required, for example for research or in patients with moderate regurgitation of uncertain significance, planimetry of the area of turbulence caused by a regurgitant jet is probably the best method, as long as the jet is not very eccentric. The area of a regurgitant jet (related to the area of the left atrium) correlates quite well with the severity of regurgitation on left ventriculography (69), although neither factor is a particularly good index of regurgitant volume (70). The introduction of biplane probes means that it is now possible to map jets in multiple planes and reconstruct their shapes and sizes in three dimensions. At present, such calculations are laborious and time-consuming, and it has not yet been reported if the resulting estimates are more accurate than existing ones, or if they confer any significant clinical gain over other simpler but more tried methods.

TRICUSPID VALVAR DISEASE

The tricuspid valve is seen best on transoesophageal echocardiography in the four-chamber views that are obtained when the transducer is at the level of the left atrium. In this plane, the septal and anterosuperior leaflets are demonstrated. Using a transducer that images in transverse planes, it is difficult to study all three leaflets and to analyse the whole of the zone of coaptation, except in those rare patients in whom the orifice of the tricuspid valve is seen in short axis as the probe is withdrawn from the stomach. With the longitudinal probe, however, the mural leaflet is shown clearly. Another problem arises because the flow of blood across the tricuspid valve is more from right to left, across the anterior part of the heart (that is, almost in a true coronal plane), than from the back of the heart towards the front. This means that it is not easy to obtain colour flow maps of high quality, or accurate pulsed-Doppler traces, from the oesophagus, unless corrections are made for the angle of incidence of the beam of ultrasound, because the feasible imaging planes are not well aligned for Doppler studies.

TRICUSPID STENOSIS

In many countries, organic tricuspid stenosis of rheumatic aetiology is now rare. It almost never occurs as an isolated lesion, but is found in a small proportion (3–5%) of patients with mitral stenosis (71). The diagnostic value of transoesophageal echocardiography in tricuspid stenosis has not been reported, but it is likely that a biplane probe will provide most information. If conventional transthoracic imaging is difficult, transoesophageal imaging could be used, for example to assess if the commissures are fused. The severity of tricuspid stenosis should be assessed with Doppler studies from the precordium (7,72).

TRICUSPID REGURGITATION

Tricuspid regurgitation occurs as a normal phenomenon in most healthy people (73). Its reported prevalence appears to be related to the sensitivity of the techniques that are used to elicit it. As anticipated, therefore, an early whiff of tricuspid regurgitation is found very frequently on transoesophageal echocardiography, although it is of no significance. Mild tricuspid regurgitation may be detected in patients who have intrinsically normal valves but some other cause for regurgitation, such as a permanent pacemaker wire that crosses the tricuspid valve.

The most common form of tricuspid valvar disease is regurgitation caused by a dilated atrioventricular junction. This is readily appreciated on transoesophageal echocardiography (Fig. 6.24). As with mitral regurgitation, a colour M-mode recording is helpful for assessing its timing and significance. There have been few reports of the transoesophageal grading of tricuspid regurgitation, but simplified systems modified from precordial ultrasound studies (74) can be used to code the depth to which a jet invades the right atrium.

EBSTEIN'S MALFORMATION

In Ebstein's malformation, the leaflets of the tricuspid valve are abnormal and their attachments to the right ventricle are displaced towards the apex (75). The septal leaflet is often absent or else tightly tethered to the septum. The mural (or inferior) leaflet is also involved and is displaced to a variable extent towards the apex. The anatomical atrioventricular junction remains at the atrioventricular groove, but the orifice of the functional valve is very low. Between these sites, a considerable portion of the right ventricle becomes 'atrialized' as it lies in the functional right atrium. The ventricular myocardium in this segment of the right heart is often thinned, and its function is poor. A further important anatomical feature is the degree of apical tethering of the anterosuperior leaflet which is, however, not usually displaced from the atrioventricular junction.

Patients with Ebstein's malformation often have other lesions, such as an atrial septal defect or right-to-left shunting through a patent oval foramen, and a ventricu-

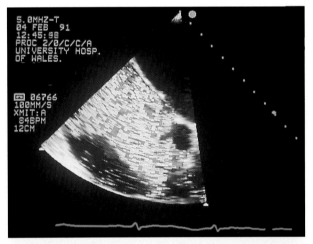

Fig. 6.24 Severe central tricuspid regurgitation in a patient with dilatation of the right atrioventricular junction.

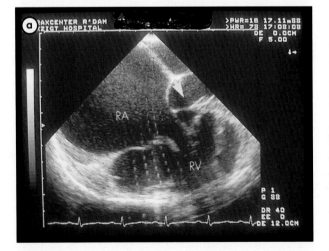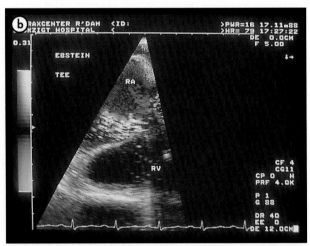

Fig. 6.25 (a) Intraoperative transoesophageal echocardiographic image in a patient with Ebstein's malformation. The lines are created by artefact during diathermy. The right atrium is enlarged and the leaflets of the tricuspid valve are displaced towards the apex of the right ventricle. There is a ventricular septal defect (arrowed) and tethering of the septal leaflet. (b) Colour flow mapping confirms that there is a broad regurgitant jet through the tricuspid valve. The turbulence, just visible within the left atrium in this image, is caused by a right-to-left shunt through a patent oval foramen.

lar septal defect (Fig. 6.25a). There may be abnormally sited papillary muscles giving rise to obstruction from a muscular 'shelf' within the right ventricular cavity (75). This causes turbulence on colour flow mapping. These features can be recognized from the oesophagus, but it is not possible to assess intraventricular or infundibular gradients with pulsed or continuous wave Doppler.

The main haemodynamic problem in most patients with Ebstein's malformation is tricuspid regurgitation (Fig. 6.25b). Often, this is severe and pansystolic through a large regurgitant orifice. It may be absolutely free regurgitation if there is no effective valvar function. Such regurgitation may occur at low velocity and be laminar so that it is not readily appreciated with colour flow imaging. The colour M-mode display can be used to confirm that there is retrograde flow above the tricuspid orifice during systole.

REFERENCES

1. Carpentier A, Chauvaud S, Fabiani JN *et al.* Reconstructive surgery of mitral valve incompetence: ten-year appraisal. *J Thorac Cardiovasc Surg* 1980;**79**:338–48.

2. Cosgrove DM, Stewart WJ. Mitral valvuloplasty. *Curr Probl in Cardiol* 1989;**14**:359–415.

3. Inoue K, Owani T, Nakamura T *et al.* Clinical application of transvenous mitral commissurotomy by a new balloon catheter. *J Thorac Cardiovasc Surg* 1984;**87**:394–402.

4. Lock JE, Khalilullah M, Shrivastava S *et al.* Percutaneous catheter commissurotomy in rheumatic mitral stenosis. *N Engl J Med* 1985;**313**:1515–8.

5. Fraser AG, Stümper OFW, van Herwerden LA *et al.* Anatomy of imaging planes used to study the mitral valve: advantages of biplane transesophageal echocardiography. *Circulation* 1990;**82**:III-668.

6. Hatle L, Brubakk A, Tromsdal A, Angelsen B. Noninvasive assessment of pressure drop in mitral stenosis by Doppler ultrasound. *Br Heart J* 1978;**40**:131–40.

7. Veyrat C, Kalmanson D, Farjon M *et al.* Noninvasive diagnosis and assessment of tricuspid regurgitation and stenosis using one and two-dimensional echo pulsed Doppler. *Br Heart J* 1982;**47**:596.

8. Stümper OFW, Fraser AG, Ho SY *et al.* Transoesophageal echocardiographic imaging in the longitudinal axis: a correlative echocardiographic — anatomic study and its clinical implications. *Br Heart J* 1990;**64**:282–8.

9. Levine RA, Handschumacher MD, Sanfilippo AJ *et al.* Three-dimensional echocardiographic reconstruction of the mitral valve, with implications for the diagnosis of mitral valve prolapse. *Circulation* 1989;**80**:589–98.

10. Levy D, Savage D. Prevalence and clinical features of mitral valve prolapse. *Am Heart J* 1987;**113**:1281–90.

11. Gillam LD, Radford MJ, Schulman P *et al.* Mitral valve prolapse: a disease in need of universal diagnostic criteria [Abstract]. *Circulation* 1987;**76**:IV-530.

12. Levine RA, Stathogiannidis E, Newell JB *et al.* Reconsideration of echocardiographic standards for mitral valve prolapse: lack of association between leaflet displacement isolated to the apical four chamber view and independent echocardiographic evidence of abnormality. *J Am Coll Cardiol* 1988;**11**:1010–9.

13. Zenker G, Erbel R, Kramer G *et al.* Transesophageal two-dimensional echocardiography in young patients with cerebral ischemic events. *Stroke* 1988;**19**:345–8.

14. Gueret P, Lacroix P, Bensaid J. Assessment of mitral valve prolapse by transesophageal echocardiography [Abstract]. *J Am Coll Cardiol* 1990;**15**:94a.

15. Fraser AG, van Herwerden LA, van Daele MERM *et al.* Is a combination of epicardial and transoesophageal echocardiography the best technique to monitor mitral valve repair? *Europ Heart J* 1989;**10**(Abstract supplement):33.

16. Grube E, Gerckens U, Cattelaens N. Is the quantification of mitral stenosis and aortic stenosis by transesophageal echocardiography feasible? In: Erbel R *et al*, eds. *Transesophageal Echocardiography.* Berlin: *Springer–Verlag*, 1989:59–65.

17. Casale PM, Whitlow P, Currie PJ, Stewart WJ. Transesophageal echocardiography in percutaneous balloon valvuloplasty for mitral stenosis. *Cleve Clin J Med* 1989;**56**:597–600.

18. Aschenberg W, Schlüter M, Kremer P *et al.* Transesophageal two-dimensional echocardiography for the detection of left atrial appendage thrombus. *J Am Coll Cardiol* 1986;**7**:163–6.

19. Chen YT, Kan MN, Chen JS *et al.* Contributing factors to formation of left atrial spontaneous echo contrast in mitral valvular disease. *J Ultrasound Med* 1990;**9**:151–5.

20. Daniel WG, Nellessen U, Schröder E *et al.* Left atrial spontaneous contrast in mitral valve disease: an indicator for an increased thromboembolic risk. *J Am Coll Cardiol* 1988;**11**:1204–11.

21. Beppu S, Nimura Y, Sakakibara H *et al.* Smoke-like echo in left atrial cavity in mitral valve disease: its feature and significance. *J Am Coll Cardiol* 1985;**6**:744–9.

22. Wilkins GT, Weyman AE, Abascal VM *et al.* Percutaneous balloon dilatation of the mitral valve: an analysis of echocardiographic variables related to outcome and the mechanism of dilatation. *Br Heart J* 1988;**60**:299–308.

23. Chen CG, Wang X, Wang Y, Lan Y. Value of two-dimensional echocardiography in selecting patients and balloon sizes for percutaneous balloon mitral valvuloplasty. *J Am Coll Cardiol* 1989;**14**:1651–8.

24. Thomas JD, Wilkins GT, Choony CYP *et al.* Inaccuracy of mitral pressure half-time immediately after percutaneous mitral valvotomy. Dependence on transmitral gradient and left atrial and ventricular compliance. *Circulation* 1988;**78**:980–93.

25. Orihashi K, Matsuura Y, Ishihara H *et al.* Transvenous mitral commissurotomy examined with transesophageal echocardiography. *Heart Vessels* 1987;**3**:209–13.

26. Kronzon I, Tunick PA, Schwinger VE *et al.* Transesophageal echocardiography during percutaneous mitral valvuloplasty. *J Am Soc Echocardiogr* 1989;**2**:380–85.

27. Herrmann HC, Kleaveland JP, Hill J *et al.* The M-Heart percutaneous balloon mitral valvuloplasty registry: initial results and early follow-up. *J Am Coll Cardiol* 1990;**15**:1221–6.

28. Yoshida K, Yoshikawa J, Akasaka T *et al.* Assessment of left-to-right atrial shunting after percutaneous mitral valvuloplasty by transesophageal color Doppler flow-mapping. *Circulation* 1989;**80**:1521–6.

29. Casale P, Block PC, O'Shea JP, Palacios IF. Atrial septal defect after percutaneous mitral balloon valvuloplasty: immediate results and follow-up. *J Am Coll Cardiol* 1990;**15**:1300–4.

30. van Herwerden LA, Fraser AG, Gussenhoven EJ *et al.* Echocardiographic analysis of regurgitant mitral valves: intraoperative functional anatomy and its relation to valve reconstruction. Submitted for publication.

31. Fraser AG, McAlpine L, Chow SY *et al.* Abnormal apposition as the cause of mitral regurgitation in patients with intact leaflet coaptation. *Circulation* 1990;**82**:III-241.

32. Smyllie JH, Sutherland GR, Geuskens R *et al.* Doppler colour flow

mapping in the diagnosis of ventricular septal rupture and acute mitral regurgitation after myocardial infarction. *J Am Coll Cardiol* 1990;**15**:1449–55.

33. Patel AM, Miller FA, Khandheria BK *et al.* Role of transesophageal echocardiography in the diagnosis of papillary muscle rupture secondary to myocardial infarction. *Am Heart J* 1989;**118**:1330–3.

34. Koenig K, Kasper W, Hofmann T *et al.* Transesophageal echocardiography for diagnosis of rupture of the ventricular septum or left ventricular papillary muscle during acute myocardial infarction. *Am J Cardiol* 1987;**59**:362.

35. Schlüter M, Kremer P, Hanrath P. Transesophageal 2-D echocardiographic feature of flail mitral leaflet due to ruptured chordae tendineae. *Am Heart J* 1984;**108**:609–10.

36. Joh Y, Yoshikawa J, Yoshida K *et al.* [Transesophageal echocardiographic findings of mitral valve prolapse.] *J Cardiol* 1989;**18**:85–91.

37. Miyatake K, Yamamoto K, Park YD *et al.* Diagnosis of mitral valve perforation by real-time two-dimensional Doppler flow imaging technique. *J Am Coll Cardiol* 1986;**8**:1235–9.

38. Bansal RC, Graham BM, Jutzy KR *et al.* Left ventricular outflow tract to left atrial communication secondary to rupture of mitral-aortic intervalvular fibrosa in infective endocarditis: diagnosis by transesophageal echocardiography and color flow imaging. *J Am Coll Cardiol* 1990;**15** :499–504.

39. Hasegawa I, Sakamoto T, Hada Y *et al.* Relationship between mitral regurgitation and left ventricular outflow obstruction in hypertrophic cardiomyopathy. *J Am Soc Echocardiogr* 1989;**2**:177–186.

40. Smallhorn JF, De Leval M, Stark J *et al.* Isolated anterior mitral cleft: two dimensional echocardiographic assessment and differentiation from "clefts" associated with atrioventricular septal defect. *Br Heart J* 1982;**48**:109–16.

41. Di Segni E, Bass JL, Lucas RV, Einzig S. Isolated cleft mitral valve: a variety of congenital mitral regurgitation identified by 2-dimensional echocardiography. *Am J Cardiol* 1983;**51**:927–31.

42. Barlow JB, Pocock WA. Billowing, floppy, prolapsed or flail mitral valves? *Am J Cardiol* 1985;**55**:501–2.

43. Perloff JK, Child JS, Edwards JE. New guidelines for the clinical diagnosis of mitral valve prolapse. *Am J Cardiol* 1986;**57**:1124–9.

44. Krivokapich J, Child JS, Dadourian BJ, Perloff JK. Reassessment of echocardiographic criteria for diagnosis of mitral valve prolapse. *Am J Cardiol* 1988;**61**:131–5.

45. Gutgesell HP, Bricker JT, Colvin EV *et al.* Atrioventricular valve anular diameter: two-dimensional echocardiographic — autopsy correlation. *Am J Cardiol* 1984;**53**:1652–5.

46. Ormiston JA, Shah PM, Tei C, Wong M. Size and motion of the mitral valve annulus in man. I. A two-dimensional echocardiographic method and findings in normal subjects. *Circulation* 1981;**64**:113–20.

47. Kaul S, Pearlman JD, Touchstone DA, Esquival L. Prevalence and mechanisms of mitral regurgitation in the absence of intrinsic abnormalities of the mitral leaflets. *Am Heart J* 1989;**118**:963–72.

48. Yoshikawa J, Yoshida K, Akasaka T *et al.* Limitations of color

Doppler flow mapping in the detection and semiquantification of valvular regurgitation. *Int J Card Imaging* 1987;**2**:85–91.

49. Schlüter M, Langenstein BA, Hanrath P *et al.* Assessment of transesophageal pulsed Doppler echocardiography in the detection of mitral regurgitation. *Circulation* 1982;**66**:784–9.

50. Wilcox I, Fletcher PJ, Bailey BP. Colour Doppler echocardiographic assessment of regurgitant flow in mitral valve prolapse. *Eur Heart J* 1989;**10**:872–9.

51. Yoshida K, Yoshikawa J, Yamaura Y *et al.* Value of acceleration flows and regurgitant jet direction by color Doppler flow mapping in the evaluation of mitral valve prolapse. *Circulation* 1990;**81**:879–85.

52. Becher H, Mintert C, Grube E, Luderitz B. Beurteilung des Schweregrades einer Mitralinsuffizienz mittels Farbdoppler-Echokardiographie. *Z Kardiol* 1989;**78**:764–70.

53. Sahn DJ. Instrumentation and physical factors related to visualization of stenotic and regurgitant jets by Doppler color flow mapping. *J Am Coll Cardiol* 1988;**12**:1354–65.

54. Stevenson JG. Two-dimensional color Doppler estimation of the severity of atrioventricular valve regurgitation: important effects of instrument gain setting, pulse repetition frequency, and carrier frequency. *J Am Soc Echocardiogr* 1989;**2**:1–10.

55. Wong M, Matsumura M, Suzuki K, Omoto R. Technical and biologic sources of variability in the mapping of aortic mitral and tricuspid color flow jets. *Am J Cardiol* 1987;**60**:847–51.

56. Chao K, Moises V, Shandas R, Sahn DJ. Surface adherence (the Coanda effect) reduces regurgitant jet size: studies by color Doppler in an *in-vitro* model [Abstract]. *J Am Coll Cardiol* 1990;**15**:121a.

57. Chen C, Rodriguez L, Vlahakes GJ *et al.* In vivo assessment of the effect of adjacent solid boundaries on the size of regurgitant jets by color Doppler flow mapping [Abstract]. *J Am Coll Cardiol* 1990;**14**:1458.

58. Taams MA, Gussenhoven EJ, Cahalan MK *et al.* Transesophageal Doppler color flow imaging in the detection of native and Bjork–Shiley mitral valve regurgitation. *J Am Coll Cardiol* 1989;**13**:95–9.

59. Klein AL, Burstow DJ, Tajik AJ *et al.* Age-related prevalence of valvular regurgitation in normal subjects: a comprehensive color flow examination of 118 volunteers. *J Am Soc Echocardiogr* 1990;**3**:54–63.

60. Come PC, Riley MF, Carl LV, Nakao S. Pulsed Doppler echocardiographic evaluation of valvular regurgitation in patients with mitral valve prolapse: comparison with normal subjects. *J Am Coll Cardiol* 1986;**8**:1355–64.

61. Miyatake K, Izumi S, Okamoto M *et al.* Semiquantitative grading of severity of mitral regurgitation by real-time two-dimensional Doppler flow imaging technique. *J Am Coll Cardiol* 1986;**7**:82–8.

62. Maurer G, Czer LSC, Chaux A *et al.* Intraoperative Doppler color flow mapping for assessment of valve repair for mitral regurgitation. *Am J Cardiol* 1987;**60**:333–7.

63. Kleinman JP, Czer LS, DeRobertis M *et al.* A quantitative comparison of transesophageal and epicardial color Doppler echocardiography in the intraoperative assessment of mitral

regurgitation. *Am J Cardiol* 1989;**64**:1168–72.

64. Nimura Y, Miyatake K, Izumi S. Physiological regurgitation identified by Doppler techniques. *Echocardiography* 1989;**6**:385–92.

65. Cape EG, Yoganathan AP, Rodriguez L *et al.* The proximal flow convergence method can be extended to calculate regurgitant stroke volume: *in vitro* application of the color Doppler M-mode [Abstract]. *J Am Coll Cardiol* 1990;**15**:109a.

66. Pearson AC, Castello R, Wallace PM, Labovitz AJ. Effect of mitral regurgitation on pulmonary venous velocities derived by transesophageal echocardiography [Abstract]. *Circulation* 1989;**80**:II-571.

67. Kreis A, Lambertz H, Gerich N, Hanrath P. Value of the transesophageal echocardiographic pulmonary venous flow in classification of mitral insufficiency [Abstract]. *Circulation* 1989;**80**:II-577.

68. Fraser AG, Tuccillo B, van der Borden S *et al.* Pulmonary venous flow in mitral regurgitation and after successful valve reconstruction [Abstract]. *J Am Coll Cardiol* 1990;**15**:74a.

69. Helmcke F, Nanda NC, Hsiung MC *et al.* Color Doppler assessment of mitral regurgitation with orthogonal planes. *Circulation* 1987;**75**:175–83.

70. Spain MG, Smith MD, Grayburn PA *et al.* Quantitative assessment of mitral regurgitation by Doppler color flow imaging: angiographic and hemodynamic correlations. *J Am Coll Cardiol* 1989;**13**:585–90.

71. Kitchin A, Turner R. Diagnosis and treatment of tricuspid stenosis. *Br Heart J* 1964;**26**:354.

72. Fawzy ME, Mercer EN, Dunn B *et al.* Doppler echocardiography in the evaluation of tricuspid stenosis. *Eur Heart J* 1989;**10**:985–90.

73. Wittlich N, Erbel R, Drexler M *et al.* Color-Doppler flow mapping of the heart in normal subjects. Echocardiography 1988;**5**:157–72.

74. Suzuki Y, Kambara H, Kadota K *et al.* Detection and evaluation of tricuspid regurgitation using a real-time, two-dimensional, color-coded Doppler flow imaging system: comparison with contrast two-dimensional echocardiography and right ventriculography. *Am J Cardiol* 1986;**57**:811–5.

75. Leung MP, Baker EJ, Anderson RH, Zuberbuhler JR. Cineangiographic spectrum of Ebstein's malformation: its relevance to clinical presentation and outcome. *J Am Coll Cardiol* 1988;**11**:154–61.

7

Lesions of the aortic valve and the left ventricular outflow tract

George R Sutherland

INTRODUCTION

Transoesophageal echocardiography varies considerably in the range of information it can provide when used to evaluate the wide spectrum of obstructive lesions that may be present within the left ventricular outflow tract. While it can supply new and unique information in the older patient with either discrete fibromuscular obstruction or a subaortic tunnel, it normally provides little valuable new information in patients with aortic valvar disease. Little is, as yet, known of any potential role it may play in the detailed evaluation of the varied sites and forms of obstruction that are associated with hypertrophic cardiomyopathy.

THE AORTIC VALVE

Although the left ventricular outflow tract is better demonstrated by transoesophageal echocardiography than by precordial echocardiography, the same does not hold true for the aortic valve. In some patients, it is not possible to image the aortic valve from the precordium because of a poor precordial ultrasound window, but in most patients the valve and its leaflets can be identified from the parasternal approach. The transthoracic approach is superior to the transoesophageal approach in terms of Doppler interrogation since it allows much better alignment to flow for either pulsed or continuous wave Doppler studies of velocities within the outflow tract and over the aortic valve. Thus, neither aortic stenosis nor regurgitation, either as isolated lesions or in combination, normally constitutes an indication for a transoesophageal study. Nevertheless, if a transoesophageal investigation is indicated for concomitant pathology, or if aortic valvar disease is an incidental finding, some useful information can be obtained on aortic valvar morphology and function. The main value of transoesophageal echocardiography in aortic valvar abnormalities, however, remains in the study of complicated or unusual lesions (for example, when there is clinical suspicion of infective endocarditis), or when aortic regurgitation complicates an acute aortic dissection. These lesions are discussed in *Chapters 9* and *10*, respectively.

AORTIC STENOSIS

Transverse transoesophageal imaging planes scan the aortic valve tangentially, and do not usually demonstrate the three leaflets simultaneously in a single symmetrical cross section. All three leaflets are visible from the oesophagus but it is not always possible to manipulate the tip of the probe so that all three commissures of the valve are seen in a single plane (Fig. 7.1).

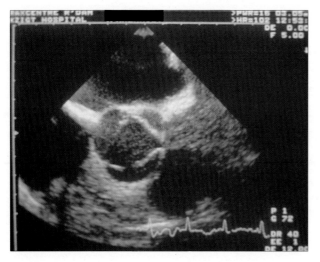

Fig. 7.1 A transoesophageal image of the aortic valve. Often, two leaflets of the valve are visualized together, when imaging in transverse planes. Sometimes, as in this patient, all three leaflets can be seen.

Thus, it can be difficult using the transoesophageal approach to determine whether the aortic valve has two or three leaflets. As with precordial investigations, the determination of aortic valvar morphology is particularly difficult if the valve is heavily calcified. Another disadvantage of single transverse imaging from the oesophagus is that the available sectioning planes are not sufficiently well aligned to detect stenosis in the situation where the bodies of the aortic leaflets remain mobile but where there is either fusion of the commissures or a tight orificial stenosis. In both these instances, the motion of the leaflets, as viewed from the oesophagus when they dome towards the aorta in systole, may be misleading and interpreted erroneously as indicating normal function. In contrast, it is easy to detect the combination of calcification in the aortic valve, restricted motion of the leaflets, and a narrowed orifice that is diagnostic of severe calcific aortic stenosis. One potential problem with the transoesophageal approach is that heavy calcification in the posterior wall of the proximal aorta can cause such bright and re-duplicated echoes, which can mask or mimic disease in the valve it-

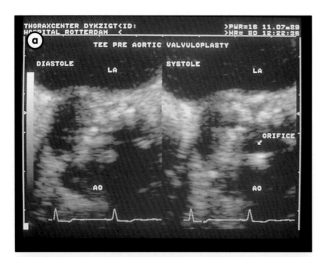

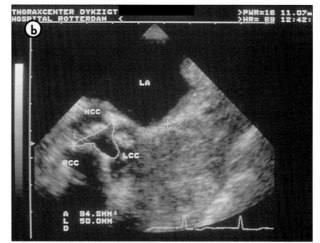

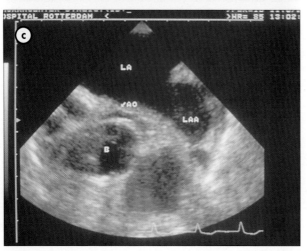

Fig. 7.2 Transoesophageal images obtained while monitoring an aortic valvuloplasty procedure in an elderly patient with severe calcific valvar aortic stenosis. (a) The transoesophageal images in both diastole and systole immediately prior to balloon aortic valvuloplasty. Note the valvar orifice is poorly seen due to the mass of calcium in the valve leaflets. (b) It is possible to estimate the area of the valvar orifice by planimetry, but the value of this technique is uncertain. (c) An image recorded during balloon insufflation. The balloon (B) is now seen as an echo-lucent area within the aortic root. In our experience, transoesophageal monitoring was of most value during such procedures in the immediate evaluation of acquired aortic regurgitation.

self. In spite of these inherent problems, transoesophageal echocardiography has been used to study patients with isolated aortic stenosis. It has been reported that valvar orificial areas, calculated from cross-sectional images obtained in this way, correlate well with either those calculated from invasively derived haemodynamic data using the Gorlin formula, or with estimates derived from the use of the continuity equation using Doppler data obtained from the precordium. No convincing case has as yet been made, however, to justify the use of transoesophageal echocardiography as a primary diagnostic technique in patients with aortic stenosis. In addition, the transoesophageal Doppler beam is poorly aligned to flow across the aortic valve, and thus accurate estimates of the severity of valvar stenosis cannot be made. In any case, the peak velocities of flow across a stenotic aortic valve will exceed the limit which can be measured unambiguously using pulsed Doppler, while continuous wave facilities are not available with most probes currently in use.

One potential application where it is conceivable that transoesophageal echocardiography may be useful in patients with aortic stenosis is in the guidance and monitoring of aortic valvuloplasty in the cardiac catheterization laboratory (Fig. 7.2). Some preliminary reports suggest that the technique can be used to monitor increases in the area of the orifice after successive dilatations, and also to demonstrate whether or not the treatment has caused, or exacerbated, aortic regurgitation. During inflation of the balloon, the probe can be used to monitor left ventricular function; this may be helpful in patients with a precarious circulation and little reserve. Changes in left ventricular volume are a rough guide of the degree to which the inflated balloon is reducing or obstructing the orifice, and hence, to how long the balloon can safely be kept inflated.

AORTIC REGURGITATION

Transoesophageal colour flow mapping is a very sensitive technique for detecting aortic regurgitation. In normal subjects, it may demonstrate a very early diastolic jet of regurgitation, which is localized to the area immediately beneath the leaflets. In patients with pathologic regurgitation, it clearly demonstrates the presence of the regurgitant jet in the left ventricular outflow tract, although it may not be able to delineate the entire extension of the jet towards the apex (Fig. 7.3). The severity of aortic regurgitation, as judged by ultrasound, has been shown to correlate best with clinical and angiographic information when the width or area of the jet just below the valvar leaflets (measured as a proportion of relative out-

flow tract dimension) is calculated as the index. This information is readily obtained from the transoesophageal approach. Occasionally, it can be difficult, in real time, to distinguish aortic incompetence from turbulent systolic flow in the outflow tract due, for example, to hypertrophic cardiomyopathy or systolic anterior movement of the mitral apparatus, and so the colour M-mode display is most useful for establishing the correct timing of flow patterns beneath the aortic valve. Since the sampling rate of the colour M-mode display is much faster than the cross-sectional colour flow map, it also provides much better delineation of the width of a regurgitant jet, which is helpful when attempting to quantify the severity of the lesion.

THE LEFT VENTRICULAR OUTFLOW TRACT

Morphologic considerations

The immediate subvalvar portion of the left ventricular outflow tract is well aligned in its long axis to the transoesophageal transducer, and the structures that form its borders from the midventricular level to the aortic root can be scanned. The spatial relationships of the mitral valvar leaflets and their subvalvar cords and papillary muscles, with the trabecular and membranous components of the ventricular septum, are readily appreciated, as is the degree of separation of the atrioventricular and ventriculoarterial valvar orifices (Fig. 7.4). The thick trabecular portion of the interventricular septum can easily be distinguished from the thin, subaortic, fibrous membranous septum. The morphologic distinction between these two ventricular septal components is far more readily apparent in a transoesophageal image than in a precordial one.

Technical factors influencing Doppler assessment

Neither a transoesophageal pulsed nor a continuous wave Doppler examination can reliably measure a gradient within the left ventricular outflow tract, because of the inherent poor alignment of the Doppler beam to the direction of flow. Furthermore, the appropriate use of pulsed Doppler sampling within the left ventricular outflow tract, however, can allow the identification of normal velocity laminar flow and also indicate the level at which any obstruction commences by determining the level at which aliasing occurs. A much more practical approach to the determination of the sites of obstruction within the outflow tract is to use colour flow

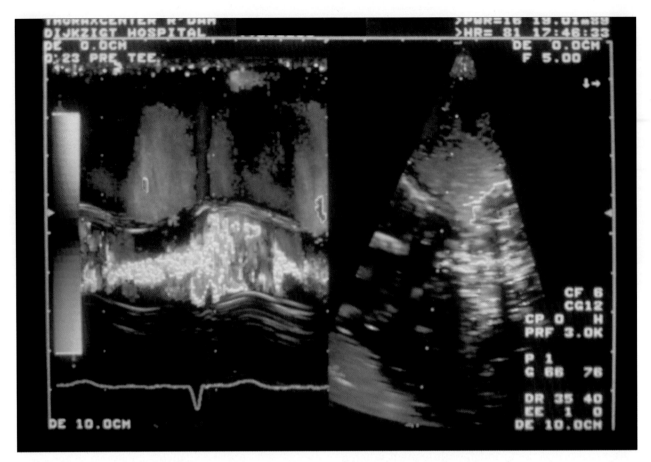

Fig. 7.3 Transoesophageal colour flow maps (cross-sectional and M-mode) recorded from a patient with moderate aortic regurgitation. The cross-sectional image (right-hand panel) has been recorded using the foreshortened four-chamber plane that includes the aortic root. In this projection, the turbulent jet of aortic regurgitation is seen to mix with the mitral inflow. On the left-hand panel, the colour M-mode from the same patient is shown. Both jet width and duration within the left ventricular outflow tract are much better evaluated because of the better temporal and spatial resolution inherent in this technique. In our opinion, such colour M-mode studies should be a routine part of the transoesophageal evaluation of aortic regurgitation. The precordial approach, nonetheless, will normally give much more information as to the causative pathologic mechanism and the site of origin of the regurgitant jet(s). In addition, the inherent foreshortened view of the regurgitant jet from the oesophagus and the inability of the single transverse plane probes to scan the complete apical extent of any jet, means that jet volumes cannot be accurately evaluated from the oesophageal approach. These problems in the analysis of aortic regurgitation may, in part, be circumvented by the introduction of biplane or multiplane probes.

mapping. Flow within the normal left ventricular outflow tract is laminar. Flow towards the aortic valve is encoded in velocity related shades of red, and flow away from the aortic valve in shades of blue. No turbulent flow is present at normal heart rates and cardiac outputs. Turbulence (mimicking obstructive flow) can occur within the normal outflow tract when either the cardiac output is increased, or where there is a tachycardia.

Discrete subaortic obstruction

Discrete subaortic fibromuscular obstruction (frequently referred to in the cardiac literature as a 'subaortic membrane') is a relatively common finding in children with a suspected clinical diagnosis of an obstructive lesion within the left ventricular outflow tract. Discrete subaortic fibromuscular obstruction has been reported to occur either as an isolated lesion or in combination with other lesions (for example, aortic coarctation, ventricular septal defect) (1), or as part of a more complex abnormality (2). It is frequently associated with congenital malformations of the aortic valve. Some degree of aortic regurgitation is almost invariably present, even in cases where the aortic valve is found to be morphologically normal at surgical inspection. In addition, associated mitral valvar abnormalities have been reported in approximately 10% of cases. Previous pathologic studies (mainly carried out in the paediatric age range)

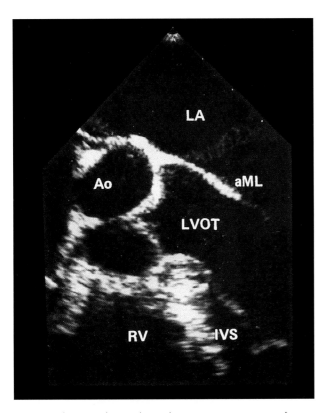

Fig. 7.4 The normal oesophageal imaging appearances of the left ventricular outflow tract. This region is well aligned to interrogation from the oesophagus, and only minimal foreshortening of the image occurs.

have demonstrated that the most constant morphology of subaortic fibromuscular obstructions is that of a virtually complete ring of fibro-elastic tissue encircling the left ventricular outflow tract situated some 0.5–1cm below the aortic valve (3). This fibromuscular protrusion into the left ventricular outflow tract is normally more prominent on its medial aspect. Single or multiple insertions of this fibromuscular tissue into leaflets of the aortic and mitral valves, and into a discrete area of thickened myocardium at the upper end of the septum, have all been reported. In the paediatric population, nonetheless, morphologic studies have suggested that such complex forms, with multiple fibromuscular insertions into the structures that either form or border onto the left ventricular outflow tract, are relatively rare (4–7).

Discrete subaortic obstruction is normally classified as a congenital lesion, the inference being that the underlying left ventricular outflow tract morphology is to some degree abnormal from birth. It is well established that the lesion may be progressive in some cases (a fact well illustrated by the incidence of regrowth of the lesion following incomplete surgical enucleation). The diagnosis in the paediatric age range (when the precordial ultrasound window normally allows high-resolution

ultrasound imaging) is normally confirmed by cross-sectional echocardiography without recourse to angiography, by the identification of the typical imaging features associated with this form of subaortic obstruction (8). Previous correlative precordial cross-sectional imaging and angiographic studies in paediatric patients with subsequent surgically proven, discrete fibromuscular subaortic obstruction, have demonstrated the inherent higher diagnostic accuracy of cross-sectional imaging versus angiography in defining the presence of this morphologic entity. The medial part of the subaortic fibromuscular obstruction is normally relatively constant in position and sited at the area of fusion of the trabecular and fibrous components of the ventricular septum. This medial subaortic 'shelf-like' structure, protruding from the upper portion of the ventricular septum into the left ventricular outflow tract, is best visualized using a precordial cross-sectional imaging left ventricular long-axis view. The lateral insertion of the obstruction is much thinner and is frequently only visualized with difficulty on precordial ultrasound imaging even in paediatric patients. Both surgical and pathologic studies have suggested, however, that in the paediatric age group, the site of the lateral insertion is relatively constant in both morphology and position, this insertion being into the area of aortomitral fibrous continuity that lies immediately superior to the base of the aortic leaflet of the mitral valve. Multiple abnormal lateral insertions into either the aortic or mural leaflets of the valve or cords have seldom been reported in the paediatric age group.

Continuous wave Doppler studies in this group of patients have shown that discrete fibromuscular subaortic obstruction is almost invariably associated with an isolated fixed obstructive waveform of varying peak velocity. In addition, continuous wave Doppler studies have been shown to reflect accurately, the peak instantaneous gradient over the lesion. Colour flow mapping has been used in such cases to identify the site(s) of the related subaortic turbulence and the co-existence of aortic or mitral valvar regurgitation. Such diagnostic accuracy using high-resolution cross-sectional imaging is normally only possible in the paediatric age group. In the adolescent or adult population, ultrasonic transducers of lower frequency (<5MHz) are usually required to obtain adequate precordial images. Furthermore, there are frequent ultrasound imaging problems in such older patients related to lung disease, obesity, prior thoracotomy, or chest deformities. In such patients, adequate visualization of a thin, 'membrane-like' fibrous structure within the left ventricular outflow tract may be almost impossible. High-resolution ultrasound imaging of intracardiac morphology from the oesophagus

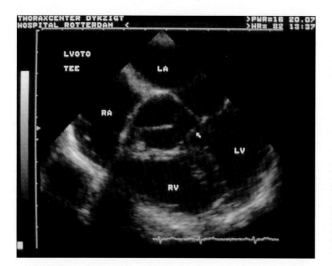

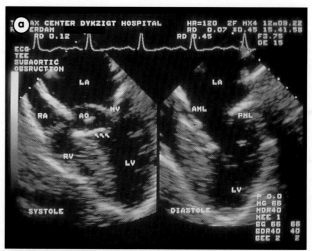

Fig. 7.5 The characteristic appearances on transoesophageal echocardiography of a discrete fibromuscular subaortic obstruction in an adult patient. In this case, the 'membrane' had only single medial and lateral insertions. The fibromuscular structure is seen to take origin medially from the region of contiguity of the membranous and trabecular portions of the ventricular septum, and to insert laterally into the area of aorto–mitral continuity. No other medial or lateral fibrous implantations were identified during the transoesophageal study.

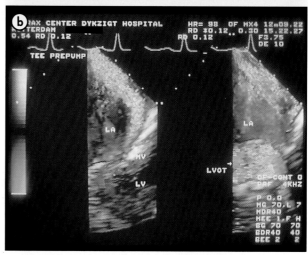

Fig. 7.6 Frames from a transoesophageal study of an adolescent patient. (a) Systolic and diastolic frames from an adolescent patient with a combination of asymmetrical septal hypertrophy and a well-formed single discrete subaortic fibromuscular obstruction (arrowed in the systolic frame). This combination may be much more common than previously suspected. The co-existing septal hypertrophy is well visualized in both the systolic and diastolic frames. (b) Early systolic (left-hand panel) and midsystolic (right-hand panel) frames. In the early systolic frame, a jet of mitral regurgitation that is directed laterally and superiorly is seen. This jet morphology would be in-keeping with abnormal coaptation or prolapse of the aortic leaflet of the mitral valve as a consequence of the involvement of this leaflet by the fibromuscular obstruction. The midsystolic frame demonstrates the widespread turbulence within the left ventricular outflow tract, which is a consequence of the combined obstructive lesions.

(allied to haemodynamic information derived from colour flow mapping) now provides an alternative ultrasound window (9,10).

The transoesophageal approach can reveal a whole range of left ventricular outflow tract pathology that may be missed from the precordium (Figs. 7.5–7.9). Multiple fibromuscular attachments may be present within the outflow tract with single or multiple insertions into the septum, the leaflets of the aortic and mitral valves, and into the cords and papillary muscles of the mitral valve. Our own experience at the Thoraxcentre in studying a large series of such patients would suggest that complex forms of fibromuscular obstruction occur in approximately half the patients (11). This is in marked contrast to the relatively simple morphology of such lesions encountered in the paediatric age group. In a series of 28 patients with suspected subaortic fibromuscular obstruction who underwent comparative precordial and transoesophageal studies, 27 were subsequently proven to have such a lesion (Fig. 7.10). In the remaining case, a false-positive diagnosis was made. In this case, precordial, transoesophageal, and intraoperative epicardial ultrasound studies all suggested the presence of a calcified subaortic fibromuscular shelf. The patient had severe calcific aortic valvar stenosis, with a calcified spur extending downward into the

left ventricular outflow tract. Of the 27 patients, precordial ultrasound gave the correct diagnosis in only 24 patients. Transoesophageal imaging was correct in every case. Of these 27 patients, simple (that is, single) fibromuscular obstruction was present in only 15

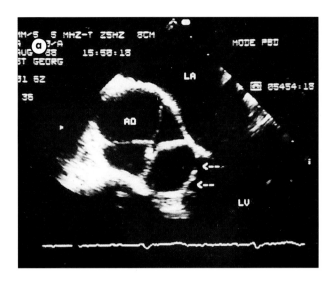

Fig. 7.7 Frames from a transoesophageal study. (a) A diastolic frame from a patient who, at first glance, had a single discrete fibromuscular obstruction (arrowed). (b) Further observation demonstrated this to be a much more complex lesion. A series of still-frame images recorded during systole (left-hand panels) and corresponding still frames from the colour flow maps (right-hand panels) are shown. The images obtained during systole demonstrate that the apparently discrete fibromuscular shelf has further implantations into the right leaflet of the aortic valve. As systole progresses, this complex mass of fibromuscular tissue wraps itself up into an obstructive ball. There was no evidence of any associated re-duplication of mitral valvar tissue in this patient. (Courtesy of Professor Peter Hanrath).

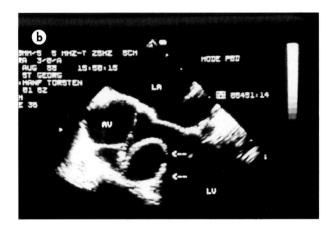

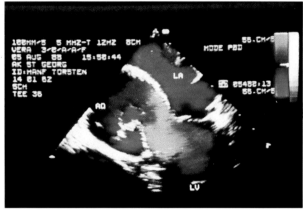

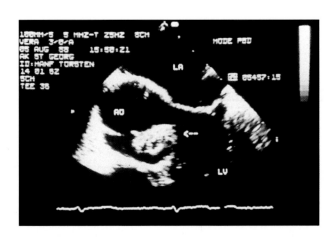

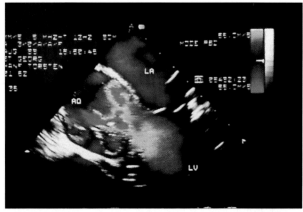

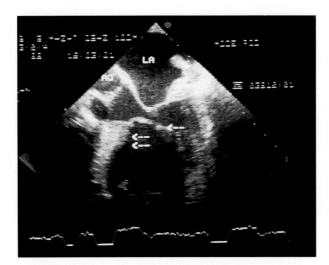

Fig. 7.8 A transoesophageal image demonstrating a lateral insertion of a discrete fibromuscular obstruction into the cords and papillary muscles of the aortic leaflet of the mitral valve. There is a single septal insertion into the upper trabecular septum (which in this case had a co-existing localized area of asymmetric hypertrophy).

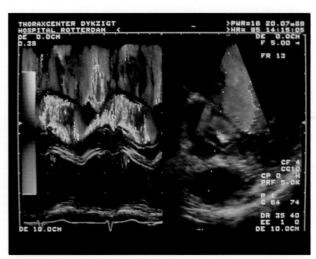

Fig. 7.9 A transoesophageal colour M-mode study from a patient with a single discrete subaortic fibromuscular obstruction. This demonstrates the characteristic findings in such a lesion. In systole, the left ventricular outflow tract is full of turbulence. In diastole, there is a very narrow jet of aortic regurgitation localized to the medial wall of the outflow tract.

Fibromuscular Subaortic Obstruction			
Morphology	Clinical diagnosis on referral	Diagnosis following precordial echocardiography	Diagnosis following transoesophageal echocardiography
isolated aortic valvar disease	9	0	0
aortic valvar stenosis + discrete fibromuscular obstruction	0	4*	4*
isolated discrete fibromuscular obstruction	12	20	23
isolated hypertrophic cardiomyopathy	4	0	0
hypertrophic cardiomyopathy + discrete fibromuscular obstruction	0	4	1
ventricular septal defect + aortic regurgitation	3	0	0
total	28	28	28
* = 1 false-positive diagnosis			

Fig. 7.10 Clinical versus precordial and transoesophageal echocardiographic findings in 28 patients with suspected subaortic fibromuscular obstruction.

patients, and multiple insertions were present in 12 patients (Fig. 7.11). The morphology of the multiple fibromuscular insertions was remarkably variable and could only be analysed from the oesophagus. Four patients had associated asymmetric septal hypertrophy. The interrelationships of this entity and the multiple fibromuscular shelves were again only appreciated on oesophageal imaging. In addition, the associated haemodynamic lesions were also much better characterized from the oesophagus. In three patients in the study group, precordial continuous wave Doppler examination had identified the presence only of a dynamic obstructive waveform within the left ventricular outflow tract (Fig. 7.12). This was an unusual finding in this group of patients since discrete fibromuscular obstruction normally is associated with a fixed obstructive waveform. Only transoesophageal imaging demonstrated the complex interactions of the aortic leaflet of the mitral valve and the multiple fibromuscular strands inserted between that leaflet and the septum that caused prolonged systolic apposition of leaflet and the interventricular septum. In these cases, the fibromuscular

Fibromuscular Subaortic Obstruction		
	Septal insertion	Lateral insertion
	identified in 19 patients	identified in 10 patients
precordial echocardiography	single 17 multiple 2	single 8 multiple 2
	identified in 27 patients	identified in 27 patients
transoesophageal echocardiography	single 21 multiple 6	single 15 multiple 12

Fig. 7.11 Definition of septal and lateral insertions in 27 patients with discrete fibromuscular obstruction: Precordial versus transoesophageal echocardiography.

Fibromuscular Subaortic Obstruction						
	Continuous wave Doppler waveform			Colour flow mapping		
	Fixed obstruction	Dynamic obstruction	Fixed + dynamic obstruction	Left ventricular outflow tract turbulence	Aortic regurgitation	Mitral regurgitation
precordial echocardiography	23	3	1	26	20	6
transoesophageal echocardiography	not applicable	not applicable	not applicable	27	27	22

Fig. 7.12 Spectral Doppler and colour flow mapping: Comparison of precordial versus transoesophageal echocardiography in 27 patients with discrete fibromuscular obstruction.

insertions were creating a mechanism of obstruction virtually identical to that observed in a subgroup of patients with hypertrophic cardiomyopathy. Thus, the isolated dynamic waveform could be explained.

Colour flow mapping in discrete subaortic fibromuscular obstruction

Aortic regurgitation was better defined in a small subset of patients using the oesophageal approach, but the main diagnostic benefit from the use of colour flow mapping studies was in the identification and analysis of associated mitral regurgitation. Mitral regurgitation of varying severity was identified by transoesophageal imaging in 81% of cases, compared to some 22% when using the precordial approach. Both the imaging appearances of prolapse of the aortic leaflet of the mitral valve and the associated laterally directed jet of mitral regurgitation associated with the prolapsing leaflet, were better defined from the oesophagus.

HYPERTROPHIC OBSTRUCTIVE CARDIOMYOPATHY

Most of the morphologic and haemodynamic abnormalities that characterize hypertrophic obstructive cardiomyopathy are well defined by precordial ultrasound studies. Where precordial cross-sectional image quality is good, and excellent Doppler velocity waveforms are obtained over both the mitral valve and the left ventricular outflow tract, then little may be added in purely diagnostic terms from a transoesophageal study (Fig. 7.13). Our own experience would suggest that the main benefit of such a study would be the information which may be gained on the precise mechanism that is causing the outflow tract obstruction. The systolic interactions of the aortic leaflet of the mitral valve, the cords, and the papillary muscles, with the septum, are frequently better analysed from this approach. Furthermore, associated abnormalities that can give rise to obstruction (such as co-existing discrete fibromuscular obstruction, re-duplication of the aortic leaflet of the mitral valve, and anomalous insertion of cords into the left ventricular

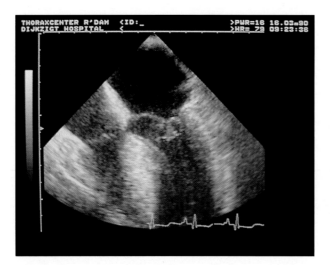

Fig. 7.13 The transoesophageal echo appearance of the left ventricular outflow tract and septum and mitral valve in a patient with hypertrophic obstructive cardiomyopathy. Both the abnormal septal hypertrophy and the 'buckling' of the mitral subvalve apparatus within the outflow tract are well visualized.

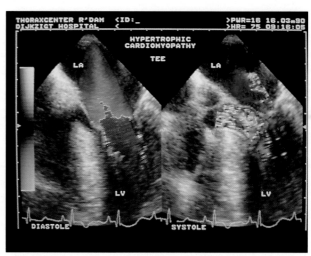

Fig. 7.14 Diastolic and systolic frames from a transoesophageal colour flow map taken from a patient with hypertrophic obstructive cardiomyopathy. In diastole, (left panel) mitral inflow is normal. In systole, the left ventricular outflow tract is filled with turbulent flow, and a jet of mitral regurgitation is seen. Mitral regurgitation is a virtual constant finding on transoesophageal studies in this lesion and is much more often detected when compared to precordial findings.

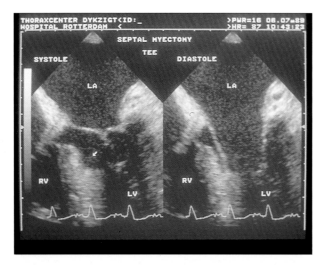

Fig. 7.15 An intraoperative transoesophageal study in a patient immediately following a septal myectomy for severe hypertrophic obstructive cardiomyopathy. Both systolic and diastolic frames are shown. The extent of the muscle resection is easily appreciated (arrowed).

outflow tract) are better excluded by transoesophageal imaging. All these latter entities may be relevant in surgical decision-making if such management is contemplated, and thus a detailed transoesophageal study may be relevant prior to contemplating surgery in this group of patients.

Precordial colour flow mapping studies are of great value in determining the site(s) of obstruction in this lesion, since these may vary in position from the left ventricular apex to the area of septal apposition of the aortic leaflet of the mitral valve within the left ventricular outflow tract. Associated lesions, such as the presence of co-existing discrete fibromuscular obstruction or the presence of significant mitral regurgitation, are often not well defined using the precordial approach. Transoesophageal colour flow mapping studies will normally provide little new information when compared to the precordial studies. Indeed, sites of obstruction towards the ventricular apex may be missed on the colour flow map, either because these apical areas cannot be normally be visualized by the current generation of single transverse plane probes, or because of the inadequate colour flow mapping information at depth, inherent in the use of 5.6-MHz transducers. Colour flow mapping may also provide new insight into both the severity and underlying pathologic mechanism of any co-existing mitral regurgitation (Fig. 7.14). The pulsed Doppler interrogation of pulmonary venous flow, taken in combination with a pulsed Doppler registration of diastolic mitral flow, can provide valuable new information on abnormalities of diastolic function of the left ventricle.

The precise location of the minimal width of the outflow tract is better appreciated, as is the presence and the mechanism of mitral regurgitation. Where a prior surgical myectomy has been carried out, the extent of muscle resected is easily appreciated (Fig. 7.15).

In our experience, the transoesophageal approach is the only way to exclude the co-existence of discrete fibromuscular obstruction in this group of patients. What then are the inherent disadvantages in using the transoesophageal approach in the evaluation of patients with this condition? The mid- to apical portion of the septum and ventricular free walls are frequently poorly visualized and thus obstruction within this portion of the ventricle cannot be excluded. In addition, imaging from the oesophagus gives sections of the septum, which are parallel to its long axis. This frequently can give rise to a false impression of both septal thickness and geometry. Septal thickness is often underestimated when imaging from the oesophagus.

REFERENCES

1. Somerville J. Aortic stenosis and incompetence. In: Anderson R H, Macartney F J, Shinebourne E A, Tynan M, eds. *Paediatric cardiology*. Edinburgh: Churchill Livingstone, 1988:987–1000.

2. Shone JD, Sellers RD, Anderson RC *et al*. The developmental complex of 'parachute mitral valve', supravalvular ring of left atrium, subaortic stenosis, and coarctation of aorta. *Am J Cardiol* 1963;**6**:714–25.

3. Edwards JE. Pathology of left ventricular outflow obstruction. *Circulation* 1965;**31**:586–99.

4. Freedom RM, Fowler RS, Duncan WJ. Rapid evolution from 'normal' left ventricular outflow tract to fatal subaortic stenosis in infancy. *Br Heart J* 1981;**45**:605–9.

5. Freedom RM, Pelech A, Brand A *et al*. The progressive nature of subaortic stenosis in congenital heart disease. *Int J Cardiol* 1985;**8**:137–43.

6. Sung CS, Price EC, Cooley DA. Discrete subaortic stenosis in adults. *Am J Cardiol* 1978;**42**:283–90.

7. Leichter DA, Sullivan I, Gersony WM. 'Acquired' discrete subvalvular aortic stenosis: natural history and hemodynamics. *J Am Coll Cardiol* 1989;**14** (6):1539–44.

8. ten Cate FJ, van Dorp WG, Hugenholtz PG, Roelandt J. Fixed subaortic stenosis:value of echocardiography for diagnosis and differentiation between various types. *Br Heart J* 1979;**41**:159.

9. Poppele G, Krüger W, Langenstein B, Hanrath P. Membranöse subvalvuläre Aortenstenose. Nachweis mittels transthorakaler und transösophagealer 2-D Dopplerechokardiographie. *Dtsch Med Wochenschr* 1988;**113** (31–32):1224–8.

10. Mügge A, Daniel WG, Wolpers HG *et al*. Improved visualisation of discrete subvalvular aortic stenosis by transesophageal color–coded Doppler echocardiography. *Am J Cardiol* 1989;**117**:474–5.

11. Sutherland GR, Schneider B, Smyllie JH *et al*. Transoesophageal echocardiography — an improved diagnostic technique for 'discrete' fibromuscular subaortic obstruction in the adolescent and adult population. *Circulation*; (in press).

Prosthetic heart valves

Jos R T C Roelandt
George R Sutherland

INTRODUCTION

Documentation of the clinical performance of prosthetic heart valves has been possible for more than 25 years. Compared to normal native valves, all prosthetic heart valves are haemodynamically abnormal. The ideal substitute for a native valve is still to be developed. More than 100 different types of prosthetic valves have been, or are presently being, implanted. The popularity of any one particular model waxes and wanes, attesting to the fact that no single prosthesis has proven to be an ideal substitute. Prosthetic valves can be categorized according to the number of their leaflets or occluders, to the types of materials used, or to their flow characteristics. The last classification is particularly relevant when using colour Doppler to evaluate valves, since it shows peripheral, eccentric, and central patterns of flow. A recent review has provided a concise overview of clinical experience with different types of valves (1).

All prosthetic heart valves are subject to the development of a wide variety of complications, including thrombosis, thromboembolism, infection, structural deterioration, dehiscence, prosthetic and paraprosthetic regurgitation, and obstruction. Some of these complications cause minimal complaints, while others may present as a catastrophic illness. An accurate noninvasive technique for studying prosthetic heart valves, therefore, would be particularly useful in view of the difficulty and risks associated with cardiac catheteriza-

tion in these patients. In this respect, the advantages and major limitations of phonocardiography, fluoroscopy, and M-mode echocardiography have all been recognized (2). Precordial cross-sectional imaging also has major limitations when used in the evaluation of the function of prosthetic valves. It can provide useful information, however, on the presence of dehiscence by identifying instability of the prosthetic ring, or it can detect abnormalities of the motion of the mechanical occluder, or of the valve leaflets, when studying a bioprosthesis.

Many instances of valvar dysfunction, however, go undetected when assessed by standard precordial cross-sectional imaging alone. This is because of the abnormal echo reflectivity of the prosthetic materials used in the construction of such valves, which causes reverberations, shadowing, and side lobes within the ultrasound image. These artefacts make it difficult to interpret images of the valves and to detect complications such as vegetations, thrombus, or the ingrowth of pannus.

Before Doppler modalities were introduced into clinical practice, virtually all patients suspected of having dysfunction of a prosthetic valve underwent haemodynamic evaluation by cardiac catheterization. The introduction of pulsed and continuous wave Doppler, and colour flow mapping, was a major advance for the assessment of prosthetic valvar function because these techniques can demonstrate unique haemodynamic information on the direction and velocity of blood flow, thereby allowing an accurate evaluation of its hydraulic function. The normal characteristics of flow for a variety of different prostheses have been summarized in recent papers (3–5).

PRECORDIAL ULTRASONIC EVALUATION OF PROSTHETIC VALVAR FUNCTION

In order to evaluate the function of any prosthetic valve, the ultrasonic beam must be able to interrogate flow throughout the whole cardiac cycle, on both sides of the valve, and over its entire orifice and sewing ring. Valves that contain prosthetic material, cast variable shadows on their distal aspect, into which little or no ultrasound can penetrate. This means that flow over prosthetic valves must be interrogated from both aspects of the valve if a complete evaluation of systolic and diastolic function is to be effected. This is perfectly possible for valves in the aortic and pulmonary positions using the precordial approach, as prevalvar flow within the respective outflow tracts can be interrogated from an apical or parasternal position, and postvalvar flow can be interrogated from either a high parasternal or a suprasternal transducer position. Problems are encountered, however, when attempting to study prosthetic atrioventricular valves. From the precordium, mitral and tricuspid flow can only be studied on the ventricular aspect of the valves, since flow within the respective atrium is, to a large extent, masked by the prosthetic material. No high precordial or suprasternal transducer position will normally allow the interrogation of flows on the atrial side of atrioventricular valves. This is not to say that no information can be acquired on prosthetic atrioventricular valves using all the Doppler modalities from a series of precordial transducer positions. Where significant mitral prosthetic regurgitation exists, whether through the centre of the orifice, or paravalvar, a careful continuous wave study can, in our experience at the Thoraxcentre, identify both an increased peak velocity of forward flow across the prosthesis and also a mitral regurgitant waveform in the majority of patients. The problem is that a precordial study cannot exclude the diagnosis when no regurgitant waveform is identified. Even when a regurgitant waveform is identified on a continuous wave Doppler study, it is frequently impossible to distinguish a central regurgitant jet from a paravalvar leak, or to determine the number of leakages if there is more than one.

Careful pulsed Doppler studies may provide additional information in this respect by detecting the site(s) of systolic aliased flow around the sewing ring of the valves, which extends into the atrium. Precordial colour flow mapping may give additional information on the sites of regurgitation in such cases by determining the flow characteristics on the ventricular aspect of the valve during systole. Areas of systolic convergence of flow will indicate the region where a leak is present. Such colour flow information is complex to analyse, and may give misleading information, particularly where there is co-existing turbulent flow within the left ventricular outflow tract.

Prosthetic tricuspid regurgitation is less difficult to diagnose than prosthetic mitral regurgitation, since marked reversal of systolic flow within the hepatic veins is easily demonstrated using pulsed wave Doppler from either a precordial or subcostal transducer position, without problems arising from prosthetic shadowing.

FLOW CHARACTERISTICS OF PROSTHETIC VALVES

In vitro studies have provided colour Doppler maps of flow characteristics of various types of prosthetic valves that are useful for their clinical evaluation (6). Each model of prosthetic heart valve has its own typical patterns of flow in systole and diastole. Tissue valves have a single central orifice, so that diastolic inflow is almost the same as it is in a healthy native valve. Single tilting-disc prostheses, such as the Björk–Shiley and Medtronic Hall valves, have two orifices (the major and minor apertures), while bileaflet prostheses such as the St Jude valve, have three orifices. The Starr–Edwards valve (ball in cage) has no central orifice but has considerable turbulence since blood flows around the central ball and past the struts of the cage into the left ventricle. The patterns of normal flow into these orifices have been studied in experimental systems *in vitro*.

All mechanical prostheses require some degree of regurgitation to effect closure of the valve. This is termed 'dynamic-closure' regurgitation. With the exception of Starr–Edwards ball prostheses, all mechanical prostheses also have some built-in leakage, defined as 'static' regurgitation, which persists throughout valvar closure and which has the function of maintaining the occluding device in the closed position (4–8). Each type of mechanical valvar prosthesis has its own unique pattern of dynamic-closure regurgitation and static regurgitation, and these individual patterns of 'physiologic regurgitation' should be appreciated before a particular valve is studied in an individual patient. It should be realized, however, that conventional precordial Doppler studies rarely detect these very localized 'physiological' regurgitant jets because of their relatively poor signal-to-noise ratio. When studying prosthetic valves in the aortic and pulmonary positions, localized diastolic jets of 'physiologic regurgitation' can be detected in a small number of patients using precordial colour flow mapping beneath the valve. The timing of such jets is best evaluated by using the enhanced temporal resolution available from colour M-mode interrogation. The physiological regurgitant jets of prosthetic valves in the mitral and tricuspid positions are virtually never identified from the precordium since they lie within the acoustic shadow generated by the prosthetic material. They can, however, be readily detected using oesophageal imaging. The number of regurgitant jets varies from prosthesis to prosthesis. When viewed from the oesophagus, Björk–Shiley prostheses in the mitral position have two physiologic regurgitant jets that are holosystolic. The origins of these jets are located within the sewing ring, are discrete and nonturbulent, and extend only some 2–3cm back into the atrial cavity. St Jude valves in the mitral position, again viewed from the oesophagus, can have up to five similar localized holosystolic jets within the sewing ring. As yet, the normal regurgitant characteristics of other prosthetic valves, as viewed from the oesophagus, have not been reported.

TRANSOESOPHAGEAL EVALUATION OF PROSTHETIC VALVAR FUNCTION

Pulmonary, tricuspid, aortic, and conduit prostheses

Transoesophageal imaging with colour flow mapping studies has been a major advance in the noninvasive assessment of prosthetic valvar function. Its main impact has been in the evaluation of mitral valve prostheses. Prosthetic valves can be visualized from the oesophagus in all four standard positions, although they are not all visualized with the same degree of ease. In particular, prostheses in the pulmonary position are difficult to interrogate from within the oesophagus, and superior information is normally available from the precordium. Tricuspid prostheses are somewhat easier to visualize from the oesophagus but optimal imaging is not always possible, and again more information is normally obtained from the precordium. The transoesophageal approach is, nonetheless, the optimal method for scanning the atrial aspect of prosthetic tricuspid valves when attempting to exclude infective vegetations, thrombus, or pannus.

The long-term results of tricuspid valvar replacement have been disappointing. These prostheses have a relatively large orifice and thus only small pressure gradients are generated across them in diastole. This results in a low mean velocity of flow across such valves

and the risk of valvar thrombosis is high even when anticoagulation is very well controlled. Transoesophageal echocardiography may therefore be of special value in patients with mechanical tricuspid prostheses in whom dysfunction is suspected, but experience is, as yet, limited. Where tissue valves have been placed in the tricuspid position, flow on both sides of the valve can usually be assessed from the precordium. As with mitral valvar prostheses, transoesophageal echocardiography has an important role in diagnosis when adequate images cannot be obtained from the precordium and where dysfunction of the valve or a paraprosthetic leak is suspected.

Aortic prostheses lie somewhat obliquely in the standard transoesophageal planes so that they can rarely be interrogated *en face*; thus, little information can be obtained on events happening within the valve ring. Flow patterns within the left ventricular outflow tract, including the site of origin and initial jet width of any regurgitant jets, and the presence or absence of any posterior or lateral para-aortic infective cavity, are frequently better assessed from the oesophagus (Figs. 8.1 and 8.2). Colour flow mapping can be used to visualize flow within the proximal ascending aorta, but this is invariably turbulent when there is a mechanical prosthesis *in situ*, and so it contributes no information about the function of the valve. The turbulent flow may also extend into the proximal coronary arteries. Continuous wave Doppler is poorly aligned to ascending aortic flow when using the oesophageal approach and thus cannot be used to determine the pressure gradient across a prosthetic aortic valve.

In patients with congenital heart disease, the function of valvar prostheses sited within conduits is frequently difficult to evaluate from the precordium because of the abnormal position of such conduits, the prosthetic material that forms the anterior conduit wall, and the three-dimensional nature of the connexion in which the conduit is placed. Transoesophageal imaging has theoretical advantages over precordial imaging in this respect, as in many cases the conduit has no prosthetic material in its posterior aspect. Unfortunately, the current generation of single plane transoesophageal probes that image in the transverse plane, only rarely visualize (and then only in short axis) conduits placed anteriorly that are used to by-pass the tricuspid valve or the right ventricular outflow tract. Little information is obtained from such studies. The posterior atrio-pulmonary connexion of a Fontan circulation is, nonetheless, well seen from the oesophagus, and useful information on flow characteristics within the conduit can be obtained from an appropriate transoesophageal study (see *Chapter 15*). The study of

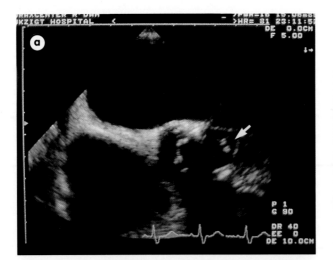

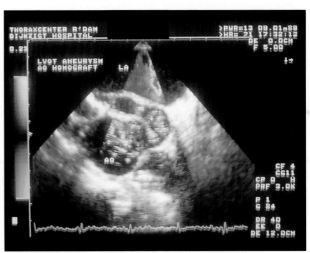

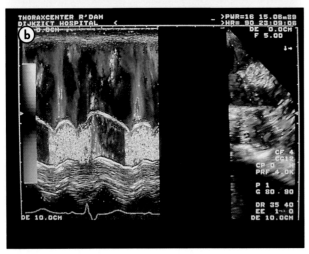

Fig. 8.2 Transoesophageal colour flow image of a patient with a homograft in the aortic position. Precordial cross-sectional echocardiography did not provide adequate images for interpretation. There is an abscess between the aortic root and the left atrium which is septated into interconnected compartments. Turbulent blood flow is visualized in one of the compartments, indicating a connexion with an intravascular space; this represents a mycotic aneurysm.

Fig. 8.1 Patient with a Hancock bioprosthesis in the aortic position and clinical signs of severe aortic regurgitation. Details of the valve could not be obtained from the precordial examination. (a) The transoesophageal cross-sectional imaging study demonstrated one cusp to be flail (arrowed). (b) The colour flow study in the same patient demonstrated turbulence in the left ventricular outflow tract during diastole (not shown), indicating aortic regurgitation. The colour M-mode recording (on the left, cursor aligned as shown on the right) shows the turbulence in the left ventricular outflow tract during diastole and clearly indicates the holodiastolic nature of the turbulent jet that completely fills the ventricular outflow tract. This indicates severe aortic regurgitation.

prosthetic valvar function within conduits may well be facilitated by the introduction of multiplane imaging probes.

The assessment of mitral prostheses

The major breakthrough for noninvasive assessment of prosthetic heart valves was the introduction of transoesophageal echocardiography combined with colour flow imaging (9–12), overcoming virtually all problems related to the precordial approach.

Firstly, we now obtain excellent images with high resolution in patients who are difficult to image from the precordium because of chest-wall abnormalities, obesity, and chronic lung disease (13). Secondly, there are fewer problems as a result of signal attenuation due to distance and, thirdly, flow-masking problems and reverberations related to the prosthetic materials are overcome (Fig. 8.3) (14).

The first step in assessing the function of a mitral prosthesis is to carry out a careful cross-sectional imaging study. An attempt should be made to assess whether the sewing ring of the valve is stable or moves more than expected. Mitral prostheses are normally visualized in their long axis from the oesophagus but, in patients with an extremely dilated left atrium, the valve may be seen *en face*. The valvar structures should be scanned, and an attempt made to exclude the presence of either thrombus or vegetations on the atrial aspect. It may be extremely difficult in the acute postoperative period to differentiate between extraneous suture material around the sewing ring of the valve and small vegetations. This is not generally a problem in the late postoperative period when an early transoesophageal study has been performed and is available for comparison.

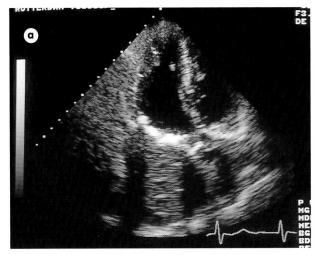

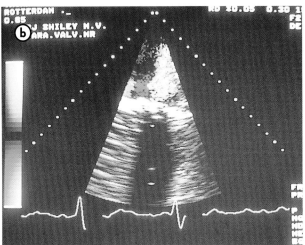

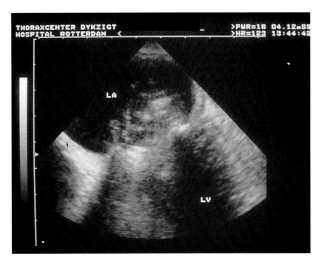

Fig. 8.4 Thrombosis of a Björk–Shiley prosthesis in the mitral position. The patient presented with shortness of breath. Precordial cross-sectional echocardiography did not show specific abnormalities of the prosthesis. The pressure half-time was prolonged and had increased since the previous examination. Transoesophageal echocardiography was performed, and a large thrombus was found at the atrial side of the prosthesis.

Fig. 8.3 (a) Precordial cross-sectional echocardiogram of the apical long-axis view of a patient with a Björk–Shiley prosthesis in the mitral position. Note the shadowing posterior to the sewing ring, and the reverberations in the left atrium caused by the disk. As a result, atrial structures, morphologic abnormalities, and blood flow, are not imaged posterior to the prosthesis.
(b) Transoesophageal colour flow imaging shows a large jet with a mosaic of colours in the left atrium. This paraprosthetic regurgitant jet went undetected from the precordial approach because of blood flow 'masking' due to the mechanical prosthesis.

Associated complications, such as atrial thrombus, are also more readily recognized by transoesophageal echocardiography (Fig. 8.4). Since it has excellent resolution, transoesophageal imaging is the method of choice for diagnosing small vegetations or ring abscesses in prosthetic endocarditis. The findings often supplement clinical and microbiological data (15); occasionally, the transoesophageal findings can confirm the

diagnosis when blood cultures are negative. The presence or absence of spontaneous contrast echoes within the atrium should be noted since, if present, these may be indicative of a tendency to formation of thrombus. The left atrial appendage, when it has been retained, should be scanned routinely for thrombus. Thereafter, a complete colour flow mapping and pulsed Doppler study should be carried out. Such studies have greatly improved our ability to evaluate the function of a mitral prosthesis (9).

When using colour flow mapping to study a normal mitral prosthesis from the oesophageal approach, the velocity of blood flow in diastole will be seen to accelerate as it approaches the atrial side of the mitral prosthetic orifice. This is represented by increasing degrees of aliasing on the colour flow map, and occurs because such valves are intrinsically stenotic. During systole, small jets of 'physiological' regurgitation are seen. The identification of these jets is unique to transoesophageal colour flow imaging. Physiological regurgitant jets are more prominent during early systole (dynamic-closure regurgitation) but in most cases they can be shown to be holosystolic. They are usually nonturbulent and are visualized as red 'flame-like' jets originating within the sewing ring of the valve and extending a short distance back into the atrium. Their timing is

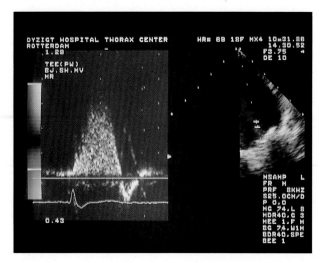

Fig. 8.5 A transoesophageal colour flow image (on the right) of a patient with a normally functioning Björk–Shiley mitral valve prosthesis and a central small regurgitant jet in the left atrium. Pulsed Doppler interrogation demonstrates the holosystolic nature of the jet (on the left). These central jets behind a mechanical prosthesis cannot be visualized or interrogated from the precordium. They represent both the dynamic (for disc closure) and static regurgitation (blood volume passing between the disc and housing during systole) that is inherent to the design of the prosthesis and can be as high as 10% of the forward flow.

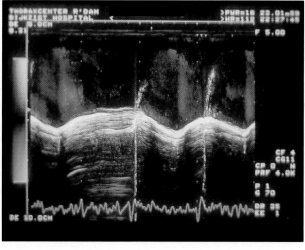

Fig. 8.6 Transoesophageal colour M-mode recording of a St Jude Medical prosthesis in the mitral valve position. This shows a very transient early systolic regurgitant jet with a high velocity (colour reversal indicates aliasing). This jet represents the normal closing 'puff' seen with a mechanical valve prosthesis. During mid- and late systole, regurgitant signals that have a lower velocity and represent minimal static regurgitation, are recorded.

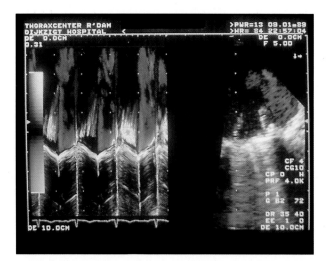

Fig. 8.7 Small regurgitant jets with turbulence recorded behind a Björk–Shiley prosthesis in mitral position. The jets have a length of less than 2cm. Colour M-mode recording demonstrates their holosystolic nature, and they most likely represent static 'physiologic' regurgitation.

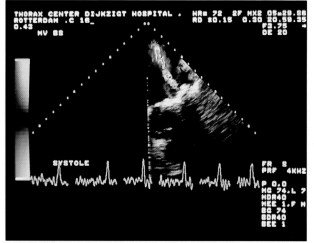

Fig. 8.8 Transoesophageal colour flow image of a patient with a Björk–Shiley mitral valvar prosthesis and a central systolic jet that is short in length and without turbulence. In addition to the 'physiologic' regurgitation, a paraprosthetic turbulent regurgitant jet is seen as a mosaic of colours.

best analysed from the colour M-mode recording (Figs. 8.5, 8.6, and 8.7).

Problems can arise when it is necessary to distinguish between 'physiological' and pathological regurgitant jets. In most cases, however, a careful transoesophageal study will allow the differentiation to be made (Fig. 8.8). Pathological regurgitant jets are also holosystolic, but they are turbulent and normally extend far into the atrial cavity (Figs. 8.8 and 8.9). If they are seen to arise outwith the sewing ring, they can be presumed to be paraprosthetic leaks, but in some cases the distinction between paravalvar and central leaks

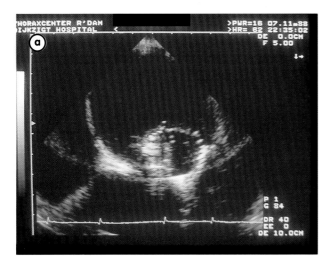

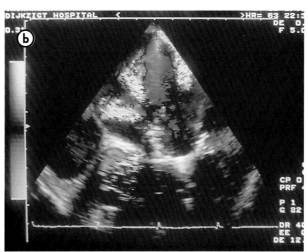

Fig. 8.9 (a) Transoesophageal cross-sectional echocardiogram of a patient with a Björk–Shiley prosthesis in the mitral position and a history of infective endocarditis. Clinically, mitral prosthetic regurgitation was present. Note the dilated left atrium. (b) The systolic transoesophageal colour flow image demonstrated four paraprosthetic regurgitant jets in the left atrium. In this frame, three of the jets are seen as a mosaic of colours resulting from turbulence.

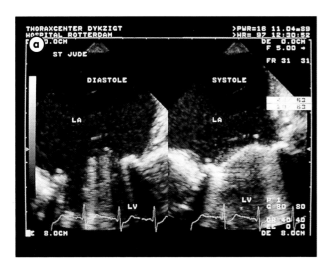

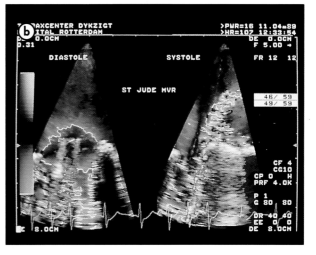

Fig. 8.10 (a) Transoesophageal cross-sectional echocardiograms (on the left) showing the opened bileaflet prosthesis (St Jude Medical) and the three orifices in diastole. On the right, the image during systole shows the closed valve. (b) The transoesophageal colour flow images show the transprosthetic flow dynamics during diastole. Note the flow convergence region in the left atrium proximal to the prosthesis and the turbulence in the orifices and left ventricle. On the right panel, during systole, a turbulent paraprosthetic regurgitant jet is seen.

cannot be made. The regurgitant jets associated with paraprosthetic leakage are most commonly directed directly upwards towards the roof of the atrium, but may be eccentrically directed towards either the atrial septum or lateral atrial wall (Fig. 8.10). These latter jets frequently have a crescent-shaped appearance produced by their adherence to the left atrial wall. In order to visualize any regurgitant jet in its entirety, the left atrium needs to interrogated meticulously by moving the transducer up and down within the oesophagus while flexing and retroflexing the tip of the probe. Careful scanning around the sewing ring will normally demonstrate the number and site of the pathological regurgitant jets. Pathological regurgitation through a prosthetic mitral valve may also be through the central part of the valve if motion of the occluder is restricted or impeded, for example by thrombus. The jet will then arise at the same site as a 'normal' regurgitant jet, but its duration will be significantly longer, and it will be turbulent. There may also be associated structural abnormalities visualized on cross-sectional imaging. Colour M-mode recording, with its high temporal resolution, may be of great help in analysing the characteristics of the jet and thus distinguishing between physiological and pathological leakage.

Attempts have been made to grade the severity of prosthetic regurgitation using the method previously described for native valves, which is based on the measurement of the area of the jet (see *Chapter 6*). This method is semiquantitative at best and can give rise to major errors. In the future, the evaluation of the volume of a jet using the three-dimensional information potentially available from biplane or multiplane probes may provide a more accurate assessment. The analysis of the patterns of flow in the pulmonary veins should also be used to evaluate the severity of the regurgitation (see *Chapter 5*).

REFERENCES

1. Jamieson WRE. Prosthetic heart valves. *Curr Opinion in Cardiol* 1989;**4**:264–8.

2. Mintz GS, Carlson EB, Kotler MN. Comparison of noninvasive techniques in evaluation of the non-tissue cardiac valve prosthesis. *Am J Cardiol* 1982;**49**:39–44.

3. Heldman D, Gardin J. Evaluation of prosthetic valves by Doppler echocardiography. *Echocardiography* 1989;**6**:63–77.

4. Cooper DM, Stewart WJ, Schiavone WA *et al.* Evaluation of normal prosthetic valve function by Doppler echocardiography. *Am Heart J* 1987;**114**:576–82.

5. Alan M, Rosman HS, Lakies JB *et al.* Doppler and echocardiographic features of normal and dysfunctioning bioprosthetic valves. *J Am Coll Cardiol* 1987;**10**:851–8.

6. Jones M, McMillan ST, Eidbo EE *et al.* Evaluation of prosthetic heart valves by Doppler flow imaging. *Echocardiography* 1986;**6**:513–25.

7. Ramirez ML, Wong M, Sadler N, Shah PM. Doppler evaluation of bioprosthetic and mechanical aortic valves: data from four models in 107 stable, ambulatory patients. *Am Heart J* 1988;**115**:418–24.

8. Van den Brink RBA, Visser CA, Bassart DCG *et al.* Comparison of transthoracic and transesophageal color Doppler flow imaging in patients with mechanical prostheses in the mitral valve position. *Am J Cardiol* 1989,**63**:1471–4.

9. Currie PJ, Schiavone WA, Stewart WJ *et al.* Evaluation of mitral prosthetic dysfunction with transesophageal color flow Doppler in ambulatory patients [Abstract]. Circulation 1987;**76** (suppl 4):39.

10. Roelandt JRTC, Fraser AG, Tuccillo B *et al.* Transesophageal color flow imaging. *Cardiovasc Imag* 1989;**1**(4):5–12.

11. Taams MA, Gussenhoven EJ, Cahalan MK *et al.* Transesophageal Doppler color flow imaging in the detection of native and Björk–Shiley mitral valve regurgitation. *J Am Coll Cardiol* 1989;**13**:95–9.

12. Nellesen V, Schnittger I, Appleton CP *et al.* Transesophageal two-dimensional echocardiography and color Doppler flow velocity mapping in the evaluation of valve prostheses. *Circulation* 1988;**78**:848–55.

13. Roelandt J, Sutherland GR. Oesophageal echocardiography. *Brit Heart J* 1988;**60**:1–3.

14. Sprecher DL, Adamick R, Adams D *et al. In vitro* color flow pulsed and continuous wave Doppler ultrasound masking or flow by prosthetic valves. *J Am Coll Cardiol* 1987;**9**:1306–10.

15. Daniel WG, Schröder E, Lichtlen PR. Transesophageal echocardiography in infective endocarditis. *Am J Cardiac Imaging* 1988;**2**:78–85.

Endocarditis

John H Smyllie
Jos RTC Roelandt

INTRODUCTION

Over the past 20 years, the incidence of infective endocarditis has increased and, associated with this, there has been a significant change in the clinical presentation of the disease (Fig. 9.1) (1–4). This change has occurred for three main reasons. Firstly, there has been a shift in the patient population 'at risk'. Patients are presenting with endocarditis at a much older age so that they are more likely to have underlying degenerative valvar disease than rheumatic heart disease. Many patients with complex congenital heart disease are now surviving into adulthood after corrective or palliative surgery. Furthermore, there is an increasing number of patients with intracardiac prosthetic devices including valves, pacemakers, and semipermanent intravenous lines. There are also more intravenous drug abusers, and more patients undergoing endoscopic examinations, particularly of the urinary tract. Secondly, a much broader spectrum of micro-organisms is now implicated in the causation of infective endocarditis. This is, in part, due to the widespread use (and misuse) of antibiotics, and to an increase in the number of immunocompromised patients. As a result, the number of nonbacterial and commensal bacterial organisms that are cultured from these patients with infective endocarditis has increased. For similar reasons, there has also been a rise in the number of patients reported to have negative blood cultures. Thirdly, a gradual change

in the classical clinical features of endocarditis has occurred over the years, with less patients presenting with fever, skin lesions, and splenomegaly, and more developing cardiac failure due to the haemodynamic consequences of intracardiac infection.

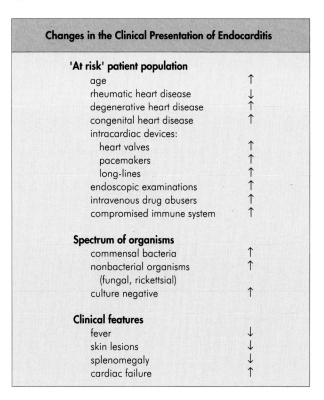

Changes in the Clinical Presentation of Endocarditis	
'At risk' patient population	
age	↑
rheumatic heart disease	↓
degenerative heart disease	↑
congenital heart disease	↑
intracardiac devices:	
heart valves	↑
pacemakers	↑
long-lines	↑
endoscopic examinations	↑
intravenous drug abusers	↑
compromised immune system	↑
Spectrum of organisms	
commensal bacteria	↑
nonbacterial organisms (fungal, rickettsial)	↑
culture negative	↑
Clinical features	
fever	↓
skin lesions	↓
splenomegaly	↓
cardiac failure	↑

Fig. 9.1 Changes in the clinical presentation of endocarditis.

Although the majority of patients with infective endocarditis are still diagnosed using clinical and bacteriological findings, this is becoming increasingly difficult, for the reasons already mentioned. With recent technical advances in the field of cardiac ultrasound, particularly with the introduction of transoesophageal echocardiography, more diagnostic reliance is now placed on echocardiographic findings (5).

THE ROLE OF ULTRASOUND IN THE DIAGNOSIS AND MANAGEMENT OF INFECTIVE ENDOCARDITIS

A definite diagnosis of infective endocarditis can be made with echocardiography either by visualizing new vegetations, or by demonstrating acquired infective complications such as abscesses, local mycotic aneurysms, or fistulas. The successful management of endocarditis, and in particular decisions concerning the need for, or the timing of surgery, depend on detecting and treating significant haemodynamic complications. This is achieved best by regular clinical assessment, together with serial echocardiography using both the precordial and the transoesophageal approaches.

Visualization of vegetations: Precordial or transoesophageal technique?

The vegetations detected by echocardiography are usually situated on one of the cardiac valves or, in the case of atrioventricular valves, on their subvalvar apparatus, but they may also occur on the edge of a septal defect, attached to pacing wires (6) or be adherent to endocardium — usually where an infected jet lesion strikes its surface (7). Aortic vegetations (Figs. 9.2 and 9.3) may be attached to either side of the valvar leaflets, whereas vegetations of both native and prosthetic valves in the mitral position are usually attached to the atrial aspect of the leaflets (Figs. 9.4 and 9.5). Vegetations of the size that can be visualized by precordial echocardiography (usually greater than 3mm) are detected in approximately 70–80% of such cases using precordial imaging (8–10). In contrast, transoesophageal echocardiography can detect vegetations as small as 1mm in size. Thus, vegetations can now be detected in the majority of patients who are subsequently proven to have infective endocarditis (Fig. 9.6) (11–13). The improved overall diagnostic yield in disease of both native and prosthetic valves (confirmed now by a number of authors) is related to the higher resolution of intracardiac structures obtained when imaging from the

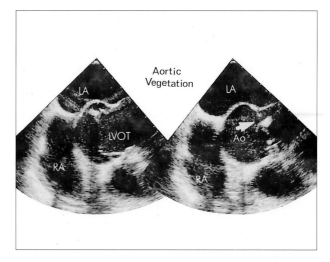

Fig. 9.2 Transoesophageal echocardiogram recorded at the level of the aortic valve in systole and diastole. There is a vegetation on the noncoronary leaflet. In diastole (right-hand panel), a perforation of the leaflet can be identified (arrowed).

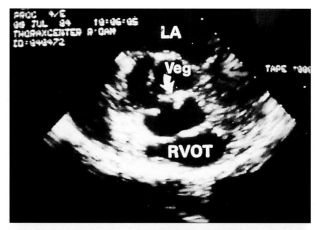

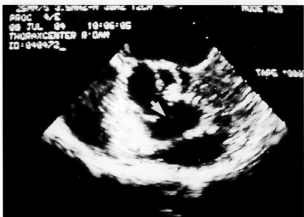

Fig. 9.3 Transoesophageal echocardiogram through the left atrium at the level of the aortic root and right ventricular outflow tract in systole (top) and diastole (bottom). There is a vegetation on the right coronary leaflet (broad arrow) and there is a cavity between the aortic root and the right ventricular outflow tract, which are in communication (thin arrow). By definition, the cavity is not an abscess but a mycotic aneurysm.

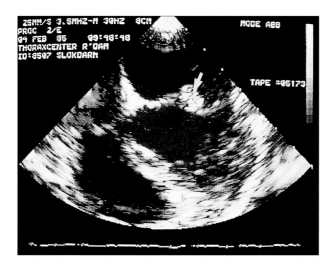

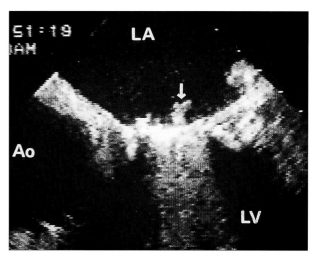

Fig. 9.4 Transoesophageal echocardiogram in the four-chamber view. There is a mass lesion (vegetation) on the left atrial side of the mural leaflet of the mitral valve (arrowed). The precordial echocardiogram from the same patient was of poor quality and nondiagnostic.

Fig. 9.5 Transoesophageal echocardiogram at the level of the aortic root and left atrioventricular junction. A tilting-disc prosthetic valve is in the mitral position, which casts a shadow within the left ventricle. There is a vegetation (arrowed) on the left atrial side of the prosthesis, becoming visible in systole (as shown) and disappearing within the prosthetic shadow in diastole.

Visualization of Vegetations on Native Valves				
Author	Year	Number of patients	Precordial echocardiography (%)	Transoesophageal echocardiography (%)
Erbel *et al* (11)	1988	20	55	100
Daniel *et al* (12)	1988	66	71	98
Taams *et al* (13)	1990	21	43	86

Fig. 9.6 Visualization of vegetations on native valves.

Visualization of Vegetations on Prosthetic Valves				
Author	Year	Number of patients	Precordial echocardiography (%)	Transoesophageal echocardiography (%)
Daniel *et al* (12)	1988	22	27	82
Taams *et al* (13)	1990	12	0	33

Fig. 9.7 Visualization of vegetations on prosthetic valves.

oesophagus. When comparing the diagnostic accuracies for both native and prosthetic endocarditis, the visualization of vegetations on prosthetic valves is a far more difficult problem (Fig. 9.7). Although the numbers of patients studied are small, an initial report (12) suggested that transoesophageal echocardiography can correctly predict the presence of vegetations in over three-quarters of patients with prosthetic valvar endocarditis, whereas, using the precordial approach, only one-quarter were detected in the same group of patients. This point is illustrated in *Fig. 9.5*. In this case, the transoesophageal study demonstrated a small vegetation on a tilting disc which was not visualized on the precordial echocardiogram. Recent work at the Thoraxcentre does not accord with this finding. In a study of 12 consecutive patients with clinically proven prosthetic valvar endocarditis, vegetations were detected by transoesophageal echocardiography in only 33% of patients (13). In our experience, the diagnosis of prosthetic endocarditis relies as much on the recognition of the infective complications, as on the presence of vegetations themselves.

It must be remembered that, theoretically, a false-positive diagnosis of vegetations can occur with transoesophageal echocardiography (14). The differential diagnosis of a valvar mass is either a vegetation, a thrombus, a ruptured cord or, rarely, a fibroelastoma. When the transoesophageal findings are taken in conjunction with the clinical picture, there is usually no difficulty in distinguishing these entities.

Not all vegetations detected by transoesophageal echocardiography are necessarily active. Previous follow-up studies have shown that, although the morphology of vegetations may change considerably during the acute phase of an infection, up to two-thirds of vegetations subsequently remain unchanged over many years, despite successful antibiotic therapy (15). The echocardiographic diagnosis of recurrent endocarditis, therefore, must be made with care in patients with pre-existing vegetations. A logical corollary of this would be that repeated transoesophageal studies should be performed throughout the period of antibiotic treatment so that acute changes in the morphology of vegetations can be monitored, and their final chronic state can be recorded for future reference. At the Thoraxcentre, patients with endocarditis undergo, on average, 2–3 transoesophageal studies while receiving antibiotic therapy.

Visualization of complications of the infective process

A further advantage of the transoesophageal approach in the management of patients with endocarditis is the recognition of local infective complications. These include paravalvar cavities (including abscesses), perforation of leaflets, intracardiac fistulas, cordal rupture, and dehiscence of prosthetic valves (13,16,17). The recognition of these complications is important, not only in aiding in the diagnosis of infective endocarditis in patients without visible vegetations, but also in making the appropriate decisions in terms of management, especially when considering the timing of surgical intervention.

PARAVALVAR CAVITIES

Echocardiographically, an abscess is defined as an extra vascular 'echo-lucent' infective cavity that lacks communication with the intravascular space. The walls of such abscesses are usually thick, and necrotic material can often be seen in their centre (Fig. 9.8). A mycotic aneurysm, in contrast, is an 'echo-free' infected cavity that communicates with the intravascular space (Fig. 9.9). Such cavities are usually thin walled and rarely contain necrotic material. The term 'infective cavity' is used at the Thoraxcentre to encompass both pathological entities.

The majority of infective cavities result from endocarditis involving the aortic valve. They are, therefore, situated around the aortic root and in the anterior septum. Transoesophageal echocardiography provides an excellent technique for imaging the aortic root and its surrounding tissues. The lateral and posterior aspects of the aortic root can be readily scanned. Infective cavities located medially and anteriorly can be difficult to scan from the oesophagus. Echocardiographic 'blind areas' are a major problem when using the transoesophageal approach to interrogate a prosthetic aortic valve for evidence of endocarditis. In this clinical context, precordial imaging will be the investigative technique of choice since any large anterior infective cavity within the septum should be visualized using the parasternal short-axis view. Complete echocardiographic evaluation of patients with endocarditis of an aortic

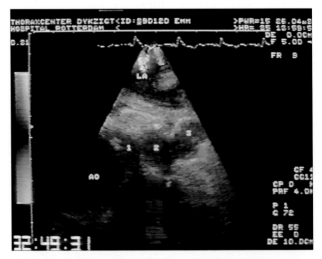

Fig. 9.8 Transoesophageal echocardiogram with colour flow mapping recorded at the level of the ascending aorta. There is a large, lobulated cavity (labelled 1,2, and 3), the walls of which appear thick. The surrounding tissue is oedematous, producing bright echoes. There is no appreciable flow within the cavity, suggesting that this is an abscess.

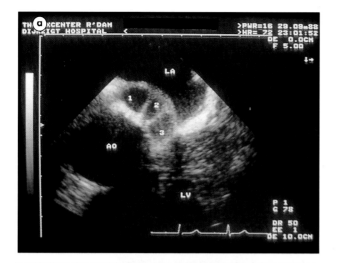

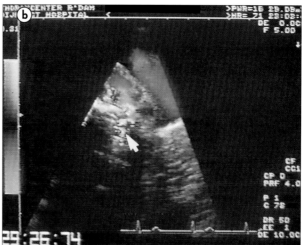

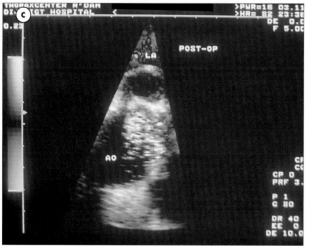

Fig. 9.9 (a) Transoesophageal echocardiogram through the left atrium at the level of the left atrial appendage and aortic root. There is a cavity between the aortic root and the left atrium, which is divided into three components (labelled 1, 2, and 3). The diagnosis was not appreciated from the precordial echocardiogram. (b) Colour flow mapping study in a similar view, recorded in systole. There is turbulent flow within the cavity, confirming its communication with the vascular space. The site of the communication (arrowed) was below the aortic valve, in the left ventricular outflow tract. (c) Another transoesophageal study recorded in the same patient after aortic valvar replacement and closure of the mycotic aneurysm. The cavity persists, although there is now no flow within it.

prosthesis, therefore, is incomplete without the use of combined transoesophageal and precordial imaging.

In our experience, the most frequent site of an infective cavity around the aortic root is within the potential extracardiac space that lies between its posterior aspect and the left atrial wall (see *Fig 3.36* and Figs. 9.8 and 9.9). Cavities at this site can be either abscesses or mycotic aneurysms. The cause of mycotic aneurysms is presumed to be rupture of an abscess into the left ventricular outflow tract, or rupture of the aortic sinus into the extracardiac space. In most cases, the walls of the resulting cavity are thin, suggesting that it has been formed from an outward rupture of the vascular wall. The entry point may lie within the left ventricular outflow tract or the aortic root. Cavities arising from these sites can be distinguished by colour flow mapping since they fill and expand during systole and diastole, respectively. Transoesophageal colour flow mapping demonstrates both turbulent flow within the cavity and its site of communication with the outflow tract (Fig. 9.9b) or

aorta. Infective cavities occur in the area of the transverse sinus. Care must therefore be taken not to misinterpret the normal finding of fluid within the transverse sinus, in some patients, as a cavity of the aortic root. The demonstration of blood flow within the cavity should prevent any diagnostic confusion.

PARAPROSTHETIC REGURGITATION

The diagnosis of prosthetic valvar endocarditis is an increasing clinical problem. Cultures from many patients prove negative and, therefore, the diagnosis must be made on the echocardiographic findings. Transoesophageal echocardiography should always be considered in patients with suspected prosthetic endocarditis. Firstly, the diagnosis can be confirmed if vegetations are visualized. Secondly, using colour flow mapping, the presence of new or increasing paravalvar regurgitation (Fig. 9.10), or valvar dehiscence, is strong although not conclusive, evidence in favour of a diagnosis of endocarditis. In patients with mitral prostheses, the recognition an acquired regurgitant jet from the precordium may be impeded by the masking effects of the prosthesis (18). This obscures the degree of regurgitation in mitral prosthetic dysfunction, irrespective of the presence or absence of endocarditis. From the oesophagus, colour flow mapping can detect paravalvar regurgitant jets within the left atrium without impedance from the mechanical prosthesis (Fig. 9.10). A clear distinction between 'normal' regurgitation across the seating of the prosthesis and paravalvar regurgitation can also be made from the transoesophageal approach by determining both the degree of turbulence of the jet and its systolic timing. The demonstration of aortic prosthetic paravalvar regurgitation is not a particular problem from the precordium since the colour-encoded regurgitant jets may be visualized without impedance from both the apical and parasternal views.

As stated above, the diagnosis of endocarditis can only be inferred when paraprosthetic regurgitation is detected since this can occur in the absence of endocarditis. Diagnostic difficulties could be avoided by performing immediate postoperative and/or predischarge transoesophageal imaging with colour flow mapping, in order to determine the haemodynamic characteristics of each newly implanted prosthesis; special emphasis would be placed on the identification of any paravalvar regurgitant jets. If a patient returns soon after replacement of a valve with a low-grade fever, and a further transoesophageal colour flow mapping demonstrates newly acquired paraprosthetic regurgitant jets, then the diagnosis of prosthetic endocarditis can reliably be made. It should be noted, nevertheless, that the natural history of mitral prosthetic dysfunction is, as yet, unknown. Precordial Doppler and colour flow mapping studies are limited and further studies using transoesophageal colour flow mapping are required to determine the normal history of mitral prosthetic valves.

In our experience, the transoesophageal study has been completely negative in a few patients with bacteriologically proven prosthetic endocarditis (13). Small vegetations can sometimes be missed around the sewing ring of the prosthetic valve. In the case of an aortic prosthesis, it may be due to masking of flow or vegetations on the left ventricular side of the ring. In the case of a mitral prosthesis, it is due to the difficulty of imaging the entire sewing ring, especially its superior and inferior portions. We recommend repeating the transoesophageal studies so that the development of an infective complication can be detected, and the timing of surgery can be planned. It is likely that biplane transoeophageal echocardiography will overcome many of the limitations associated with using a transducer that images only in transverse planes.

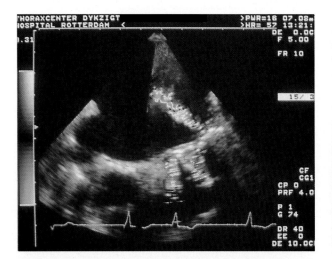

Fig. 9.10 Transoesophageal colour flow map, recorded at the level of the mitral valve in systole. The patient has a mechanical prosthesis and suspected endocarditis. An initial transoesophageal study was negative. The repeat study, shown above, demonstrated a new paraprosthetic regurgitant jet, and the diagnosis of endocarditis was confirmed.

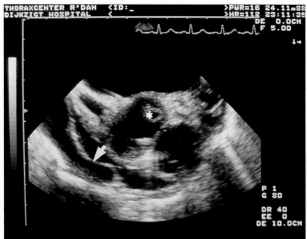

Fig. 9.11 Transoesophageal echocardiogram through the left atrium at the level of the aortic root. This oblique sector through the aortic valve revealed a circular echo near the coronary cusp (*) suggesting perforation of the leaflet; this was confirmed at surgery: there is a venous line within the right atrium (arrowed).

PERFORATION OF LEAFLETS AND INTRACARDIAC FISTULAS

Other complications, such as perforated leaflets (see *Fig. 9.2* and Fig. 9.11) and the presence of intracardiac fistulas, are readily visualized from the transoesophageal approach. The addition of colour flow mapping is particularly useful for identifying the presence and site of perforations in the valvar leaflets (Fig. 9.12).

In this way, it is possible to differentiate a perforation from central regurgitation (Fig. 9.13) — lesions that are indistinguishable using either clinical criteria or ventriculography. Recognition of perforations in the aortic leaflets may be more difficult because of the oblique cross section obtained when scanning the aortic valve from the oesophagus. Intracardiac fistulas are also readily identified using combined imaging and colour flow mapping (Fig. 9.14).

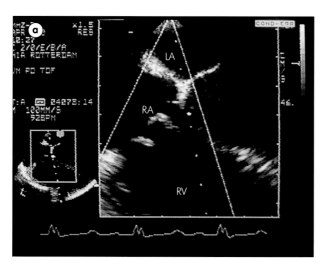

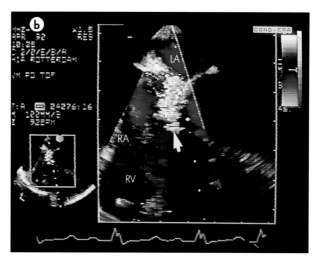

Fig. 9.12 Echoes recorded in the four-chamber view in systole, from a patient with endocarditis involving a patch over a ventricular septal defect, and the tricuspid valve. (a) Cross-sectional image. There are several areas of 'echo' dropout in the tricuspid valve, which might represent perforations of the leaflets. (b) The corresponding colour flow map demonstrates a jet of tricuspid regurgitation through a perforation in the septal leaflet (arrowed).

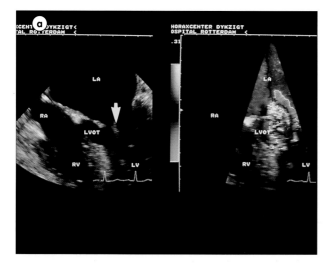

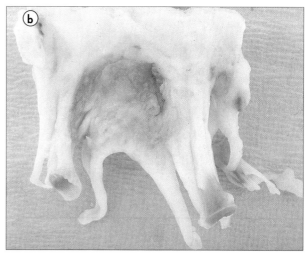

Fig. 9.13 Transoesophageal echocardiogram with colour flow mapping and pathologic correlation from a patient with hypertrophic cardiomyopathy and infective endocarditis of the mitral valve. (a) Left panel: The impression of a perforation in the aortic leaflet of the mitral valve (arrowed). Right panel: The colour flow mapping study confirms the perforation by demonstrating a turbulent jet in systole through the defect. (b) The aortic leaflet of the mitral valve from the same patient. The perforation is clearly visible.

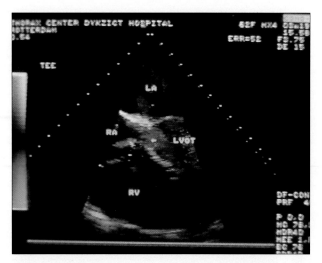

Fig. 9.14 Systolic frame of a transoesophageal colour flow map recorded in the four-chamber view, just inferior to the aortic valve. The patient had aortic valve endocarditis with cardiac failure. There is a turbulent jet traversing the left ventricular outflow tract and entering the right atrium. This fistula from the left ventricular outflow tract to the right atrial was not suspected after the initial precordial study and was later confirmed at surgery.

Transoesophageal echocardiography as a possible cause of infective endocarditis

Transoesophageal echocardiography is a semi-invasive procedure in which there is a potential risk of causing infective endocarditis as a result of transient bacteriaemia. To date, this technique has not been implicated in a single case of infective endocarditis reported worldwide. There have been several studies, however, which have demonstrated that a small but significant number of patients develop bacteraemia following uncomplicated oesophageal intubation (19,20). The bacteria cultured from these patients have been commensal organisms. This has led to the recommendation that antibiotic prophylaxis should be given to patients at 'high risk' of developing endocarditis. These include patients with prosthetic valves, patients with recurrent infection, and patients with a compromised immune system. In 'high-risk' patients who present with suspected endocarditis, the balance between giving prophylactic antibiotics and negating subsequent blood cultures, and the small risk of inducing endocarditis, must be weighed individually for each patient. In this situation, if a transoesophageal study is considered essential and cannot be delayed to allow sufficient cultures to be taken, then it is our recommendation that prophylactic antibiotics are withheld.

CONCLUSION

Transoesophageal echocardiography is of great value in the diagnosis and management of infective endocarditis. Although it is a safe procedure, it is not without some discomfort for the patients. In this light, we advise that transoesophageal echocardiography is used, firstly, for patients with a high clinical suspicion of endocarditis of a native mitral valve, in whom bacteriological and transthoracic echocardiographic studies have been negative, secondly, for patients with suspected endocarditis of a prosthetic mitral valve, and thirdly, for patients with suspected abscesses or fistulas associated with endocarditis of native or prosthetic aortic valves.

REFERENCES

1. Gahl K, Muegge A, Nonnast-Daniel B, Daniel WG. Infective endocarditis: changing clinical features in a changing time. *Eur Heart J* 1987;**8** (suppl I):279–82.

2. Bain RJ, Geddes AM, Littler WA, McKinlay AW. The clinical and echocardiographic diagnosis of infective endocarditis. *J Antimicrob Chemother* 1987;**20** (suppl A):17–27.

3. McKinsey DS, Ratts TE, Bisno AL. Underlying cardiac lesions in adults with infective endocarditis. The changing spectrum. *Am J Med* 1987;**82**:681–8.

4. Kaye D. Changing pattern of infective endocarditis. *Am J Med* 1985;**78** (suppl 6B):157–62.

5. Smyllie JH, Sutherland GR, Roelandt JRTC. The changing role of echocardiography in the diagnosis and management of infective endocarditis. *Int J Cardiol* 1989;**23**:291–301.

6. Zehender M, Buchner C, Geibel A *et al.* Diagnosis of hidden pacemaker lead sepsis by transesophageal echocardiography and a new technique for lead extraction. *Am Heart J* 1989;**118**:1050–3.

7. Zijlstra F, Fioretti P, Roelandt JRTC. Echocardiographic demonstration of free wall vegetative endocarditis complicated by a pulmonary embolism in a patient with ventricular septal defect. *Br Heart J* 1986;**55**:497–9.

8. Martin RP, Meltzer RS, Chia BL *et al.* Clinical utility of two-dimensional echocardiography in infective endocarditis. *Am J Cardiol* 1980;**46**:379.

9. Croney D, Chandraratna PAN, Wishnow RM *et al.* Clinical implications of large vegetation in infective endocarditis. *Arch Int Med* 1983;**143**:1874–7.

10. Strom J, Becker R, Davis R *et al.* Echocardiographic and surgical correlation in bacterial endocarditis. *Circulation* 1980;**62** (suppl I):I-164.

11. Erbel R, Rohmann S, Drexler M *et al.* Improved diagnostic value of echocardiography in patients with infective endocarditis by transesophageal approach. *Eur Heart J* 1988;**9**:43–53.

12. Daniel WG, Schroeder E, Muegge A, Lichtlen PR. Transesophageal echocardiography in infective endocarditis. *Am J Cardiac Imaging* 1988;**2**:78–85.

13. Taams MA, Gussenhoven EJ, Bos E *et al.* Enhanced morphological diagnosis in infective endocarditis by transoesophageal echocardiography. *Brit Heart J* 1990;**63**:109–13.

14. Mugge A, Daniel WG, Frank G, Lichtlen PR. Echocardiography in infective endocarditis: reassessment of prognostic implications of vegetation size determined by the transthoracic and the transesophageal approach. *J Am Coll Cardiol* 1989;**14**:631–8.

15. Stewart JA, Silimperi D, Harris P *et al.* Echocardiographic documentation of vegetative lesions in infective endocarditis: Clinical implications. *Circulation* 1980;**61**;374-80.

16. Gussenhoven WJ, van Herwerden LA, Roelandt J *et al.* Detailed analysis of aortic valve endocarditis: comparison of precordial, esophageal and epicardial two-dimensional echocardiography with surgical findings. *JCU* 1986;**14**:209–11.

17. Polak PE, Gussenhoven WJ, Roelandt JRTC. Transesophageal cross-sectional echocardiographic recognition of an aortic valve ring abscess and a subannular mycotic aneurysm. *Eur Heart J* 1987;**8**:664–6.

18. Sprecker DL, Adamick R, Adams D, Kisslo J. *In vitro* color flow, pulsed and continuous wave Doppler ultrasound masking of flow by prosthetic valves. *J Am Coll Cardiol* 1987;**9**:1306–10.

19. Dennig K, Sedlmayr V, Seling B, Rudolph W. Bacteremia with transesophageal echocardiography [Abstract]. *Circulation* 1989;**80** (suppl II):II-473.

20. Görge G, Erbel R, Henrichs J *et al.* Positive blood cultures during transoesophageal echocardiography [Abstract]. *J Am Coll Cardiol* 1990;**15**:62a.

Diseases of the thoracic aorta

Alan G Fraser
Meindert A Taams

INTRODUCTION

In most adults, the only part of the ascending aorta that can be studied with ultrasound from the standard left parasternal approach is the proximal segment above the aortic valve. The remainder of the ascending aorta and the whole of the arch cannot be imaged. Occasionally, the lower half of the descending thoracic aorta is identified behind the heart. These limitations of the transthoracic approach can be overcome in most younger patients by imaging the aortic arch from a suprasternal or supraclavicular approach; in older patients, this is often difficult. The abdominal aorta is accessible on ultrasonic scanning of the abdomen, although the quality of the images is poor if the gut contains a large amount of air. Thus, in elderly patients in whom aortic disease is most prevalent, most of the thoracic aorta cannot be demonstrated by traditional ultrasonic techniques.

The transoesophageal approach represents a major advance in the echocardiographic study of the thoracic aorta (1,2). With experience and care, the aorta can be examined from the aortic valve to just below the diaphragm, with the exception of the upper part of the ascending aorta and the proximal part of the aortic arch. These areas are almost invariably hidden from the oesophageal view by the right main bronchus and the trachea (Fig. 10.1) (see *Chapter 3*). Fewer segments than normal may be imaged in patients with very tortuous aortas since displacement of the aorta from the oesophagus results in loss of ultrasonic contact.

An oesophageal transducer that produces longitudinal planes of scanning is useful for assessing pathology of the aorta because it complements the transverse planar

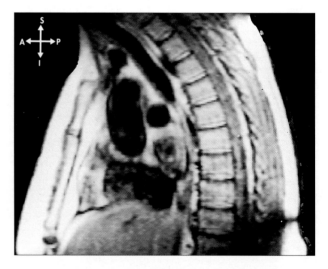

Fig. 10.1 Magnetic-resonance image of the upper thorax in a midline sagittal scan, which displays the whole of the ascending aorta. The larynx, and then the trachea as far as its bifurcation, are also demonstrated. The oesophagus is not clearly shown but it lies between the trachea and the vertebral bodies. It is clear that the upper third of the ascending aorta cannot be imaged from the oesophagus using a standard transducer that only images in transverse planes.

views. Together, these approaches make it easier to demonstrate and understand complex pathology. The longitudinal transducer images a long segment of the ascending aorta (see *Fig. 3.69*) and, therefore, overcomes one of the disadvantages of imaging only in transverse planes (3). It also demonstrates the origins of the head and neck arteries when imaging the arch of the aorta (4). These cannot be shown with the transverse transducer. With the biplane probe, nevertheless, the proximal part of the aortic arch remains inaccessible to study in most patients.

ATHEROSCLEROTIC CHANGES

The aorta lies very close to the oesophagus, and oesophageal transducers use relatively high frequencies of ultrasound (such as 5.6MHz). For both reasons, when the overall gain and grey scale are appropriately adjusted (Fig. 10.2), the aortic wall is demonstrated in considerable detail. Problems arise only from 'near-field' artefacts affecting the posteromedial part of the aortic wall which is closest to the transducer.

Atherosclerotic plaques are identified as irregular or smooth and rounded protuberances projecting into the aortic lumen (5). They may occur singly, or be widespread. It is usually impossible to demonstrate the different constituents or the internal structure of an atherosclerotic plaque, except for the presence of deposits of calcium, which cast very strong echoes and cause masking of all more distant structures (Fig. 10.3). Thrombus may be found on the surface of a large plaque.

At present, the practical applications of identifying atherosclerotic plaques are few. Particular imaging planes cannot be reproduced on repeated studies with sufficient precision for the technique to be reliable for the serial quantification of atherosclerotic lesions. It is not yet possible, therefore, to use transoesophageal echocardiography to assess treatment designed to cause regression of atherosclerosis. In any case, the technique does not allow ultrasonic access to the small plaques in small arteries such as the coronary arteries, which are most likely to cause clinical problems.

ANNULOAORTIC ECTASIA

In patients who have annuloaortic ectasia, a larger than usual segment of the ascending aorta is demonstrated on transoesophageal imaging because the proximal aorta passes more horizontally and to the right than is normal (see *Fig. 10.14a*). In basal transverse planes, therefore, the aorta is seen apparently along its long axis when the transducer is withdrawn above the level of the aortic valve. In reality, the ascending aorta is seen in a long tangential section.

The oesophageal approach is often better than the

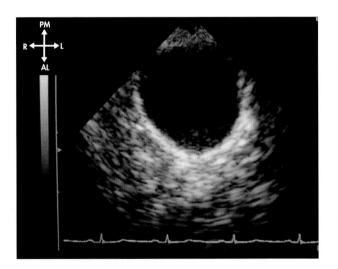

Fig. 10.2 Transoesophageal image of a normal descending thoracic aorta. The level of gain has been increased until some echoes are detected within the lumen, but it is not so high that the sharp delineation of the wall of the aorta is obliterated by artefacts.

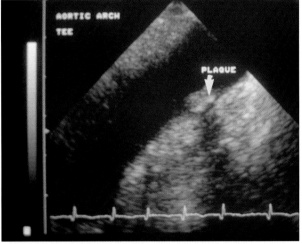

Fig. 10.3 Cross-sectional image of the arch of the aorta, obtained by retroflexing the tip of the probe and rotating it in a clockwise direction (to the right) once the transducer has been positioned opposite the upper end of the descending thoracic aorta. The image is normal, apart from a large calcified atherosclerotic plaque (arrowed) that casts an acoustic shadow.

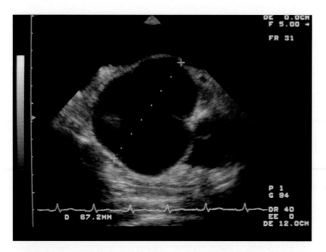

Fig. 10.4 Transverse-axis scan through the proximal ascending aorta at the level of the sinutubular ridge in a patient with Marfan's disease. The diameter of the aorta has been measured with calipers and is 6.7cm. The commissure between the left-facing and right-facing leaflets of the pulmonary valve is also seen in this image.

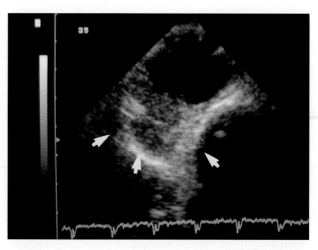

Fig. 10.5 Saccular aneurysm (arrowed) located near the junction of the aortic arch and the descending thoracic aorta. Its lumen is completely filled by thrombus. Part of the left pulmonary artery is also seen.

precordial one for assessing the anatomy and size of the aortic root, especially in patients with dilated aortas. It is a useful method of investigating patients with Marfan's disease since it circumvents the problems for transthoracic imaging caused by deformities of the chest wall, such as pectus carinatus. The diameter of the aorta can be measured at serial studies (Fig. 10.4), allowing surgery to be considered when this diameter increases. The rate of complications is higher when the aorta above the level of the coronary sinuses is enlarged (6), but it is not yet certain what absolute size of the aorta, or what rate of increase in its diameter, indicates that surgery is advisable. The normal diameter of the aortic root at the sinuses of Valsalva does not exceed 2.1cm/m^2 (7) and, in the past, surgery has been advised when the aortic diameter exceeds 6cm (8). Prospective studies using transoesophageal echocardiography may help to answer these questions. In Marfan's disease, the technique is also excellent for assessing associated lesions such as regurgitation across a myxomatous mitral valve and aortic regurgitation secondary to dilatation of the ventriculo-aortic junction (aortic annulus). When a patient with Marfan's disease complains of sudden severe chest pain, an emergency transoesophageal study should be performed to exclude aortic dissection, unless there is another obvious cause.

In elderly patients with aortic valvar disease and enlargement of the aortic root, transoesophageal echocardiography may be useful when precordial studies are technically difficult. Measurements of the dimensions of the aorta can be obtained and may be used when

making clinical decisions about possible surgery.

AORTIC ANEURYSM

Transoesophageal echocardiography readily demonstrates localized or extensive aneurysms involving the segments of the aorta that are accessible to imaging (1,9).

Saccular aneurysms have a relatively narrow orifice and, beyond this, a dumb-bell shaped cavity that protrudes asymmetrically from the circumference of the aorta (Fig. 10.5) (10). They often contain laminar thrombus, within which there may be patches of calcification. Colour flow mapping shows that flow, both into and out of the cavity, occurs through the single orifice, unlike a dissection where entry to, and re-entry from, the false lumen are usually (but not invariably) through separate intimal tears. Another distinction is that flow into a saccular aneurysm is often laminar, while in dissections it is usually turbulent. Large saccular aneurysms may present as a mediastinal mass on radiography of the chest. In such patients, transoesophageal echocardiography with colour flow mapping demonstrates if the mass is vascular or not, and whether it arises from the aorta or from another vessel. It may also demonstrate complications caused by a saccular aneurysm that compresses adjacent structures such as the pulmonary artery (10).

Fusiform aneurysms involve the whole circumference of the aorta, and the transition from a noninvolved to an aneurysmal segment is marked by a gradual increase

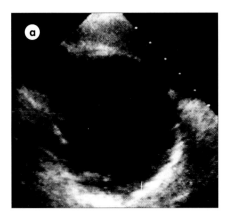
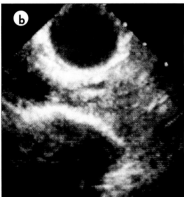
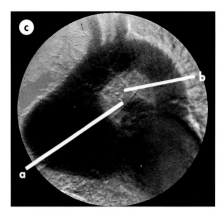

Fig. 10.6 Transverse planar images of the ascending (a) and descending (b) thoracic aorta, compared with a digital subtraction aortogram (c) in the same patient. There is a very large fusiform aneurysm of the proximal half of the ascending aorta, with a smooth transition to normal. The echocardiographic image of the descending aorta is normal.

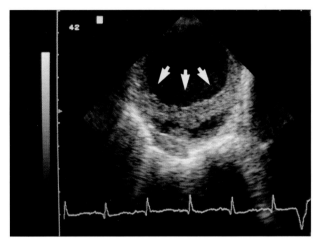

Fig. 10.7 Fusiform aneurysm of the descending thoracic aorta (42cm from the incisors) with a maximal diameter of approximately 6cm. There is laminar thrombus (arrowed) within the aorta, which has become lifted off from the aortic wall. This could be distinguished from a dissection because in more proximal imaging planes, the upper end of the thrombus was identified in the centre of the aortic lumen and there was no overlying intimal flap. This image also shows some calcium in the aortic wall.

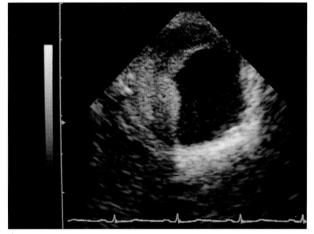

Fig. 10.8 Cross-sectional image of the descending thoracic aorta, demonstrating a thrombus occupying one-half of its circumference. Its surface is irregular.

in the diameter of the aorta (Fig. 10.6). This is recognized during a transoesophageal study by scanning in sequential transverse planes while the probe is advanced or withdrawn, and at the same time rotated to keep the aorta in view. During such an examination, it is helpful for subsequent reporting, and for comparison with serial follow-up studies, to record on the video screen how far the tip of the probe is from the incisors while particular images are being obtained. As with saccular aneurysms, thrombus commonly forms within a fusiform aneurysm (Fig. 10.7), and spontaneous echo contrast may be seen. The thrombus may be so extensive that the central lumen of the aorta becomes narrow

and irregular, resulting in turbulent flow. The irregular luminal surface of a thrombus within the aorta (Fig. 10.8) helps to distinguish it from a dissection with a completely thrombosed false lumen, since the latter is usually covered by a smooth intimal flap (1).

AORTIC DISSECTION

Transoesophageal echocardiography with colour flow mapping is now the investigation of choice for the immediate assessment of patients who present with symptoms that might be caused by dissection of the aorta (11,12). In patients with acute dissection, the early mortality is more than 2% per hour (13) and so rapid diagnosis and prompt treatment are crucial to improving survival. Alternative investigations, such as computed tomography and angiography, are much more time-consuming, and angiography may be dangerous. In addition, diagnostic problems may not be solved by these investigations since they give occasional false-negative results (14–16). Magnetic resonance imaging excellently demonstrates dissections, but the technique is not widely available and it cannot be performed in acutely ill patients. Transoesophageal echocardiography is better at identifying intimal tears and distinguishing between the true and false lumens (17,18). No investigative technique is ideal for the diagnosis of aortic dissection, but the sensitivity and specificity of transoesophageal echocardiography (99% and 98%, respectively, in a multicentre study of 164 patients) are higher than those achieved by angiography or computed tomography (Fig. 10.9) (19).

Standard precordial echocardiography should be performed before embarking on a transoesophageal study in a patient with suspected dissection (9). From a parasternal window, this may reveal a pericardial effusion complicating a dissection involving the ascending aorta, and it can indicate the presence and severity of associated aortic incompetence. An intimal flap in the proximal ascending aorta can be identified (20,21), although false-positive findings are possible in patients with dilated aortas in whom a reverberation artefact may mimic an intimal flap (2). The same artefact occa-

sionally causes problems on transoesophageal echocardiography (1,19). Precordial colour flow mapping is very useful (22), but transoesophageal studies are more sensitive than transthoracic ones (23). Ultrasonic studies should also be performed from the supraclavicular and suprasternal windows (24) in order to examine the aortic arch and the origins of the head and neck vessels. In patients with dissection extending beyond the diaphragm, it is possible to use cardiac transducers to study the abdominal aorta, although linear-array probes designed for abdominal scanning are preferred.

A stressful transoesophageal echocardiographic study induces an adrenergic response with the risk that any increases in heart rate and blood pressure will exacerbate or extend a dissection. It may not be possible to prevent this in patients who are hypotensive before the study is started, since this means that they cannot be given sedation. Instead, blood pressure should be monitored closely (for example, using an intra-arterial line), and if it is not already being given, parenteral hypotensive treatment (such as nitroprusside or a beta adrenoceptor antagonist given intravenously) should be available for instant use.

The priority during a transoesophageal study in a patient with suspected dissection is to establish whether or not this is the diagnosis. An attempt should be made to delineate the extent of dissection by following, for example, the classification of De Bakey (Fig. 10.10) (25). In inexperienced hands, the study may be difficult to perform in extremely ill and restless patients, but if it

Comparison of Investigations for Aortic Dissection			
	TE	ANGIO	CT
sensitivity (%)	99	88	83
specificity (%)	98	94	100
positive predictive value (%)	98	96	100
negative predictive value (%)	99	84	86
TE = transoesophageal echocardiography ANGIO = aortography CT = computed tomography with contrast enhancement			

Fig. 10.9 Comparison of the diagnostic sensitivities and specificities of the common definitive investigations for aortic dissection. Adapted from Erbel R, Engberding R, Daniel W et al. Echocardiography in diagnosis of aortic dissection. *Lancet* 1989;**i**:457–61.

De Bakey Classification of Aortic Dissection	
Type I	involves the ascending aorta, and extends into the aortic arch +/− the descending thoracic aorta +/− the abdominal aorta
Type II	limited to the ascending aorta
Type III	limited to the descending thoracic aorta (beyond the origin of the left subclavian artery) +/− the abdominal aorta

Fig. 10.10 Definitions of the types of dissection based on their extent, according to the criteria of De Bakey (25).

can be established whether or not the ascending aorta, the aortic arch, and the descending aorta are involved, it is then possible to decide about treatment without performing other investigations (11). In dissections of the descending aorta, it is important to identify if the aorta is involved proximal to the left subclavian artery since this determines the surgical approach. Unfortunately, it is not possible to obtain this information in every case.

A scheme for investigating and managing patients with suspected dissection is given in Fig. 10.11. Undue time and trouble should not be expended in ill patients to produce ideal images of a dissection if the diagnosis and its broad details can be established quickly. If necessary, more precise information (such as the sites of entry or re-entry tears) can be obtained by repeating the study in the operating room once the patient has been anaesthetized. Before cardiopulmonary bypass, epivascular imaging and colour flow mapping can also be performed (26). As discussed in *Chapter 13*, these techniques are particularly useful for studying the upper part of the ascending aorta, which cannot be

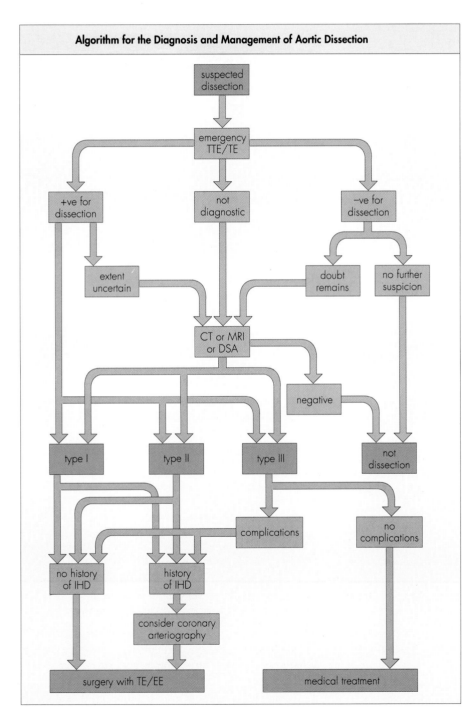

Fig. 10.11 Clinical algorithm for the emergency diagnosis and management of patients with suspected dissection of the aorta.
TTE = transthoracic echocardiography;
TE = transoesophageal echocardiography;
CT = computed tomography;
MRI = magnetic resonance imaging;
DSA = digital subtraction angiography;
IHD = ischaemic heart disease;
EE = epicardial and epivascular echocardiography.
Type I, type II and type III refer to De Bakey classification of dissection.

Comparison of Value of Different Investigations in Aortic Dissection				
	TE	**ANGIO**	**CT**	**MRI**
involvement by dissection				
ascending aorta	++	++	++	+++
aortic arch	++	++	++	+++
descending aorta	+++	++	+++	+++
head and neck arteries	+	++	++	+++
abdominal aorta,				
renal arteries	0	+++	++	++
orifices of coronary arteries	++	+	0	+
coronary arteries	0	+++	0	0
morphology of dissection				
identification of intimal tears	+++	+	+	+
false versus true lumen	+++	++	+	++
flow pattern in false lumen	+++	+	0	+
thrombus in false lumen	+++	0	++	+++
detection of complications				
abnormal LV wall motion	++	+	0	+
aortic incompetence	+++	+++	0	+
pericardial effusion	+++	+	+++	+++

TE = transoesophageal echocardiography (single or biplane)
ANGIO = cardiac catheterization with aortography and coronary arteriography
CT = conventional computed tomography and contrast enhancement
MRI = magnetic resonance imaging
0 = impossible to obtain information
+ = some information available but many limitations
++ = good technique, but still some limitations
+++ = excellent technique providing diagnostic information

Fig. 10.12 Comparison of the relative values of the different investigations commonly used to diagnose dissection of the aorta.

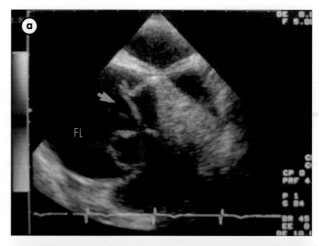

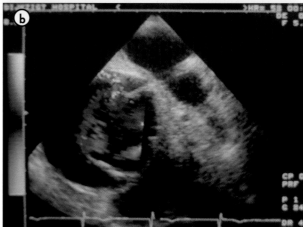

Fig. 10.13 (a) Cross-sectional image in diastole, and (b) colour flow map in systole, of the proximal ascending aorta in a patient with acute dissection (De Bakey, type I). In diastole, the large false lumen occupies most of the area of the aorta and the intimal flap appears folded. There is a suggestion of intimal tears (red arrows) at the sites where the flap lies parallel with the beam of ultrasound, but the interruption of the flap, which is demonstrated most clearly (blue arrow), is near its posterior border. Colour flow mapping confirms that there is flow across the intimal flap only at this last site. The rest of the flap is now under tension, and there are no other areas of turbulent flow. This patient has a prominent pectinate muscle within the left atrial appendage, which is a normal variant.

imaged from the oesophagus.

A negative transoesophageal study does not absolutely exclude a diagnosis of dissection. The disease may be missed by transoesophageal echocardiography if it is restricted to the upper ascending aorta (De Bakey, type II), but this 'blind spot' can be reduced by using a biplane probe (27). If there is strong clinical suspicion of dissection, which is not confirmed by transoesophageal echocardiography, then other investigations are recommended. Depending on clinical urgency and local availability, a computed-tomographic study with contrast enhancement, angiography, or a magnetic-resonance scan, may be invaluable. Our assessment at the Thoraxcentre of the relative strengths and weaknesses of these techniques, compared with transoesophageal echocardiography, is presented in Fig. 10.12.

Identification of the morphology of a dissection

As first reported in 1984 (28), a diagnosis of dissection of the aorta is confirmed by transoesophageal echocardiography when a linear structure, representing an intimal flap, is identified within the aortic lumen (Fig. 10.13a). In acute or recent dissections, this is usually a thin structure that is very mobile, particularly near the site of an intimal tear. Occasionally, a flap may be missed if the gain is too low (Fig. 10.14a). In older or chronic dissections, the intimal flap may be considerably thickened (see for example, *Fig. 10.17*), and virtually immobile.

An intimal flap produces double lumens within the aor-

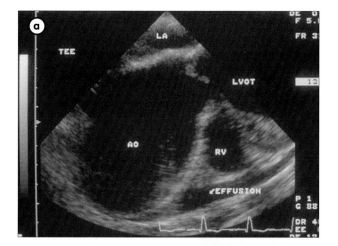

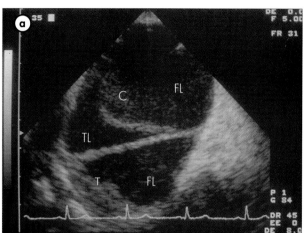

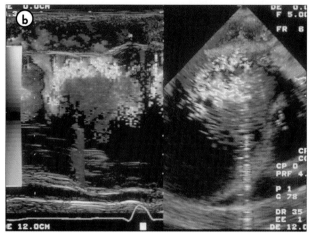

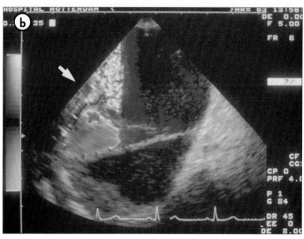

Fig. 10.14 (a) Cross-sectional image of a dilated proximal ascending aorta in a patient with suspected dissection. There is a small pericardial effusion, seen anterior to the right ventricle. Within the aortic lumen, it is possible that there is an intimal flap anteriorly but the level of gain is low, and the appearances are not diagnostic for dissection. (b) The colour flow map (on the right) demonstrates turbulent flow that is localized to the posterior part of the aortic root. Subsequent surgical inspection confirmed that this was the site of an intimal tear. The colour M-mode recording that has been obtained through the left ventricular outflow tract just beneath the aortic valve, shows that this patient has an eccentric jet of aortic regurgitation.

Fig. 10.15 (a) Cross-sectional image and (b) colour flow map of the descending thoracic aorta (35cm from the teeth) in a patient with a dissection of the thoracic and abdominal aorta (De Bakey, type III). At this level, there are two intimal flaps and three aortic lumens. Within the false lumen, there is spontaneous contrast (C) and some thrombus (T). The central lumen is the true one, and an intimal tear is shown both by the pattern of flow of spontaneous contrast and by a turbulent jet on colour flow mapping (arrowed). Flow within the true lumen is laminar. In these images, no branches of the aorta have been demonstrated, but it is possible that the intimal flap is 'tethered' posterolaterally by the origin of an intercostal artery.

ta. The smaller one is usually the true lumen. The false lumen is often considerably larger in cross-sectional area, and it may form a crescent-shaped structure that almost completely surrounds the true lumen. Occasionally, two intimal flaps and three separate luminal areas may be identified in a single echocardiographic image. This 'triple-lumen sign' usually indicates that an arterial branch arising from the aorta in the same region is still supplied from the true lumen through a sleeve-like intimal projection that is sur-rounded by false lumen. Thus, the central lumen is the true one and the others are both parts of an extensive false lumen (Fig. 10.15).

An important objective of the transoesophageal study in a patient with dissection is to identify, if possible, the sites of all intimal tears, and to determine which are the entry and re-entry tears. Extreme mobility of the intimal flap can imply that there is an intimal tear in the vicinity of the imaging plane, although sometimes the opposite is true: the flap at the entry

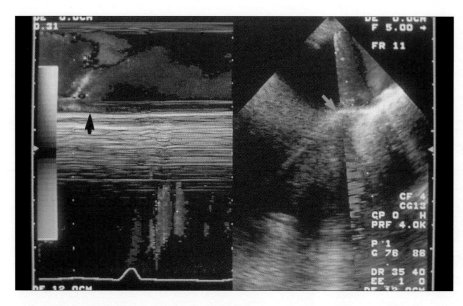

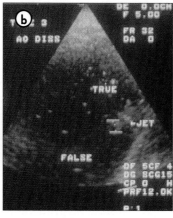

Fig. 10.16 In this patient with proximal aortic dissection, an irregularity was observed in the anterior aortic wall at the junction of the distal arch with the upper descending thoracic aorta (blue arrow), but it was not clear if this was part of the dissection or an atherosclerotic plaque. The colour flow map (right-hand panel) was not diagnostic, whereas the colour M-mode showed diastolic flow within a small echo-free cavity (red arrow). It also showed a diastolic jet from the false lumen into the centre of the true lumen of the aorta, suggesting that this was the site of a re-entry tear.

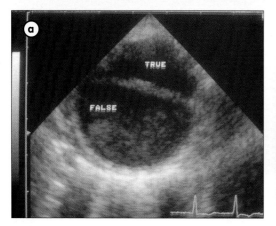

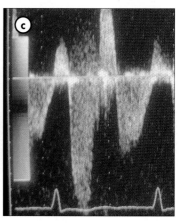

Fig. 10.17 (a) This patient has a thickened and relatively immobile intimal flap in the descending thoracic aorta. The larger lumen is the false one, and it contains some spontaneous contrast. On imaging, there is no obvious intimal perforation. (b) Colour flow mapping suggests that there is flow across the intimal flap posterolaterally. In diastole, there is a laminar jet towards the true lumen. (c) Pulsed Doppler sampling within this jet shows a phasic and bidirectional pattern of flow between the false and true lumens. This intimal tear is the site both of 'entry' and 're-entry'.

tear may be almost stationary, while the intima projecting beyond it ripples in waves of ever- increased amplitude, rather like the appearances of a whip being cracked. When an intimal flap is not under tension (for example, during diastole), it may become folded on itself. Imaging may then suggest that there is an intimal tear at the apex of a fold (see *Fig. 10.13a*). This is, however, more likely to be a false-positive, rather than a real finding, because continuity of echoes from a flap is lost where it lies parallel to the beam of ultrasound. Thus, colour flow mapping should always be used to confirm or refute the diagnosis of an intimal tear (Figs. 10.13b, 10.14b, and 10.15b) (29). Occasionally, the pattern of flow of spontaneous contrast can be used to confirm the site of an intimal tear if contrast is seen streaming

into the true lumen or if there is a negative contrast effect within the false lumen. The colour M-mode display gives greater temporal and spatial resolution of patterns of flow and so it can help to clarify whether or not there is an intimal tear (Fig. 10.16). It is also useful to sample flow across a tear with pulsed Doppler, which may show both entry and re-entry at the same site (Fig. 10.17). A small area of laminar or turbulent flow in the vicinity of the true aortic wall may be caused by blood flowing into an intercostal artery (Fig. 10.18), which is therefore a normal finding.

When an intimal flap is found, the false and true lumens should be identified and followed along as much of their length as possible (Fig. 10.19). This information is useful when trying to understand the arterial blood

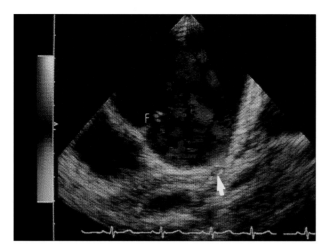

Fig. 10.18 At the lateral aspect of the descending aorta in this patient, flow is seen entering an intercostal artery (arrowed). There is aliasing due to an increase in velocity. This patient had an aortic dissection (part of the intimal flap (F) is just visible medially) and so it was important to recognize that this pattern of flow was not caused by an intimal tear.

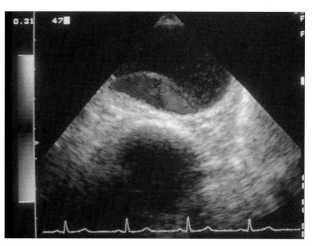

Fig. 10.20 This patient had a De Bakey type I dissection. In the distal arch, colour flow mapping shows normal flow within the small true lumen and virtually no flow within the large false one.

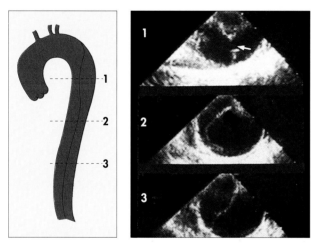

Fig. 10.19 Three images obtained at different levels of the descending aorta. An intimal tear (arrowed) was found at the upper end of this dissection (level 1), but no other tears were observed when the course of the dissection was followed to the level of the diaphragm.

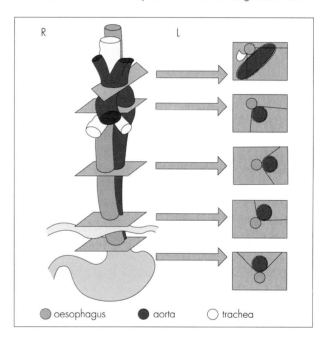

oesophagus   aorta   trachea

Fig. 10.21 Diagrammatic representation of the anatomical relationship of the oesophagus and the thoracic aorta, at different levels.

supply to the aortic branches such as the coronary arteries and the head and neck arteries. The true lumen can be identified in the proximal ascending aorta because it is always in continuity with the left ventricle through the aortic valve. Usually, it expands during systole. Colour flow mapping can also help to distinguish the false from the true lumen (Fig. 10.20) (29). Almost invariably, flow in the true lumen in the ascending aorta is in a normal antegrade direction, while that in the false lumen in the ascending aorta occurs predominant-

ly in diastole and is retrograde if the entry tear is distal. Occasionally, a dissection is spiral, with the relative positions of the true and false lumens changing at different depths. Another factor that complicates the interpretation of the echocardiographic images is that the anatomical relationship between the descending thoracic aorta and the oesophagus changes at different depths. Thus, a dissection that is straight may appear to be spiral (Fig. 10.21). These considerations are important because a patient may have more than one dissection, and it is

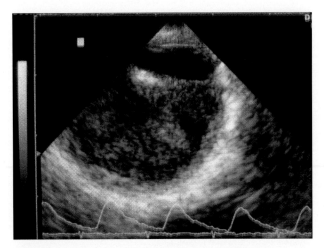

Fig. 10.22 Chronic dissection, with virtually no flow within a large false lumen that is 'filled' with spontaneous echocardiographic contrast. There is also a thin layer of thrombus within the false lumen, adjacent to the wall of the aorta, and some calcium within the intimal flap medially.

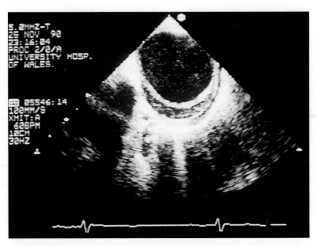

Fig. 10.23 Transverse planar image of the midthoracic descending aorta in a patient who presented with sudden severe pain in the back. The only abnormality on transoesophageal echocardiography was a crescentic intramural thrombus. No intimal tears were found.

important to determine whether a false lumen seen at one level within the aorta, connects with that seen at other levels.

Echoes may be returned from blood within both the false and the true lumens. The presence of spontaneous contrast implies that there are clumps of blood cells such as microaggregates of platelets (30). These are seen as multiple granular echoes (Fig. 10.22) that swirl slowly in the bloodstream. In general, they are associated with low velocities of flow or stagnant pools of blood, and are precursors of thrombus and a risk factor for embolism (31). In the context of aortic dissection, spontaneous contrast implies that blood is flowing slowly and that thrombosis may occur. The prognostic implications of this finding in a false lumen are not yet clear, although it suggests that the volume of flow is not great. In order to detect spontaneous contrast, it is important that the grey scale and overall gain are adjusted to ensure that echoes from within a double lumen or the bloodstream are demonstrated. Whether or not such signals are seen, also depends strongly on the frequency of ultrasound which is used. The sensitivity to detect backscatter of ultrasound from small objects increases in a nonlinear way when higher frequencies are used (32).

Thrombus is often seen within the false lumen of a dissection, especially if it is chronic or in patients who have had aortic surgery. It causes a uniform granular or 'ground-glass' appearance that may be distinguished from the adjacent aortic wall (see *Fig. 10.22*). If the thrombus is old, specks of calcification may be apparent within it. The major diagnostic difficulty arises when a small false lumen becomes completely thrombosed and

there is no other evidence of dissection. A crescentic, soft-tissue shadow around the true lumen will then be seen. It is occasionally impossible on transoesophageal echocardiography to differentiate between a small false lumen that is completely thrombosed, a small laminar thrombus in a fusiform aneurysm, and even a uniform atherosclerotic plaque or thickening of the endothelium. It has also been suggested that patients may develop spontaneous haemorrhage within the wall of the aorta, without this progressing to more extensive and frank dissection. This causes severe chest pain that is clinically indistinguishable from that caused by a larger dissection, and an intramural haematoma (Fig. 10.23) that may be difficult to recognize on transoesophageal echocardiography.

Complications of dissection

Many factors must be considered when deciding whether or not to operate in patients with acute dissection. These include not only the extent of the dissection but also the presence or absence of associated complications and their severity. Several of these can be assessed by transoesophageal echocardiography (19,33).

Pericardial effusion is readily appreciated in most transoesophageal imaging planes (see *Fig. 10.14a*), particularly the transgastric short-axis and basal four-chamber views. Right atrial and right ventricular diastolic collapse can be identified, both in cross-sectional and M-mode displays. It has been reported that these signs are not very sensitive indicators of pericardial tampon-

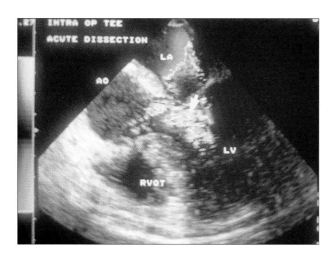

Fig. 10.24 Diastolic colour flow map in a patient with extensive dissection. The proximal aortic root is almost completely occupied by a false lumen in which no flow is demonstrated. There is a broad jet of aortic regurgitation (arrowed), which is severe since it almost completely fills the outflow tract of the left ventricle. A small pericardial effusion is seen anteriorly. Flow within the left atrium is normal.

ade, but they are quite specific (34); right ventricular diastolic collapse is probably the best indicator (35). Exaggerated respiratory variations in flow across the mitral valve (36), and presystolic closure of the aortic valve, can also be detected from the oesophagus. Since the effusion in patients with dissection is usually haemorrhagic, blood clots may be shown within it or on the free surface of the heart. Pleural effusions are also demonstrated.

A second major complication in dissections that involve the ascending aorta, is aortic incompetence. This may occur from a variety of causes, including rupture of a leaflet, dilatation of the ventriculo-aortic junction, or redundancy or prolapse of the aortic leaflets produced by bulging downwards of an intimal flap in diastole (37). Transoesophageal echocardiographic imaging of the aortic root and the valvar leaflets may identify which of these causes is responsible for regurgitation in a particular patient. Colour flow mapping provides information about the presence and severity of the regurgitation (Fig. 10.24). A colour M-mode recording through the left ventricular outflow tract, just beneath the aortic leaflets, best delineates the width of the regurgitant jet (see *Fig. 10.14b*). This should be used to grade its severity (38) since the length of an aortic regurgitant jet is an unreliable indicator. The cursor should be as perpendicular as possible to the outflow tract in order to avoid overestimating the severity of regurgitation (39).

The third potential complication that should be studied as an integral part of the transoesophageal examination is the involvement of the origins of the coronary arteries by a proximal dissection. The origin of the main stem of the left coronary artery is fairly easy to identify. The right coronary artery is less easy to see, but it is frequently involved by a proximal aortic dissection. Therefore, in patients with chest pain and electrocardiographic changes denoting inferior ischaemia or infarction, an attempt should be made to study this vessel carefully. If three lumens are identified in the vicinity of the orifice of the right coronary artery, this usually indicates that the artery is supplied from the true lumen through a sleeve of intima that is invaginated from the true lumen up to its origin. The flow of blood into the coronary artery may be obstructed in diastole if the distending pressure within the false lumen is high (40). This can cause ischaemia, even when there is no coronary atheroma.

Changes in ventricular function and abnormalities of regional wall motion resulting from ischaemia or infarction in a patient with acute dissection, are best appreciated on transgastric short-axis scans. Volume overload from aortic regurgitation, and concentric hypertrophy suggesting a history of hypertension, can also be recognized using qualitative or quantitative criteria.

Postoperative follow-up

The role of transoesophageal echocardiography during surgery for aortic dissection is discussed in *Chapter 13*. After surgery, serial transoesophageal studies are of considerable value in following up patients (41,42). The significance of various findings is still to be established, but prospective studies are being performed. At the very least, the technique establishes whether or not there is a persisting double lumen and if there are any changes in the size of the true and the residual false lumens. It may demonstrate the development of a progressive dissecting haematoma, or the complete thrombosis of a previously patent false lumen. It is now appreciated that patent double lumens persist in a large proportion of patients who have been operated upon for dissection that involves all segments of the thoracic aorta (De Bakey, type I) (41,43).

AORTIC TRANSECTION

There have been no reports of the use of transoesophageal echocardiography for the emergency diagnosis of aortic transection. This acute injury to the aorta occurs as a result of rapid deceleration, for example in road-traffic accidents. It consists of complete rupture of the aorta, with continuity of the proximal and distal aortic segments and integrity of the lumen being maintained only by the overlying and critically bulging adventitia. The usual location for this injury is the upper descending thoracic aorta, just distal to the origin of the left subclavian artery. This is the site where the aorta is subject to most strain during deceleration since it represents the junction of the mobile aortic arch and the tethered descending thoracic aorta. This region is accessible on transoesophageal echocardiography, but imaging in the transverse plane may not be the ideal approach since the aorta is transected in its short axis. Imaging in the longitudinal plane may be more useful. At present, the diagnosis is made by aortography, but transoesophageal echocardiography in the emergency department may prove to be the best and quickest investigation for detecting or excluding traumatic injuries to the thoracic aorta. Another advantage is that the echocardiographic machine can be taken to the bedside, while aortography involves moving a patient with multiple injuries to the angiographic suite.

COARCTATION

Transoesophageal echocardiography is not used to diagnose coarctation in children. In them, as in neonates, the suprasternal approach is very informative. Nevertheless, transoesophageal echocardiography can demonstrate coarctation and so it may be useful in older children or adults who are being investigated for suspected coarctation (see *Chapter 14*) or in patients who have had surgery for coarctation and present with a possible recurrence.

The most common site for a discrete coarctation is just distal to the origin of the left subclavian artery. When scanning from the descending aorta towards the arch, the diameter and cross-sectional area of the lumen of the aorta narrow concentrically as the coarctation is reached. The velocity of flow across a coarctation is not directly related to its severity, and such flow is perpendicular to the planes of imaging obtained with a transverse transoesophageal transducer. From the suprasternal approach, colour flow mapping can be very informative (44), but from the oesophagus in a patient with coarctation, its value is limited. It may be possible to distinguish very severe coarctation from aortic atresia, but imaging alone is unreliable. Collateral flow may be identified as it enters the descending thoracic aorta at right angles to its wall, distal to the coarctation.

Transoesophageal echocardiography may also be useful in patients who are undergoing dilatation of a coarctation with a balloon (45). As with other transoesophageal studies performed during interventions in the cardiac catheterization room, however, the patient must be anaesthetized. The transoesophageal probe is positioned opposite the primary or recurrent coarctation to guide the placement of the balloon and then, after inflation, to assess whether or not there has been a significant increase in the cross-sectional area of the lumen. It is also possible to demonstrate whether or not inflation of the balloon has caused a dissection (45).

ASSESSMENT OF VASCULAR FUNCTION

The lumen of the aorta is seen very clearly in most patients, and so its cross-sectional area can be digitised and calculated with considerable accuracy. When such measurements are combined with simultaneously recorded traces of arterial pressure, obtained using micromanometer-tip catheters, it is possible to derive rates of change of the aortic luminal area during systole and diastole. These calculations correspond to the compliance and elasticity of the aorta. Such techniques and measurements are time-consuming and they involve invasive methods of recording pressure. They therefore remain research applications although, in the future, similar methods could be used to assess vascular function, for example in patients with atherosclerosis, hypertension, or heart failure. M-mode traces of the diameter of the descending aorta have been used to derive similar information (46) and to demonstrate changes in aortic function during an infusion of nitrates (47).

REFERENCES

1. Taams MA, Gussenhoven WJ, Schippers LA *et al.* The value of transoesophageal echocardiography for diagnosis of thoracic aorta pathology. *Eur Heart J* 1988;**9**:1308–16.

2. Kasper W, Hofmann T, Meinertz T *et al.* Diagnostik thorakaler Aorteneurysmen und Dissektionen mit Hilfe der transosophagealen Echokardiographie. *Z Kardiol* 1986;**75**:609–15.

3. Stümper OFW, Fraser AG, Ho SY *et al.* Transoesophageal echocardiographic imaging in the longitudinal axis: a correlative echocardiographic — anatomic study and its clinical implications. *Br Heart J* 1990;**64**:282–8..

4. Takamoto S, Kyo S, Matsumura M *et al.* Observation of the aortic arch and its branches in aortic dissection by longitudinal scanning of transesophageal Doppler color flow mapping [Abstract]. *Circulation* 1989;**80**:II-475.

5. Pop G, Sutherland GR, Koudstaal PJ *et al.* Transesophageal echocardiography in the detection of intracardiac embolic sources in patients with transient ischemic attacks. *Stroke* 1990;**21**:560–5.

6. Roman MJ, Devereux RB, Kramer–Fox R, Spitzer M. Aortic root dilatation in the Marfan syndrome: patterns, familiality and short-term clinical course [Abstract]. *J Am Coll Cardiol* 1988;**11**:74a.

7. Roman Mj, Devereux RB, Kramer–Fox R, O'Loughlin J. Two-dimensional echocardiographic aortic root dimensions in normal children and adults. *Am J Cardiol* 1989;**64**:507–12.

8. Donaldson RM, Emanuel RW, Olsen EGJ, Ross DN. Management of cardiovascular complications in Marfan syndrome. *Lancet* 1980;**ii**:1178–81.

9. Engberding R, Bender F, Grosse–Heitmeyer W *et al.* Identification of dissection or aneurysm of the descending thoracic aorta by conventional and transesophageal two-dimensional echocardiography. *Am J Cardiol* 1987;**59**:717–9.

10. Taams MA, Gussenhoven WJ, Bos E, Roelandt J. Saccular aneurysm of the transverse thoracic aorta detected by transesophageal echocardiography. *Chest* 1988;**93**:436–7.

11. Laas J, Schlüter G, Daniel W *et al.* Acute type-A dissection of the aorta:which diagnostic modes remain for surgical indication? *Eur J Cardiothorac Surg* 1987;**1**:169–72.

12. Kotler MN. Is transesophageal echocardiography the new standard for diagnosing dissecting aortic aneurysms? *J Am Coll Cardiol* 1989;**14**:1263–5.

13. Harris PD, Bowman FO, Malm JR. The management of acute dissections of the thoracic aorta. *Am Heart J* 1969;**78**:419–22.

14. Shuford WH, Sybers RG, Weens HS. Problems in the aortographic diagnosis of dissecting aneurysm of the aorta. *N Eng J Med* 1969;**280**:225–31.

15. White RD, Lipton MJ, Higgins CB *et al.* Noninvasive evaluation of suspected thoracic aortic disease by contrast-enhanced computed tomography. *Am J Cardiol* 1986;**67**:282–90.

16. Erbel R, Börner N, Steller D *et al.* Detection of aortic dissection by transoesophageal echocardiography. *Br Heart J* 1987;**58**:45–51.

17. Mügge A, Daniel WG, Laas J *et al.* False-negative diagnosis of proximal aortic dissection by computed tomography or angiography and possible explanations based on transesophageal echocardiographic findings. *Am J Cardiol* 1990;**65**:527–9.

18. Sasaki S, Yoshida H, Matsui Y *et al.* [The value of recent non-invasive medical imagings in diagnosis of dissecting aortic aneurysm;further investigation on transesophageal echocardiography and MRI.] *Kyobu Geka* 1989;**42**:297–302.

19. Erbel R, Engberding R, Daniel W *et al.* Echocardiography in diagnosis of aortic dissection. *Lancet* 1989;**i**:457–61.

20. Victor MF, Mintz GS, Kotler MN *et al.* Two-dimensional echocardiographic diagnosis of aortic dissection. *Am J Cardiol* 1981;**48**:1155–9.

21. Roudaut RP, Billes MA, Gosse P et al. Accuracy of M–mode and two-dimensional echocardiography in the diagnosis of aortic dissection: an experience with 128 cases. *Clin Cardiol* 1988;**11**:553–62.

22. Iliceto S, Nanda NC, Rizzon P *et al.* Color Doppler evaluation of aortic dissection. Circulation 1987;**75**:748–55.

23. Hashimoto S, Kumada T, Osakada GA *et al.* Assessment of transesophageal Doppler echography in dissecting aortic aneurysm. *J Am Coll Cardiol* 1989;**14**:1253–62.

24. Kasper W, Meinertz T, Kersting F *et al.* Diagnosis of dissecting aortic aneurysm with suprasternal echocardiography. *Am J Cardiol* 1978;**42**:291–4.

25. DeBakey ME, Henly WS, Cooley DA *et al.* Surgical management of dissecting aneurysms of the aorta. *J Thorac Cardiovasc Surg* 1965;**49**:130–49.

26. Fraser AG, Geuskens R, van Herwerden LA *et al.* Transesophageal and intraoperative echocardiography in aortic dissection and aneurysm [Abstract]. *Circulation* 1989;**80**:II-2.

27. Shah PM, Omoto M, Adachi H *et al.* Diagnostic value of newly developed biplane transesophageal echocardiography in thoracic aortic aneurysms [Abstract]. *Circulation* 1989;**80**:II-3.

28. Börner N, Erbel R, Braun B *et al.* Diagnosis of aortic dissection by transesophageal echocardiography. *Am J Cardiol* 1984;**54**:1157–8.

29. Takamoto S, Omoto R. Visualization of thoracic dissecting aortic aneurysm by transesophageal Doppler color flow mapping. *Herz* 1987;**12**:187–93.

30. Mahony C, Evans JM, Spain C. Spontaneous contrast and circulating platelet aggregates [Abstract]. *Circulation* 1989;**80**:II-1.

31. Daniel WG, Nellessen U, Schroder E *et al.* Left atrial spontaneous echo contrast in mitral valve disease: an indicator for an increased thromboembolic risk. *J Am Coll Cardiol* 1988;**11**:1204–11.

32. Morse PM, Ingard KU. *Theoretical acoustic*s. New York: McGraw Hill, 1968:400–66.

33. Erbel R, Mohr–Kahaly S, Rennollet H *et al.* Diagnosis of aortic dissection: the value of transesophageal echocardiography. *Thorac Cardiovasc Surg* 1987;**35**:126–33.

34. Himelman RB, Kircher B, Rockey DC, Schiller NB. Inferior vena cava plethora with blunted respiratory response: a sensitive echocardiographic sign of cardiac tamponade. *J Am Coll Cardiol* 1988;**12**:1470–7.

35. Engel PJ, Hon H, Fowler NO, Plummer S. Echocardiographic study of right ventricular wall motion in cardiac tamponade. *Am J Cardiol* 1982;**50**:1018–21.

36. Appleton CP, Hatle LK, Popp RL. Cardiac tamponade and pericardial effusion: respiratory variation in transvalvular flow velocities studied by Doppler echocardiography. *J Am Coll Cardiol* 1988;**11**:1020–30.

37. Sraow JS, Desser KB, Benchimol A *et al*. Two-dimensional echocardiographic recognition of an aortic intimal flap prolapsing into the left ventricular outflow tract. *J Am Coll Cardiol* 1984;**4**:180–2.

38. Perry GJ, Helmcke F, Nanda NC *et al*. Evaluation of aortic insufficiency by Doppler color flow mapping. *J Am Coll Cardiol* 1987;**9**:952–9.

39. Baumgartner H, Kratzer H, Helmreich G, Kühn P. Quantitation of aortic regurgitation by colour coded cross-sectional Doppler echocardiography. *Eur Heart J* 1988;**9**:380–7.

40. Zotz R, Stern H, Mohr–Kahaly S *et al*. Koronarinsuffizienz bei Aortendissektion Typ II. *Z Kardiol* 1987;**76**:784–6.

41. Iwasaki M, Suzuki S, Takayama Y *et al*. [The usefulness of two-dimensional transoesophageal echocardiography in follow-up studies of dissecting aortic aneurysm.] *Nippon Kyobu Geka Gakkai Zasshi* 1989;**37**:622–30.

42. Erbel R, Engberding R, Daniel R *et al*. Follow-up of aortic dissection by TEE — A cooperative study [Abstract]. Circulation 1989;**80**:II-3.

43. Mohr–Kahaly S, Erbel R, Rennolett H *et al*. Ambulatory follow-up of aortic dissection by transesophageal two-dimensional and color-coded Doppler echocardiography. *Circulation* 1989;**80**:24–33.

44. Simpson IA, Sahn DJ, Valdes–Cruz LM *et al*. Color Doppler flow mapping in patients with coarctation of the aorta: new observations and improved evaluation with color flow diameter and proximal acceleration as predictors of severity. *Circulation* 1988;**77**:736–44.

45. Erbel R, Bednarczyk I, Pop T *et al*. Detection of dissection of the aortic intima and media after angioplasty of coarctation of the aorta. An angiographic, computer tomographic, and echocardiographic comparative study. *Circulation* 1990;**81**:805–14.

46. Michishige H, Matsuzaki M, Toma Y *et al*. Assessment of the influences of aging and hypertension on thoracic aortic wall distensibility by transesophageal echocardiography [Abstract]. *Circulation* 1989;**80**:II-3.

47. Diebold B, Py A, Abergel E, Zelinsky R. Transoesophageal echocardiographic demonstration of a muscular activity in the human thoracic aorta: effects of trinitrine [Abstract]. *J Am Coll Cardiol* 1990;**15**:62a.

11

Ischaemic heart disease

John H Smyllie
Heinz Lambertz
George R Sutherland

INTRODUCTION

Transoesophageal echocardiography has several potential applications in patients with disease of the coronary arteries. These include the direct visualization of the morphology of the proximal coronary arteries and the identification of stenotic lesions within them, the demonstration of abnormalities of regional wall motion related to ischaemia within both the left and right ventricles, both at rest and after various forms of stress, and the diagnosis and definition of the morphology of the surgical complications of myocardial infarction.

The main disadvantage inherent in the use of the transoesophageal approach in patients with ischaemic heart disease is that many areas of the ventricular myocardium cannot usually be visualized using the current generation of single-plane transducers in which the elements scan only in the transverse plane. Thus, the left ventricular apex, the left ventricular anterior and inferior walls below the level of the papillary muscles, and a large part of the antero-apical septum, cannot be visualized easily. Recent technical advances have allowed the construction of biplane imaging transducers that can image most segments of the ventricular myocardium by using the combined information derived from planes in the transverse and longitudinal axes. With the current generation of such probes, however, the quality of images must be sacrificed to allow biplane imaging.

Future technical developments may result in the availability of probes with a single multidirectional scanning head, which may allow high-resolution imaging of all myocardial segments, and thus further increase the potential applications of the transoesophageal technique in the evaluation of patients with coronary arterial disease.

VISUALIZATION OF THE ARTERIES

Transoesophageal imaging of the aortic root in the transverse plane provides only oblique cross sections of the aortic valve, the sinuses of Valsalva, and the proximal portion of the ascending aorta. As a result, the orifice and proximal portion of the left coronary arterial system can nearly always be visualized, whereas the right coronary artery is infrequently visualized in patients in whom the right ventricle is of normal size and at normal pressure.

In patients with congenital cardiac malformations, lung disease, or in whom right ventricular pressure is raised as a consequence of left heart disease, the proximal portion of the right coronary artery is more frequently imaged since the vessel is larger.

Visualization of Coronary Arteries					
Author	Number of patients	Left main stem (%)	Left anterior descending (%)	Circumflex coronary artery (%)	Right coronary artery (%)
Taams et al (1)	60	93	15	57	–
Gerckens et al (2)	62	80	72	85	15
Iliceto et al (3)	76	95	67	49	–
Reichert et al (4)	25	88	52	88	–
Samdarshi et al (5)	57	100	86	84	24

Fig. 11.1 Visualization of coronary arteries.

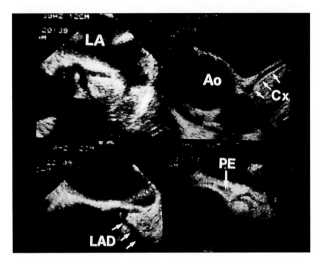

Fig. 11.2 Composite transoesophageal images of the left coronary artery. The upper left panel shows the left main stem and its bifurcation, and the lower left panel shows the proximal portion of the left anterior descending artery (LAD). The main circumflex is shown in the upper right panel, and a possible pitfall is demonstrated in the lower right panel. There is some fluid in the transverse sinus (PE), which might be mistaken for a coronary vessel. The true left coronary artery can be seen below this.

Left coronary artery

The left main stem, its bifurcation, and the proximal portion of the anterior descending and the left circumflex arteries, can be visualized in approximately 90% of patients undergoing transoesophageal studies (Fig. 11.1) (1–5). Care should always be taken to ensure that the structure that is imaged is indeed the left coronary artery; it is possible, where image quality is poor or where the operator is inexperienced, to mistake either the transverse sinus or the great cardiac vein for a portion of the left coronary artery (Fig. 11.2). Demonstration that the vessel takes origin from the aortic sinus allows confirmation that the structure imaged is the left coronary artery.

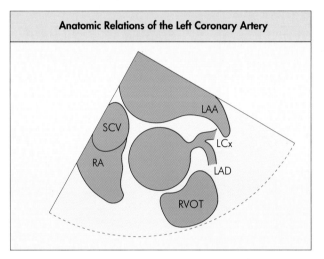

Fig. 11.3 The usual anatomic relations of the main stem of the left coronary artery and its bifurcation, as imaged during transoesophageal echocardiography.

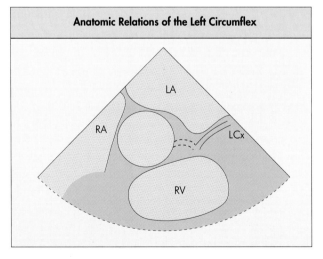

Fig. 11.4 The usual anatomic relations of the circumflex coronary artery as it passes under the left atrial appendage in the left atrioventricular groove.

Identification of Coronary Stenoses >50% Luminal Narrowing					
Author	Left main stem	Left anterior descending	Circumflex coronary artery	Right coronary artery	Overall
Taams et al (1)	15/15	1/3	9/9	–	25/27 (93%)
Gerckens et al (2)	–	–	–	–	10/37 (43%)
Reichert et al (4)	4/4	3/5	0/4	–	7/13 (54%)
Samdarshi et al (5)	7/9	2/4	1/2	1/1	11/16 (69%)

Fig. 11.5 Identification of coronary stenoses >50% luminal narrowing.

The main stem of the left coronary artery is variable in length prior to its bifurcation into the anterior descending and circumflex branches. It normally moves in and out of the imaging plane during the cardiac cycle. The anterior descending artery may be followed from the bifurcation for a short distance towards the ventricular septum by downward angulation of the tip of the transducer. It is unusual (although not impossible) to be able to follow it far enough to identify either its first major branches, the septal, or the diagonal branches. The circumflex artery may be followed laterally for a variable distance from the bifurcation by anticlockwise rotation of the probe combined with slight withdrawal (Figs. 11.3 and Fig. 11.4). In addition, a short-axis cross section of the circumflex artery may occasionally be seen in the lateral portion of the left atrioventricular groove when this region is scanned at the midmitral valve level. In our experience at the Thoraxcentre, this latter view of the circumflex artery provides no useful diagnostic information.

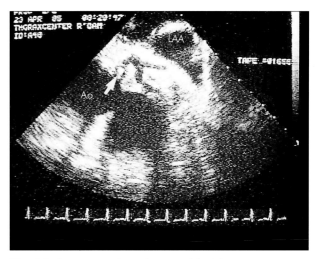

Fig. 11.6 Transoesophageal image of the left coronary artery. There is a stenotic plaque in the left main stem (arrowed).

Identification of stenotic lesions in the proximal left coronary arterial system

Noncalcific atheromatous deposits within the proximal part of the left coronary arterial system can be identified using transoesophageal imaging (Fig. 11.5); this is especially true of lesions within the main stem (Fig. 11.6). There is a poor correlation, nonetheless, between the severity of the obstruction, as judged from the echocardiographic image, when compared to quantitative evaluation of coronary arteriographic findings (2,5). This may be because stenotic lesions within coronary arteries are often eccentric and, thus, their full evaluation requires imaging from at least two planes. This is not possible using single-plane transoesophageal echocardiography. Calcified atheromatous deposits within the vessel walls are also readily identified since calcium is a strong reflector of ultrasound. Calcified lesions do not always cause significant coronary obstruction and, therefore, their identification is of limited clinical value in itself. In addition, the shadow caused by the calcium deposits can prevent the visualization of any associated luminal narrowing. Where calcium is not present within the vessel walls, the accuracy with which stenoses can be identified is increased. Problems remain in differentiating truly stenotic lesions from false-positive appearances suggestive of narrowing caused by oblique sectioning of tortuosities of the artery.

Right coronary artery

In patients with normal right ventricular pressure, volume, and myocardial function, the right coronary

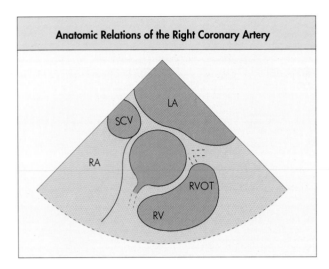

Anatomic Relations of the Right Coronary Artery

Fig. 11.7 The usual anatomic relations of the origin of the right coronary artery.

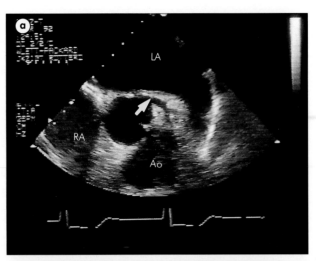

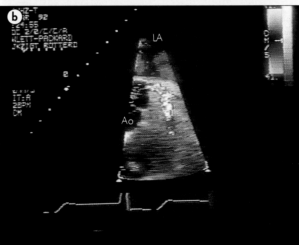

Fig. 11.8 Transoesophageal echocardiogram with colour flow mapping in a patient with normal coronary arteries. (a) Cross-sectional image showing a normal main stem (arrowed) and bifurcation, which were confirmed at angiography. (b) Colour flow map of the same image showing diastolic turbulent flow in the left anterior descending artery, starting just after the bifurcation.

artery is, in our experience, more difficult to visualize than the left (see *Fig. 11.1*). As previously stated, the proximal right coronary is more frequently imaged in conditions in which flow through it is increased. Its orifice is rarely found in the same transoesophageal cross section as the left. It can usually be visualized in a cross section of the aortic root which is slightly inferior to that in which the left coronary artery is imaged (Fig. 11.7).

Colour flow mapping of the coronary arteries

Both proximal coronary arteries are amenable to spectral Doppler interrogation and studies using colour flow mapping (6,7). In normal subjects, colour flow mapping studies demonstrate uniform laminar flow (represented by either homogeneous red or blue, depending on the direction of flow within the left main and proximal right coronary artery) (see *Chapter 3*). In theory, flow should remain laminar within the anterior descending and circumflex branches of the left system in patients with normal vessels, but this is not always the case. Both turbulent and aliased flow may occur in normal vessels (Fig. 11.8). Such abnormalities are particularly prevalent in the colour maps recorded at bifurcations and in tortuous segments of the vessels. Despite these inherent problems in using the presence of intraluminal turbulence as a marker for stenotic lesions, previous authors have claimed that the recognition of turbulent flow within the vessel can increase the diagnostic sensitivity of transoesophageal imaging for identification of a stenotic lesion (4,5).

Pulsed Doppler interrogation of coronary flow

Pulsed Doppler studies have also been used in an attempt to improve the definition and quantification of stenoses within the proximal arteries (8). Although pulsed Doppler studies can demonstrate both abnormal increases in peak velocity and altered profiles of flow associated with apparent narrowing on the imaging examination, such studies can give misleading results and are extremely difficult to perform and interpret. Further problems inherent in any pulsed Doppler interrogation of coronary arterial flow are the relatively small calibre of the vessels that must be interrogated, and the fact that these vessels are constantly moving in and out of the plane of imaging throughout the cardiac

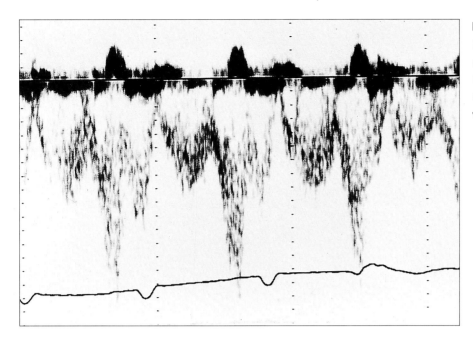

Fig. 11.9 Transoesophageal pulsed Doppler recording from a normal left anterior descending coronary artery. Coronary blood flow occurs in both systole and diastole, with the highest velocities occurring in diastole.

cycle (9). In addition, the relatively horizontal course of the proximal portions of both the left main and the circumflex arteries means that alignment of the interrogating sample volume to flow is virtually impossible, and thus estimation of the true pressure gradient in these vessels is impossible. Only information on abnormal intraluminal velocity profiles can be derived. Alignment to flow is significantly better when attempting to interrogate profiles of flow in the anterior descending artery (Fig. 11.9). Some evaluation of the severity of stenosis can then be made from observed changes in peak velocities over an apparent narrowing in the vessel. Pulsed Doppler recordings have also been demonstrated to show changes in parameters of flow induced by administration of drugs. Such reproducible semiquantitative changes in flow, which reflect drug-induced changes in the coronary vascular bed, have been noted following the administration of both dipyridamole and dobutamine. Although it is not possible to measure absolute peak velocities accurately, some authors have suggested that changes in relative peak velocities recorded after the administration of dipyridamole may be useful as indicators of coronary flow reserve (8). The clinical value of these observations is, as yet, unclear as accurate measurements of the volume of coronary flow using transoesophageal pulsed Doppler techniques would appear to be fraught with methodological problems.

Summary

It is our opinion that transoesophageal echocardiography is of limited value in the evaluation of lesions within the coronary arteries. Adequate visualization of the coronary vessels is possible only in a proportion of patients. Even where the quality of the images is excellent, only limited segments of the proximal coronary vessels can be visualized. Both false-positive and false-negative results concerning the presence or absence of stenoses are too common an occurrence to allow the accurate definition of morphology of individual vessels. Colour flow mapping studies are also of little additional value. Pulsed Doppler studies may identify changes in the velocity profiles of flow, which are associated with severe stenosis but, as yet, these have not been proven to be of clinical relevance. It would seem that the only practical value of transoesophageal studies in the evaluation of coronary arterial lesions in patients with ischaemic heart disease is in the identification of a left main stenosis as a coincidental finding, during routine transoesophageal echocardiography for other indications.

Other aspects of evaluation of the coronary arteries

Atheromatous aneurysms of the (proximal) coronary arteries have been identified by transoesophageal imaging (10). The technique may yet prove to be of value in the diagnosis and follow-up of the progressive proximal coronary arterial lesions associated with Kawasaki disease. Patients with congenital cardiac malformations, such as those with tetralogy of Fallot, who have an increased incidence of anomalous origin of the anterior descending artery from the right coronary artery, may have this anomaly excluded or confirmed as part of a routine transoesophageal study. There is, at present, no information available on any potential role the transoesophageal technique may have in the evaluation of coronary arterial fistulas (Fig. 11.10). Our experience with a number of such lesions, nonetheless, would indicate that both the origin and exit of the anomalous communication can be better visualized from the transoesophageal approach. Direct visualization of the morphology, and Doppler evaluation of the characteristics of the flow of both vein grafts and internal mammary grafts using transoesophageal imaging, are possible, but, as with coronary arterial lesions, the frequency and reliability with which these can be performed is low. It is unlikely that transoesophageal evaluation of these structures will ever become a clinically relevant investigational technique.

TRANSOESOPHAGEAL EVALUATION OF ABNORMALITIES OF LEFT VENTRICULAR REGIONAL WALL MOTION AT REST

In our opinion, at present, abnormalities of both global and regional left ventricular function are, in general, better and more appropriately assessed using precordial echocardiography. Left ventricular function can (and should) be assessed, nonetheless, as part of the standard protocol of examination in patients undergoing transoesophageal studies. The short-axis view of the left ventricle obtained by transgastric imaging provides high-quality images of both endocardial and epicardial contours. Short-axis cross sections can be obtained at both the orifice of the mitral valve and the level of its

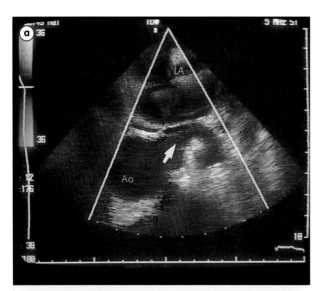

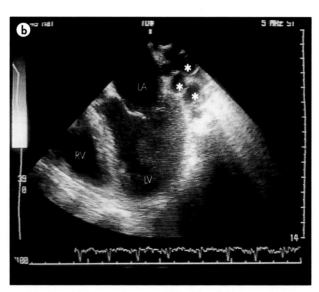

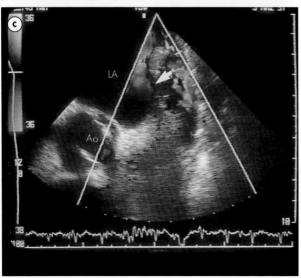

Fig. 11.10 Transoesophageal images with colour flow mapping in a patient with an unsuspected fistula from the left circumflex artery to the left atrium. (a) The first suspicion of an abnormality was the demonstration of a dilated main stem (arrowed). (b) The dilated, ectatic circumflex artery appears as a multilobular mass in the left atrioventricular groove(*). (c) The colour flow map shows flow within the abnormal coronary artery and a laminar jet in the left atrium originating from the lateral wall at the entry site of the fistula (arrowed).

papillary muscles. In these cross sections, major areas of myocardium supplied by all three main coronary arteries can be visualized. The advantage over images derived at routine precordial studies is that clear visualization of endocardium of the left ventricle is nearly always obtained by the transoesophageal technique. It can, therefore, provide images suitable for quantitative analysis of regional wall motion. This is particularly relevant for methods using computer-generated and automated techniques for detecting endocardial contours. A more detailed description on the acquisition and analysis of data, which can be used to analyse left ventricular function from transoesophageal images, can be found in *Chapter 12*.

TRANSOESOPHAGEAL STRESS ECHOCARDIOGRAPHY

Stress echocardiography has been proposed as a valuable technique for the identification of myocardial ischaemia. Several different forms of stress have been used in combination with precordial echocardiography. These are physical exercise (11–17), atrial pacing (18–20), and pharmacological interventions (21). The main disadvantages of dynamic exercise echocardiography is that, frequently, images of poor quality are obtained, due to interference from motion, both during and immediately after exercise (11,12). In addition, translation (sidewards motion) of the heart due to respiration, reduces the sensitivity of the technique in identifying abnormalities of regional wall motion.

In an attempt to provide an alternative to precordial stress echocardiography, a system has recently been developed whereby an atrial pacing facility has been incorporated into the shaft of a standard 5-MHz phased-array transoesophageal probe (Fig. 11.11). Such studies should only be carried out in patients in whom precordial imaging is of inadequate quality, or in patients who cannot perform a standard exercise test. Three circular, silver atrial pacing electrodes are installed at 7, 9, and 12cm from the tip of the transducer. The connecting wires are spirally wound around the outside of the shaft and insulated with a layer of silicone. Using a combination of two of the three electrodes (determined by trial and error), continuous pacing of the atrium during a prolonged period of study can be achieved without the need to move the transducer. The resulting left ventricular cross section that is imaged can then remain constantly in vision throughout the pacing study.

The atrial pacing protocol

In the majority of patients, stable left atrial capture can be obtained by using electrodes 1 and 2 (Fig. 11.11), with a pulse duration of 10ms and an intensity of between 7 and 20mA. A baseline recording of the transoesophageal image should be made initially at the spontaneously generated heart rate. Atrial pacing should be initiated at a rate of 100 beats/min, and then increased stepwise every two minutes by 20 beats/min, up to 85% of the maximal heart rate predicted according to the age of the patient. A 12-lead electrocardiogram should routinely be recorded throughout such studies.

The transoesophageal short-axis view of the left ventricle at the level of the middle of the papillary muscles must be recorded throughout the study. The images recorded are subsequently analysed using a continuous cine-loop format available on an off-line system of analysis processed in a microcomputer. Split-screen and quad-screen formats should be used so that endocardial motion and wall thickening at baseline, during, and after pacing, can be analysed side by side. A normal study is defined as either one in which homogeneous

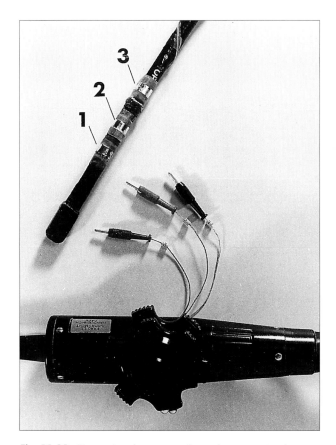

Fig. 11.11 Conventional transoesophageal cross-sectional echoscope modified for simultaneous atrial pacing. Three circular, silver pacing electrodes have been attached.

increases in wall thickening occur in all myocardial segments that are imaged, or (in the case of a pre-existing abnormality of regional wall motion) one in which no new changes in wall motion develop, either during or following the atrial pacing study. An abnormal study, in contrast, is defined as one in which atrial pacing induces the development of either a new abnormality of regional wall motion, or a further deterioration of a pre-existing one.

Initial clinical experience using transoesophageal stress echocardiography

A series of 67 patients with clinically suspected coronary arterial disease, who were referred for coronary arteriography, were studied by transoesophageal stress echocardiography (22). A standard bicycle exercise test had been performed one day prior to the pacing study in 58 patients. In 13 of the 67 patients, coronary arteriography revealed no evidence of a significant obstructive lesion

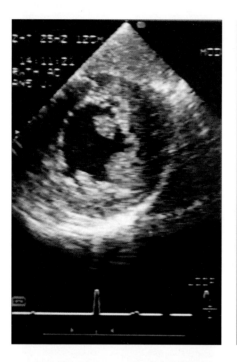
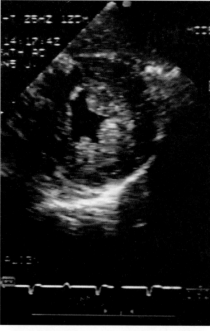

Fig. 11.12 Normal transoesophageal stress echocardiogram of a patient without coronary arterial disease. The left ventricle is imaged in the short-axis view at midpapillary level. End-systolic frames at rest (left panel) and at peak atrial pacing (right panel) are shown. On pacing, the end-systolic volume is reduced but the shape of the ventricular cross section is unchanged.

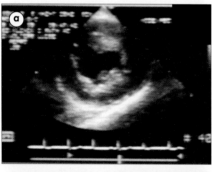
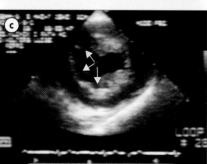
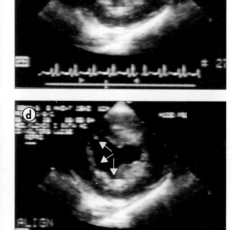

Fig. 11.13 Transoesophageal stress echocardiogram showing original 'quad' screen images at end-systole, from a patient with triple-vessel disease. Pacing-induced abnormalities of wall motion are indicated by arrows. (a) At rest, there is no regional abnormality of wall motion. (b) At maximal pacing, hypokinesis is noted in the septum. (c) Immediately after pacing, there is akinesis in the anterior wall and septum. (d) Two minutes after pacing, hypokinesis persists.

(defined as greater than 50% narrowing of the luminal diameter). All 13 patients had a normal transoesophageal stress test (Fig. 11.12). In the remaining 54 patients, 23 had single-, 19 double-, and 12 triple-vessel disease. Of these patients, 50 had an abnormal transoesophageal study (Figs. 11.13 and 11.14). A comparison of the findings generated by all the techniques, including a list of their relative diagnostic sensitivities and specificities, is outlined in Fig. 11.15.

Advantages of transoesophageal stress echocardiography

The main advantage of transoesophageal stress echocardiography would appear to be the high quality of the images obtained throughout the procedure. A remarkably high sensitivity and specificity are attained for the detection of coronary arterial disease because of this. These results are a marked improvement on the results of the precordial stress echocardiographic studies so far reported (11–21). The images derived from such transoesophageal studies also lend themselves more readily to quantitative analysis of regional left ventricular function. Other forms of transoesophageal stress echocardiography have been reported, such as physical exercise and pharmacological intervention. These are generally impractical, and the combined use of oesophageal atrial pacing and transoesophageal imaging would appear to be the best solution.

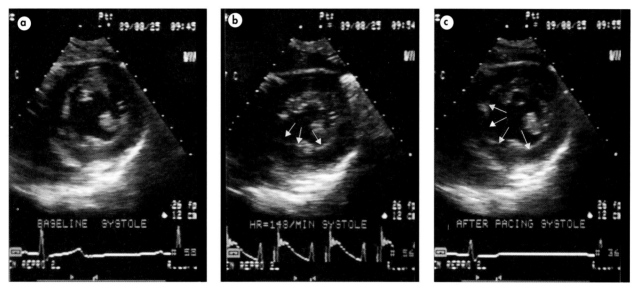

Fig. 11.14 Transoesophageal echocardiogram of a patient with double-vessel disease. End-systolic frames at rest (a), at maximal atrial pacing at 148 beats/min (b), and immediately after pacing (c) are shown. There is good left ventricular function at rest, but abnormalities of anterior and septal wall motion develop during, and after, atrial pacing (arrowed).

Diagnostic Accuracy of Bicycle Ergometry, Pacing Electrocardiogram, and Transoesophageal Stress Echocardiography					
Stress test	Specificity (%)	Sensitivity (%)			
		Overall	Vessel disease		
			1	2	3
bicycle ergometry (n=58) [12/46]	58*	57 †	40 ‡(n=20)	53 ‡(n=15)	91 (n=11)
pacing electrocardiogram (n=67) [13/54]	69*	56 †	30 ‡(n=23)	63 ‡(n=19)	92 (n=12)
transoesophageal stress echocardiography n=67 [13/54]	100	93	83 (n=23)	100 (n=19)	100 (n=12)

The figures in brackets are the number (n) of patients in each group without coronary artery disease/with coronary artery disease; * = P<0.05 vs transoesophageal stress echocardiography; † = P<0.0001 vs transoesophageal stress echocardiography; ‡ = P<0.01 vs transoesophageal stress echocardiography (Fisher's exact test).

Fig. 11.15 Specificity and sensitivity of bicycle ergometry, pacing electrocardiogram, and transoesophageal stress echocardiography for the detection of coronary arterial disease.

Disadvantages of transoesophageal stress echocardiography

The disadvantage of transoesophageal stress echocardiography lies in its semi-invasive nature. Although the procedure was generally well tolerated during initial studies, four patients suffered transient chest discomfort. This was related to the pacing procedure and was most likely caused by the high intensity of the pacing pulse. A further problem with the technique may be pacing-induced oesophageal spasm, which produces chest pain. This might result in an inappropriate cessation of the pacing study. A more important inherent disadvantage is that only one cross section of the left ventricle can be recorded during the study period. Thus, localized abnormalities of wall motion induced in the basal or apical regions may go undetected. The introduction of biplane or multidirectional scanning may overcome this limitation.

TRANSOESOPHAGEAL ECHOCARDIOGRAPHIC EVALUATION OF THE SURGICAL COMPLICATIONS OF MYOCARDIAL INFARCTION

The complications of myocardial infarction which are amenable to surgical repair include ventricular septal rupture, left ventricular aneurysm, left ventricular pseudoaneurysm, and dysfunction or rupture of the papillary muscles. In our experience, transoesophageal imaging in a single transverse plane has major limitations in the evaluation of the first three lesions, and is only consistently of value in the assessment of abnormalities of the mitral valve.

When considering the possible advantages and limitations of transoesophageal imaging in the evaluation of this diverse group of complications of infarction, it is worth remembering that the series of transverse cross-sectional planes available from either the oesophagus or from the fundus of the stomach can only image the smooth inlet and the proximal and midventricular segments of the muscular septum. Significant areas of the apical trabecular septum and of the antero-apical and infero-lateral segments of the myocardial free wall are not well visualized. Postinfarction ventricular septal defects are frequently located in the antero-apical part of the muscular septum. Left ventricular pseudoaneurysms are commonly located in the left ventricular free wall at the base of the papillary muscles. Both these myocardial regions are poorly visualized from the transoesophageal approach. Thus, it should be expected that transoesophageal echocardiography would be a less than optimal technique for their visualization.

Our own experience has confirmed limitations of the technique in studying patients with a postinfarction pseudoaneurysm. A defect in the postero-lateral left ventricular free wall has been observed (Fig. 11.16) and colour flow mapping confirmed the presence of to-and-fro flow between the left ventricle and the pericardial cavity. We have also witnessed a rupture of the anterior wall of the left ventricle (Fig. 11.17). More apically placed communications between the ventricle and the pericardial cavity, in contrast, could not be visualized. Precordial ultrasound studies had clearly

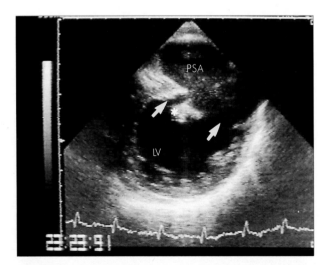

Fig. 11.16 Transoesophageal image of the transgastric short-axis view of the left ventricle. There is a posterior pseudoaneurysm (PSA), which has two entry points (arrows) either side of an infarcted posteromedial papillary muscle (*).

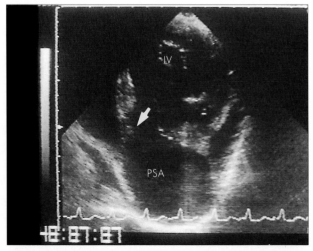

Fig. 11.17 Transoesophageal image of the transgastric short-axis view of the left ventricle. There is a rupture of the anterior wall (arrowed) with the formation of an anterior pseudoaneurysm.

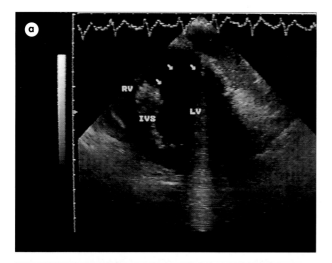

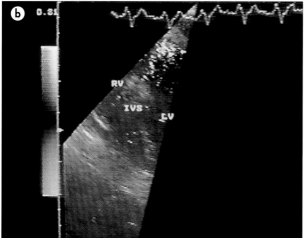

Fig. 11.18 Transoesophageal image of the transgastric short-axis view of the left ventricle. (a) Rupture of the posterior septum (arrows). (b) Corresponding colour flow map showing turbulent flow within the right ventricle.

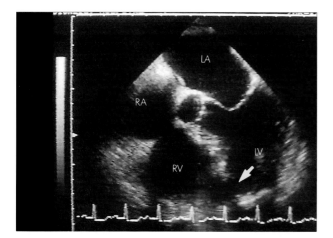

Fig. 11.19 Transoesophageal four-chamber view in a patient with a postinfarction ventricular septal rupture. There is a defect in the apical septum (arrowed), which could not be visualized by precordial echocardiography. Colour flow mapping, however, could not demonstrate any transseptal flow due to the depth of the defect from the probe.

identified the presence of the pseudoaneurysm in all cases. In the cases in which transoesophageal studies identified the defect, the information derived was clearly limited in defining the margins of the defect when compared to that obtained from the precordium.

Similar problems have been encountered when studying patients with postinfarction ventricular septal defects. In our experience, the defect can only be visualized in approximately one-third of patients. A defect in the posterior septum is shown in Fig. 11.18, and a defect in the antero-apical portion of the ventricular septum is shown in Fig. 11.19. In other patients whom we have studied, a defect was subsequently proven at surgery to be located in the apical part of the septum. In only half of these cases did colour flow mapping demonstrate the characteristic right ventricular turbulent flow associated with a restrictive ventricular septal defect (see *Fig. 11.18b*). It is likely that failure to record the disturbance of the right ventricular flow in these cases was related to the distance between the transducer and the area of interest, since the depth at which colour Doppler information can be recorded from the transoesophageal approach is limited when using a 5-MHz transducer. In all of these cases, the correct diagnosis was readily apparent from the precordial studies. Our previous experience with the use of combined precordial cross-sectional imaging and colour flow mapping has demonstrated remarkably high sensitivities and specificities for the diagnosis of both postinfarction septal defect (23) and rupture of the ventricular free wall (24). Transoesophageal echocardiography, therefore, would appear to have little additional information to offer when compared to precordial studies.

The role of transoesophageal imaging in the evaluation of both acute (25) and chronic lesions of the mitral valve is discussed in detail in *Chapter 6*.

REFERENCES

1. Taams MA, Gussenhoven WJ, Cornel JH *et al.* Detection of left coronary artery stenosis by transoesophageal echocardiography. *Eur Heart J* 1988;**9**:1162–6.

2. Gerckens U, Cattelaens N, Drinkovic N *et al.* Detection of proximal coronary artery stenosis by transesophageal echocardiography [Abstract]. *Eur Heart J* 1989;**10** (suppl):121.

3. Iliceto S, Memmola C, De Martino G, Rizzon P. Evaluation of anatomy and flow of the left coronary artery by transesophageal 2D echocardiography [Abstract]. *Eur Heart J* 1989;**10** (suppl):121.

4. Reichert S, Visser C, Koolen J *et al.* Transesophageal echocardiographic examination of the left coronary artery with a 7.5 MHz 2D and Doppler transducer [Abstract]. *Eur Heart J* 1989;**10** (suppl):122.

5. Samdarshi TE, Chang LK, Ballal RS *et al.* Transesophageal color Doppler echocardiography in assessing proximal coronary artery stenosis [Abstract]. *J Am Coll Cardiol* 1990;**15**:93a.

6. Kyo S, Takamoto S, Matsumura M *et al.* Visualization of coronary blood flow by transesophageal Doppler color flow mapping. *J Cardiogr* 1986;**16**:831–40.

7. Zwicky P, Daniel WG, Mugge A, Lichtlen PR. Imaging of the coronary arteries by color-coded transesophageal Doppler echocardiography. *Am J Cardiol* 1988;**62**:639–40.

8. Iliceto S, Marageli V, Memmola C *et al.* Assessment of coronary flow reserve by transesophageal echo-Doppler [Abstract]. *J Am Coll Cardiol* 1990;**15**:62a.

9. Yamagishi M, Miyatake K, Beppu S *et al.* Assessment of coronary blood flow by transesophageal two-dimensional pulsed Doppler echocardiography. *Am J Cardiol* 1988;**62**:641–4.

10. Tunick PA, Slater J, Pasternack P, Kronzon I. Coronary artery aneurysms: a transesophageal study. *Am Heart J* 1989;**118**:176–9.

11. Visser CA, van der Wieken RL, Kan G *et al.* Comparison of two-dimensional echocardiography with radionuclide angiography during dynamic exercise for the detection of coronary disease. *Am Heart J* 1983; **106**:528–34.

12. Crawford MH, Amon KW, Vance WS. Exercise 2-dimensional echocardiography. Quantification of left ventricular performance in patients with severe angina pectoris. *Am J Cardiol* 1983;**51**:1–6.

13. Heng MK, Simard M, Lake R, Udhoji VH. Exercise two-dimensional echocardiography for diagnosis of coronary artery disease. *Am J Cardiol* 1984;**54**:502–7.

14. Armstrong WF, O'Donnell J, Dillon JC *et al.* Complementary value of two-dimensional exercise echocardiography to routine treadmill exercise testing. *Ann Intern Med* 1986;**105**:829–35.

15. Armstrong WF, O'Donnell J, Ryan T, Feigenbaum H. Effect of prior myocardial infarction and extent and location of coronary artery disease on accuracy of exercise echocardiography. *J Am Coll Cardiol* 1987;**10**:531–8.

16. Ryan T, Vasey CG, Presti CF *et al.* Exercise echocardiography: detection of coronary artery disease in patients with normal left ventricular wall motion at rest. *J Am Coll Cardiol* 1988;**11**:993–9.

17. Robertson WS, Fiegenbaum H, Armstrong WF *et al.* Exercise echocardiography: a clinically practical addition in the evaluation of coronary artery disease. *J Am Coll Cardiol* 1983;**2**:1085–91.

18. Iliceto S, D'Ambrosio G, Sorino M *et al.* Comparison of post-exercise and transoesophageal atrial pacing two-dimensional echocardiography for the detection of coronary artery disease. *Am J Cardiol* 1986;**57**:547–53.

19. Chapman PD, Doyle TP, Troup PJ *et al.* Stress echocardiography with transoesophageal atrial pacing: preliminary report of a new method for the detection of ischemic wall motion abnormalities. *Circulation* 1984;**70**:445–50.

20. Iliceto S, Sorino M, D'Ambrosio G *et al.* Detection of coronary artery disease by two-dimensional echocardiography and transesophageal atrial pacing. *J Am Coll Cardiol* 1985;**5**:1188–97.

21. Picano E, Lattanzi F, Masini M *et al.* High dose dipyramidole echocardiography test in effort angina pectoris. *J Am Coll Cardiol* 1986;**8**:848–54.

22. Lambertz H, Kreis A, Trümper H, Hanreth T. Simultaneous transesophageal atrial pacing and transesophageal two-dimensional echocardiography: A new method of stress echocardiography. *J Am Coll Cardiol* 1990;**16**:1143–53.

23. Smyllie JH, Sutherland GR, Geuskens R *et al.* Doppler color flow mapping in the diagnosis of ventricular septal rupture and acute mitral regurgitation after myocardial infarction. *J Am Coll Cardiol* 1990;**15**:1449–55.

24. Sutherland GR, Smyllie JH, Roelandt JRTC. Advantages of colour flow imaging in the diagnosis of left ventricular pseudoaneurysm. *Br Heart J* 1989;**61**:59–64.

25. Patel AM, Miller FA, Khandheria BK *et al.* Role of transesophageal echocardiography in the diagnosis of papillary muscle rupture secondary to infarction. *Am Heart J* 1989;**118**:1330–3.

12

Intraoperative monitoring

Marc E R M van Daele
Jos R T C Roelandt

INTRODUCTION

Cardiac complications remain the most important cause of perioperative mortality, particularly in the increasing subset of older patients who undergo major general surgical procedures. Anaesthetic management of these patients at high risk has improved dramatically with the aggressive use of new inotropic and vasoactive drugs. To obtain optimal benefit from their use, however, it is essential to detect early, and sensitively, any change in cardiac function. In this respect, there are several limitations to many of the current conventional methods used to monitor cardiac function in the operating theatre.

The surface electrocardiogram has frequently been used as the sole monitoring technique for the detection of evolving myocardial ischaemia, despite its limited sensitivity in detecting early subendocardial changes (1). Moreover, since the recording of a standard 12-lead electrocardiogram is impractical during surgery, only one or two selected leads are usually recorded and then, even severe transmural ischaemia may go unnoticed (2). Invasive haemodynamic monitoring (in particular the use of the pulmonary wedge pressure) has been proposed as an alternative, or additional method, for identification of acquired ischaemia (3). Haemodynamic indices, however, can be influenced by many factors during the perioperative period, one of these factors being myocardial ischaemia. Indeed, a number of studies have shown invasive haemodynamic monitoring to be insensitive for the early detection of evolving ischaemia (4,5). The fact that severe myocardial injury results in a rise in the pulmonary wedge pressure, and a fall in systemic blood pressure, is not in dispute, but the goal of any monitoring technique should be to detect the onset of ischaemia at a stage sufficiently early to allow therapeutic intervention before the ischaemia progresses to infarction (6).

Invasive measurements are also used by the anaesthetist to assess global cardiac function during the perioperative period. Although such indices are indisputably of great value for clinical decision-making, they have inherent limitations. The pulmonary wedge pressure is commonly used as an index of preload, since it indirectly reflects the left ventricular end-diastolic pressure. The direct index of preload is, however, the end-diastolic fibre length of myocardial muscle, or its correlate, the end-diastolic volume. The use of pressure as an index of volume remains valid only if the myocardial compliance itself remains unaltered; this may not be the case during anaesthesia, since myocardial compliance can be influenced by many factors such as severe myocardial ischaemia, changes in heart rate, a variety of drugs, volatile anaesthetic agents, and 'stunning' of myocardium after cardiac surgery. In the light of all these considerations, it is clear that new monitoring modalities would be of inestimable value if they could provide additional intraoperative information on both regional and global myocardial function.

Transoesophageal echocardiography provides a modality which, for the first time, allows perioperative, on-line continuous visualization of the beating heart, without interfering with the surgical procedure. Such monitoring has been shown to be of great value in three main areas. Firstly, the technique allows accurate and reproducible identification of regional wall-motion abnormalities of the left ventricle; these are the earliest and most sensitive markers of myocardial ischaemia. Secondly, transoesophageal studies can provide direct information on changes in volume and inotropic state of the left ventricle. Thirdly, the technique has proven to be an extremely sensitive means with which to visualize intracardiac air and other sources of acute perioperative embolization. Each of these current applications and their inherent limitations are reviewed in this chapter.

SAFETY OF THE PROCEDURE

The technique of introducing the transoesophageal transducer into an anaesthetized patient differs from the procedure used in a patient who is awake. The airway should always be protected by an endotracheal tube before insertion of the probe, so as to minimize the risk of aspiration of pharyngeal or gastric contents, or of introducing the probe into the trachea. Introduction is best achieved with the patient supine and the head in midline position. By lifting the mandible, together with the tongue, with one hand, the probe can then be introduced with the other hand. For successful introduction, it is important to direct the tip of the probe towards the midline of the pharynx. It is desirable, therefore, for the endotracheal tube to have previously been fixed to one side. The depth of anaesthesia must be adequate to prevent undesirable reactions to the stress of the introduction of the probe, which is, at worst, comparable to the stress produced by tracheal intubation. Before introduction, the tip of the probe should be covered with lubricant, and the steering controls of the probe should be unlocked so that it can gently follow the contours of the pharynx. In very rare cases where blind introduction of the probe is difficult, direct visualization of the proximal oesophagus with a laryngoscope can be helpful. The technique is then almost identical to the technique of tracheal intubation and is not difficult, especially for an anaesthetist. As there is a potential risk of causing oesophageal damage, or even perforation, force should never be used when introducing the probe. Similarly, the probe should not be advanced while the tip is flexed or retroflexed. It is probably safest to retain the steering controls in an unlocked position, allowing passive motion both when advancing and retracting the probe.

Intraoperative transoesophageal echocardiography has proven to be a relatively safe procedure. The only complication reported, thus far, is transient paralysis of the vocal cords in two patients: in both cases, this probably resulted from abnormal sustained pressure on the laryngeal nerves, which occurred during long neurosurgical procedures with the patient in an upright position, the head retroflexed, and both the endotracheal tube and the echocardiographic probe in position (7). In routine perioperative monitoring, however, with the patient in a supine position and no extreme retroflexion of the head, local pressure on the pharynx should be minimal. Furthermore, local pressure of the tip of the transducer on the wall of the distal oesophagus (or the stomach) is far too little to cause any local pressure-necrosis, even after very prolonged monitoring. Contact pressure may potentially be high enough to cause local pressure-necrosis only if the transducer remains over a long period, in a fixed, completely flexed, position in the distal oesophagus (a view from which no useful image is obtained) (8).

Thermal injury is another hazard that could also occur in theory, although this has not been reported thus far. During ultrasound emission, the scanhead of the transducer produces a very small amount of heat. When the transducer is in contact with surrounding tissue, this heat is easily transmitted, without causing any rise in temperature. If, however, the scanhead is in the stomach, but makes no contact with the wall (again, no image is obtained), and transmits over a prolonged period, there is the theoretical risk of heating-up. All commercially available probes, therefore, are now equipped with a temperature sensor, which will lead to an automatic switch-off of ultrasonic transmission if the temperature of the transducer reaches 41°C. Thus, the theoretical risk of thermal injury now only exists in case of failure of this safety measure. Nevertheless, it must be remembered that, in patients who are being operated on under hypothermia, an emitting transoesophageal transducer might be an undesirable source of heat. Due to all of these considerations, we at the Thoraxcentre, believe it is a good habit to unlock the steering mechanism and switch off the transmission power when the transducer remains in location while it is not being used over a prolonged period of time.

If possible, we also prefer not to have a nasogastric tube in position during transoesophageal monitoring. Nevertheless, if such a tube is desirable, it is not a problem in our experience to have both the tube and the probe within the oesophagus of most adult patients. The nasogastric tube may occasionally be interposed between the probe and the heart and, since it contains air, can thus cause problems in imaging.

MONITORING OF REGIONAL FUNCTION AND ISCHAEMIA

For many years before the introduction of transoesophageal echocardiography, it was well known from animal experiments that a change in both systolic and diastolic wall-motion patterns is an early and very sensitive indicator of evolving myocardial ischaemia (Fig. 12.1). Indeed, such changes precede any electrocardiographic or haemodynamic changes (9–12). This knowledge was of little clinical relevance until transoesophageal echocardiography opened up the possibility of monitoring for such changes in anaesthetized patients (13,14). The usually superb resolution with which the endocardial border and large segments of the epicardium are visualized allows assessment of both centripetal motion and myocardial thickening in systole. Despite the high sensitivity of new wall-motion abnormalities, there are some limitations to the specificity, since other causative factors, other than ischaemia, have also been reported (Fig. 12.2).

Myocardial contraction is most easily studied using short-axis views of the left ventricle, since, in the dog heart at least, approximately nine-tenths of stroke volume is derived from shortening in the ventricular short axis. Very little contribution to the cardiac output results from shortening of the long axis (15). The short-axis view at the midpapillary level of the left ventricle is the best single view for routine monitoring of regional motion, since this view includes segments of myocardium supplied by each of the main coronary arteries. In cases where the precise site of a critical coronary stenosis is known from prior angiography, however, another view, which images a greater portion of the myocardium at risk, could be selected.

When imaged at a midpapillary level, all myocardial segments of the normal left ventricle move inward, and thicken during systole. If the cross section is taken at the level of the mitral valve, the outflow and membranous components of the septum may be included in this view, which could give the impression of septal hypokinesis or akinesis in a normal left ventricle. Apart from inward motion and thickening of the left ventricular wall, lateral motion, and a small degree of rotation of the whole heart, also occur in normal systole.

In subjective analysis of wall motion, based on visual inspection, the investigator has to rely on an impression of what constitutes normal or abnormal wall motion, and has to discount myocardial motion that results from translation and rotation of the whole heart. Each segment of myocardium is then scored on a scale with five grades (Fig. 12.3). As yet, there is no generally accepted nomenclature for the myocardial segments as

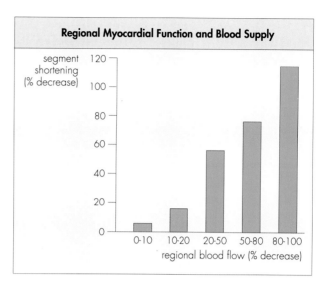

Fig. 12.1 Segments of the myocardium grouped according to the proportional decrease in regional blood flow, showing progressive decreases in myocardial function. Segments with 10–20% decreases in regional blood flow show significant decreases in function. (Reproduced by permission of the American Heart Association Inc. Vatner S F, Correlation between acute reductions in myocardial blood flow and function in conscious dogs; *Circ Res* 1980;**47**:201–7).

Nonischaemic Causes for Abnormal Left Ventricular Wall Motion
image plane through membranous septum
ventricular pacing
left bundle branch block
postischaemic myocardial stunning
postcardiac surgery myocardial stunning
prosthetic valve

Fig. 12.2 Nonischaemic causes for apparently abnormal left ventricular wall motion.

Grade	Features of wall motion	Criterion
1	normal	more than 30% estimated radial shortening, and considerable wall thickening during systole
2	mild hypokinesia	radial shortening estimated to be 10–30%, and decreased wall thickening
3	severe hypokinesia	radial shortening estimated to be less than 10%, and hardly any recognizable wall thickening
4	akinesia	no radial shortening and no wall thickening
5	dyskinesia	bulging out and thinning during systole

Fig. 12.3 Criteria commonly used for subjective grading of wall motion in a segment of the left ventricular wall.

seen in the transoesophageal short-axis view. The American Society of Echocardiography has proposed a nomenclature that divides the midpapillary cross section into octants. Most investigators, however, have used a division of quadrants (5,14,16); segments are described as septal, anterior, lateral, and inferior (posterior), and the insertion of the right ventricular free wall and the anterolateral papillary muscle are used as anatomical landmarks (Fig. 12.4). Some authors use both papillary muscles as landmarks for a division into quadrants, but it must be remembered that when such a definition is adopted, these are at an angle of approximately 130°, rather than 90°.

In most clinical studies, regional wall motion is scored by two independent and blinded observers, and the criterion for the identification of ischaemia is the deterioration of wall motion in any segment by two classes or more, as noted by both observers. The skill of the observers in detecting new regional abnormalities is essential if the method is to be reliable. Clements *et al* reported that, in their experience, this skill is easy to acquire (17). Despite such observations, it seems to us that visual interpretation and subjective grading provide little in the way of scientific data for further research on ischaemic wall motion. In particular, such an approach makes it difficult to compare different studies.

Although several clinical studies have clearly demonstrated the superior sensitivity of transoesophageal echocardiography over the electrocardiogram for the detection of myocardial ischaemia during anaesthesia, by means of new 'regional wall-motion abnormalities' (5,14), these studies all have one severe methodologic limitation, this being that analysis of wall motion was performed off line by reviewing the videotape recordings for the comparison of ventricular motion at different time periods. It is doubtful (18) whether similar sensitivities can be obtained by on-line analysis when the anaesthetist has to compare, from memory, the existing wall motion to the earlier one. It is also impractical for the anaesthetist to pay continuous attention to the echocardiographic monitoring screen, although this would be required to permit early identification of ischaemia, prior to the occurrence of electrocardiographic changes and their haemodynamic consequences. It is due to this practical problem that transoesophageal echocardiography has not yet gained widespread clinical application as a routine monitoring device. Several manufacturers of echocardiographic apparatus are trying to facilitate the on-line analysis of ventricular wall motion. This can be achieved by implementing software in the machines, which will allow storage of images of a cardiac cycle, so that at any time during an operation, the wall motion at that time can be

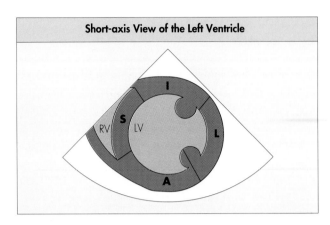

Fig. 12.4 Schematic representation of a short-axis view of the left ventricle at the level of the papillary muscles.

compared, in a side-by-side 'split-screen' display, to the wall motion at an earlier stage. Such possibilities may facilitate the on-line analysis, but do not really circumvent all limitations.

In our clinic, the current role of transoesophageal monitoring is therefore primarily in research applications, rather than in routine management of patients. This results, in part, from the practical limitation mentioned above, and also from the number of echo machines and personnel that would be required to monitor all high-risk patients.

In terms of our research, we recently compared the relative sensitivity of echocardiographic, electrocardiographic, and haemodynamic indices of ischaemia in 100 anaesthetized patients, all having angiographically documented, severe coronary arterial disease (5). All three modalities were studied simultaneously. The echocardiograpic images were graded off line, blinded to electrocardiographic or other patient data. Myocardial ischaemia was identified by transoesophageal echocardiography in 14 patients; in 11 patients, this was associated with ST-segment depression of at least 1mm on the electrocardiogram. Echocardiographic changes were always seen simultaneously with, or prior to, the electrocardiographic changes. There were two patients in this series, however, in whom electrocardiographic changes occurred without any observed change in wall motion. Both were patients who had suffered from previous myocardial infarctions and who now had ejection fractions (angiographically documented) below 0.4. Transoesophageal echocardiography, therefore, although a sensitive tool in patients with initially good ventricular function, may be difficult to interpret in patients with previously damaged and poorly contracting ventricles. Variability in subjective gradings between different observers was not a major problem. Two blinded observers, grading the wall motion on a scale with five classes, had identical gradings in 77% of cases, differed by one class in 19% of cases, and differed by two classes in only 4% of cases.

Transoesophageal echocardiographic monitoring, therefore, is a valuable method in studies that compare the incidence of myocardial ischaemia in different protocols of patient management, for example, to study the impact of different ventilatory regimens on the incidence of myocardial ischaemia in patients undergoing coronary arterial bypass surgery (16). Nevertheless, both effective clinical application and research application of transoesophageal echocardiographic monitoring of ischaemia require further development of methods that, ideally, provide rapid, quantitative, and reproducible analysis of the motion of the ventricular wall.

Quantitative analysis of wall motion has, so far, been based mainly on the comparison of end-diastolic versus end-systolic endocardial contours of the left ventricle (19). The end-diastolic and end-systolic frames are selected within one cardiac cycle, based either on electrocardiographic and phonocardiographic markers, or defined as simply the largest and smallest enclosed areas. Using a lightpen ('mouse'), the endocardial contours are traced and stored in a microcomputer system (Fig. 12.5). Subsequent comparison of these contours can provide quantitative insight into both global and re-

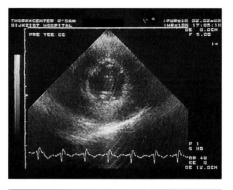
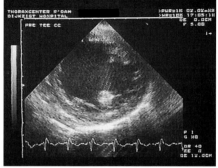
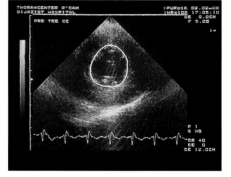
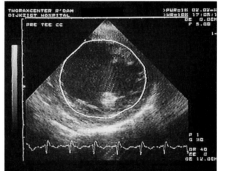
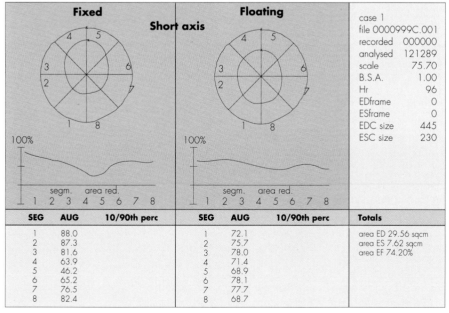

Fig. 12.5 Schematic representation of quantitative analysis of wall motion, based on end-diastolic and end-systolic echocardiographic images. Top: Selected end-diastolic and end-systolic frames. Middle: The identical frames after the endocardial border has been traced. These traces are then transmitted into a microcomputer-based analysis program. Bottom: Print-out of such computer-assisted analysis, using either a fixed-axis reference system (left) or a floating-axis reference system (right).

case 1	
file	0000999C.001
recorded	000000
analysed	121289
scale	75.70
B.S.A.	1.00
Hr	96
EDframe	0
ESframe	0
EDC size	445
ESC size	230

SEG	AUG	10/90th perc	SEG	AUG	10/90th perc	Totals
1	88.0		1	72.1		area ED 29.56 sqcm
2	87.3		2	75.7		area ES 7.62 sqcm
3	81.6		3	78.0		area EF 74.20%
4	63.9		4	71.4		
5	46.2		5	68.9		
6	65.2		6	78.1		
7	76.5		7	77.7		
8	82.4		8	68.7		

gional myocardial function, but there are also many inherent problems in such methods of analysis of wall motion. Firstly, since systolic motion is determined by both myocardial contraction and lateral motion of the whole heart relative to the transducer position, there is a problem of how to correct for the 'noncontraction' motion. In a 'fixed-axis' system of analysis, the end-diastolic and end-systolic contours are compared in their relative position to the transducer and videoscreen. Lateral motion of the whole heart on this screen during systole may then lead to false-positive observations of regional hypokinesia. Alternatively, a 'floating-axis' system of reference has been proposed. The 'centre of gravity' of both end-diastolic and end-systolic contours is computed, and, to correct for motion of the whole heart, the relative position of end-diastolic and end-systolic contours is adjusted by superimposing these centres (Fig. 12.5). Since the development of segmental dyskinesia does affect the end-systolic centre of gravity, a 'floating-axis' system tends to underestimate the extent of a regional abnormality and may result in false-negative observations. A second problem is that manual detection of contours is time-consuming and prone to subjective influences. It has yet to be proven that the results derived by this method are any more reliable than those obtained by subjective interpretation. Thirdly, the selection of only two frames from the cardiac cycle results in a loss of information. This has impact on the sensitivity of the method, since recent studies have shown that, in early myocardial ischaemia, it is not the hypokinesia itself that is the first effect of ischaemia on wall motion, but that a temporal inhomogeneity occurs in the pattern of both contraction and relaxation (20). This results in a wave-like pattern of wall motion on visual inspection, which may be missed if end-diastolic and end-systolic frames alone are studied. Zeiher et al found that, in humans, myocardial ischaemia first manifested itself as asynchronous polyphasic wall motion, rather than as a change in the amplitude of the wall excursion (21). If end-diastolic and end-systolic frames only were analysed, nearly half of the ischaemic episodes were missed when compared to the integrative analysis of wall motion throughout the entire contraction.

Frame-to-frame analysis of motion of the left ventricular wall throughout the cardiac cycle (systolic and diastolic), assisted by a computer, therefore appears to be a logical step which would, in effect, combine the advantages of both integrative analysis of wall motion and the quantification of any change in regional wall motion. Such analysis requires the development of sophisticated computer software. Ideally, a computer-assisted system for analysis of wall motion would store all images

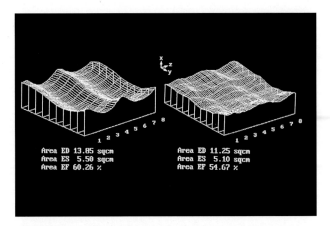

Fig. 12.6 Three-dimensional representations of endocardial motion throughout the cardiac cycle. On the Y-axis, sequential frames (25/s) are displayed, starting and ending with an end-diastolic frame. On the Z-axis, the different segments of the endocardium are displayed. The height on the X-axis represents the distance of the particular segment at a particular moment to the 'centre of gravity' of the ventricular cavity. Left-hand panel: Synchronous wall motion for all segments in a healthy volunteer during rapid atrial pacing. Right-hand panel: Inhomogeneous wall motion during rapid atrial pacing in a patient with severe coronary artery disease. In both, pacing was performed with electrodes incorporated in the imaging transoesophageal probe.

of one cardiac cycle, detect the endocardial contour in every frame, and then provide an intelligible display of the pattern of wall motion in real time (Fig. 12.6). Such a system should include the possibility of calculating any desired index of abnormal wall motion, such as, for example, a shift in the timing or the velocity of segmental motion. Automated detection of endocardial contours is essential for such a system of analysis, since manual tracing of the vast number of videoframes involved is totally impractical, even for research purposes. Several systems for such automated detection of endocardial contours are currently under development, in our institution as well as in others (22, 23).

GLOBAL LEFT VENTRICULAR FUNCTION

Assessment of global ventricular function (preload and inotropic state) is an important goal of monitoring, since it has direct consequences on perioperative decision-making in terms of the administration of fluid or vasodilatory or inotropic drugs.

Preload

Since transoesophageal echocardiography directly visualizes the heart, it has the potential to provide better indices of both end-diastolic volume and stroke volume (24). Early studies have demonstrated that volumes of the left ventricle can be assessed accurately by using several, well-defined echocardiographic cross sections, and making some permissible assumptions on three-dimensional ventricular geometry (25). A major limitation in assessing such volumes by transoesophageal echocardiography is that, usually, only a foreshortened long-axis or four-chamber view can be obtained in which the area that appears to be the apex is not the anatomical apex. Furthermore, complex models requiring many cross-sectional images and sophisticated computing, are neither feasible nor practical for routine monitoring. It therefore appears more logical to adopt a system using a single short-axis section that monitors changes in volume, rather than measures volume itself. The index to be monitored, the end-diastolic stretching of myocardial tissue, is a two-dimensional, rather than a three-dimensional, phenomenon, and is likely to be reflected in a single, constant two-dimensional image recorded from a normal-shaped ventricle. The midpapillary short-axis view used in the monitoring of regional wall-motion abnormalities, is probably best since, at this level, a small change in the position of the transducer has the smallest effect on the enclosed area of the left ventricular cavity. Several clinical studies have demonstrated that transoesophageal echocardiography provides a more reliable index of changes in left ventricular filling than does monitoring with pulmonary arterial catheters, both in cardiac and noncardiac surgery (24, 26). If, however, a single view is used as an index for changes in preload and stroke volume, it is essential that an identical level of cross section is maintained throughout the procedure, and that no regional abnormalities of the wall motion occur that would make the monitoring of preload unreliable. The transoesophageal technique thus provides a promising and practical alternative for monitoring changes in preload, but the relative values of wedge pressure versus transoesophageal echocardiography are not entirely clear; they probably provide their optimal information at the different ends of the spectrum. Our preliminary experience in patients receiving pre-operative hypervolaemic haemodilution (if refusing blood transfusion for religious reasons) suggests that, in underfilled patients, initial administration of fluid has a large impact on end-diastolic volume at the expense of a relatively small increase in wedge pressure. In contrast, once the patient is overfilled, further administration of fluid leads to insignificant changes in end-diastolic volume but a steep rise in wedge pressure. This could be explained from the simple fact that the relationship between end-diastolic pressure and end-diastolic volume is curvilinear rather than linear. As a result, transoesophageal echocardiography is probably the more sensitive index for small changes in preload in patients who are not overfilled.

Inotropic state

Real-time visualization of the beating heart allows a rapid assessment of systolic function. This can be derived either from immediate visual impressions from measures such as the ejection fraction (measured from the midpapillary muscle level), or from M-mode measurements such as the velocity of circumferential shortening. Even simple visual inspection for the assessment of inotropic state is often of great clinical value; for example, in patients with hypotension and low cardiac output following cardiopulmonary bypass, transoesophageal monitoring was demonstrated to be a very practical tool that allowed a rapid discrimination between depressed myocardial function and hypovolaemia as the causative factor (27). Such discrimination is an important guide to treatment since inotropic stimulation of a hypovolaemic, vigorously contracting small ventricle is useless and potentially harmful, as is the administration of more fluid to a patient with a depressed, hypocontractile and dilated left ventricle. In patients who are difficult to wean from cardiopulmonary bypass, however, and who were not previously instrumented with a transoesophageal transducer, epicardial echocardiography (with a standard transducer directly on the exposed heart) is, at least in our experience, an easier alternative to transoesophageal echocardiography.

INTRAOPERATIVE EMBOLIC EVENTS

Acute, intraoperative embolic events, in either the pulmonary or the systemic circulation, are rare, but potentially lethal hazards. Conventional anaesthetic monitoring for pulmonary embolization relies on the capnogram, oximetry, pulmonary arterial pressure, and other haemodynamic parameters. The factor which all these parameters have in common is that the sequel of pulmonary embolism, rather than the event itself, is monitored. The ability to monitor embolic events in the systemic circulation is even more limited, with the diagnosis normally being made after the damage is done.

Since air within the circulation has a different density to blood, it is easily visualized by echocardiography (Fig. 12.7). To a lesser degree, this is also the case for other sources of emboli. Early studies demonstrated a high sensitivity of both M-mode and cross-sectional echocardiography in detecting a variety of emboli passing through the heart, but again it is only with the introduction of transoesophageal echocardiography that continuous on-line monitoring during surgery has become practical.

Paradoxical air embolization is a well-known hazard in neurosurgical and craniofacial operations that are conducted with the patient in an upright position, since air may then easily gain access to the systemic venous circulation. Pulmonary vascular obstruction may result in cardiovascular collapse, but paradoxical embolization into the systemic circulation may occur through a patent oval foramen at an even earlier stage. Echocardiography provides an ideal method, both for the identification of patients at risk for paradoxical emboli, and for intraoperative monitoring. Pre-operative, precordial echocardiographic examination, combined with colour flow mapping or contrast injection during a Valsalva manoeuvre, may visualize an atrial septal defect or a patent oval foramen. Unfortunately, the Valsalva manoeuvre frequently impairs the quality of images in precordial echocardiography. Transoesophageal echocardiography provides the optimal window for inspection of the atrial septum, (see *Chapter 3*) and, in anaesthetized patients, a brief period of positive end-expiratory pressure is helpful for the provocation and visualization of right-to-left atrial shunting (28). A transoesophageal four-chamber view is the most appropriate in patients at risk, to visualize any emboli passing through the right atrium and ventricle and through an oval foramen. The consequence of such detection of air should be that the surgeon either finds the entry point and closes it, or that the head of the patient is lowered.

Removal of residual intracardiac air is always a concern after cardiac surgery involving any cardiotomy. The high sensitivity of transoesophageal echocardiography in detecting any residual bubbles of air in intracardiac blood makes it a potentially valuable tool for checking this prior to restoration of the normal systemic circulation. From our own experience, as well as from other literature (29), it appears that transoesophageal echocardiography is an 'oversensitive' technique for the detection of retained intracardiac air, since it very frequently detects small amounts of air which are of no clinical consequence. The most likely explanation is that the technique can detect bubbles which are so small that they dissolve in the circulation

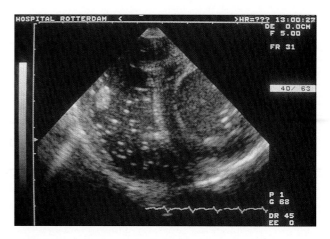

Fig. 12.7 Small amount of air emboli passing through the right heart.

before causing any damage. The technique can, nevertheless, provide a semiquantitative impression of the amount of retained intracardiac air, which may, on rare occasions, need further venting.

Transoesophageal studies can also play a role in the detection of embolic events in orthopaedic surgery. Replacement of the hip, in particular, is associated with frequent embolic events, sometimes resulting in acute circulatory collapse and death. Using transoesophageal echocardiography, such embolic events can be monitored precisely, but monitoring alone is of little clinical consequence. The major research of transoesophageal echocardiography for intraoperative monitoring is currently in this area; for example, the technique has been used to assess the impact of modifications of the surgical procedure in preventing embolic events.

CONCLUSION

Further improvements in the quality of both images and computer software are likely to allow more detailed studies of subtle changes in cardiac function in humans. Transoesophageal studies that are used to monitor ventricular function are likely to expand their role in routine monitoring and in clinical research, in both anaesthesiology and in interventional cardiology. At present, however, transoesophageal echocardiography is in various stages of development for different applications. Whereas the role of transoesophageal echocardiography as a diagnostic tool for the definition of cardiac morphology has been defined in great detail, and is gaining widespread clinical application, its role as a monitor of myocardial function is in a relatively early stage of development and application. This is likely to change and mature in the years ahead.

REFERENCES

1. Barnard RJ, Buckberg GD, Duncan HW. Limitations of the standard transthoracic electrocardiogram in detecting subendocardial ischaemia. *Am Heart J* 1980;**9**:476–82.

2. Chaitman BR, Bourassa MG, Wagmans P *et al.* Improved efficacy of treadmill exercise testing multiple lead ECG system and basic hemodynamic response. *Circulation* 1978;**57**:71–8.

3. Kaplan JA, Wells PH. Early diagnosis of myocardial ischemia using the pulmonary artery catheter. *Anesth analg* 1981;**60**:789–93.

4. Häggmark S, Hohner P, Östman M *et al.* Comparison of hemodynamic electrocardiographic, mechanical and metabolic indicators of intraoperative myocardial ischemia in patients with coronary artery disease. *Anesthesiology* 1989;**70**:19–25.

5. van Daele M, Sutherland GR, Mitchell MM *et al.* Do changes in pulmonary capillary wedge pressure adequately reflect myocardial ischemia during anesthesia? A correlative hemodynamic, electrocardiographic and transesophageal echocardiographic study. *Circulation* 1990;**81**:865–71.

6. Slogoff S, Keats AS. Does perioperative myocardial ischemia lead to postoperative myocardial infarction? *Anesthesiology* 1985;**62**:107–14.

7. Cucchiara RF, Nugent M, Sewart JB, Messick JM. Air embolism in upright neurosurgical patients: detection and localization by two-dimensional transesophageal echocardiography. *Anesthesiology* 1984;**60**:353–5.

8. Urbanowicz JH, Kernoff RS, Oppenheim G *et al.* Transesophageal echocardiography and its potential for esophageal damage. *Anesthesiology* 1990;**72**:40–3.

9. Tennant R, Wiggers CJ. The effect of coronary occlusion on myocardial contraction. *Am J Physiol* 1935;**112**:351–61.

10. Waters DD, da Luz P, Wyatt HL *et al.* Early changes in regional and global left ventricular function induced by graded reductions in regional coronary perfusion. *Am J Cardiol* 1977;**39**:537–43.

11. Vatner SF. Correlation between acute reductions in myocardial blood flow and function in conscious dogs. *Circ Res* 1980;**47**:201–7.

12. Battler A, Froelicher VF, Gallagher KP *et al.* Dissociation between regional myocardial dysfunction and ECG changes during ischemia in the conscious dog. *Circulation* 1980;**62**:735–44.

13. Beaupre PN, Kremer P, Cahalan MK *et al.* Intraoperative detection of changes in left ventricular segmental wall motion by transesophageal two-dimensional echocardiography. *Am Heart J* 1984;**107**:1021–3.

14. Smith JS, Cahalan MK, Benefiel DJ *et al.* Intraoperative detection of myocardial ischemia in high risk patients: Electrocardiography versus two-dimensional transesophageal echocardiography. *Circulation* 1985;**72**:1015–21.

15. Rankin JS, McHale PA, Arentzen CE *et al.* Three dimensional dynamic geometry of the left ventricle in the conscious dog. *Circ Res* 1976;**39**:304–13.

16. Mitchell MM, Prakash O, Rulf ENR *et al.* Nitrous oxide does not induce myocardial ischemia in patients with ischemic heart diease and poor ventricular function. *Anesthesiology* 1989;**71**:526–34.

17. Clements FM, Hill R, Kisslo J, Orchard R. How easily can we learn to recognize regional wall motion abnormalities with 2D transesophageal echocardiography? *Proc Soc Cardiovasc Anesthesiol 1986*; 7th Annual Meeting, Montreal 1986.

18. Saada M, Cahalan MK, Lee E *et al.* Real-time evaluation of echocardiograms [Abstract]. *Anesthesiology* 1989;**71**:344a.

19. Schnittger I, Fitzgerald PJ, Gordon EP *et al.* Computerized quantitative analysis of left ventricular wall motion by two-dimensional echocardiography. *Circulation* 1984;**70**:242–50.

20. Weyman AE, Franklin TD, Hogan RD *et al.* Importance of temporal heterogeneity in assessing the contraction abnormalities associated with acute myocardial ischemia. *Circulation* 1984;**70**:102–12.

21. Zeiher AM, Wollschlaeger HW, Bonzel T *et al.* Hierarchy of levels of ischemia-induced impairment in regional left ventricular systolic function in man. *Circulation* 1987;**76**:768–76.

22. Ezekiel A, Areeda JS, Garcia EV, Corday SR. Intelligent left ventricular contour detection results from two-dimensional echocardiograms. *Comp Cardiol 1987*. Long Beach, California. IEEE Computer Society 1987;603–6.

23. Bosch JG, Reiber JHC, van Burken G *et al.* Automated endocardial contour detection in short-axis 2-D echocardiograms; methodology and assessment of variability. In: Ripley K L, ed. *Proceedings of the 15th International Conference on Computers in Cardiology, Sept 1988, Washington.* Long Beach, California, 1989:137–40.

24. Beaupre PN, Cahalan MK, Kremer PF *et al.* Does pulmonary artery occlusion pressure adequately reflect left ventricular filling during anesthesia and surgery? [Abstract]. *Anesthesiology* 1983;**59**:3a.

25. Martin RW, Bashein G. Measurement of stroke volume with three-dimensional transesophageal ultrasonic scanning: comparison with thermodilution measurement. *Anesthesiology* 1989;**70**:470–6.

26. Roizen MF, Beaupre PN, Alpert RA *et al.* Monitoring with two-dimensional transesophageal echocardiography: comparison of myocardial function in patients undergoing supraceliac, suprarenal-infraceliac or infrarenal aortic occlusion. *J Vasc Surg* 1984;**1**:300–5.

27. Topol EJ, Humphrey LS, Blanck TJJ *et al.* Characterization of post-cardiopulmonary bypass hypotension with intraoperative transesophageal echocardiography [Abstract]. *Anesthesiology* 1983;**59**:2a.

28. Cucchiara RF, Seward JB, Nishimura RA *et al.* Identification of patent foramen ovale during sitting position craniotomy by transesophageal echocardiography with positive airway pressure. *Anesthesiology* 1985;**63**:107–9.

29. Topol EJ, Humphrey LS, Borkon AM *et al.* Value of intraoperative left ventricular microbubbles detected by transesophageal two-dimensional echocardiography in predicting neurologic outcome after cardiac operations. *Am J Cardiol* 1985;**56**:773–5.

13

Intraoperative assessment of surgical repair

Oliver F W Stümper
Alan G Fraser

INTRODUCTION

Cardiac surgery is now a routine and safe procedure for most patients with acquired or congenital heart disease. During the past decade, improved surgical techniques and refinements in myocardial protection have dramatically reduced intraoperative and early hospital mortality. Further improvements, therefore, now focus on achieving optimal haemodynamic results, in the expectation that these will enhance the quality of life after surgery and reduce the chance of re-operation. To achieve these goals, there is a need for intraoperative techniques that can be used to assess the structural and haemodynamic results of a cardiac operation immediately after cardiopulmonary bypass.

Intraoperative epicardial echocardiography has been performed for approximately 10 years, but it has not yet become widely accepted as a routine means of assessing the results of surgery. Initially, cross-sectional imaging was the only technique that was available (1). Even when it is combined with contrast echocardiographic studies, imaging cannot provide all the information that is required to judge the adequacy of a surgical repair (2–5). More recently, the introduction of spectral Doppler and colour flow mapping has renewed interest in intraoperative ultrasound, since these two additional modalities provide quantification of pressure gradients and real-time imaging of flow patterns (6–8). The combination of epicardial cross-sectional imaging with Doppler ultrasound techniques allows the cardiac surgeon to evaluate any surgical repair of acquired or congenital heart disease. Nevertheless, there are several limitations inherent to the epicardial approach; for example, it interferes with surgical procedures, it can cause arrhythmias, and there is a theoretical risk of causing infection.

Transoesophageal echocardiography is now available as an alternative to the epicardial approach. It can be used both for intraoperative monitoring and for the immediate assessment of surgical results at the completion of cardiopulmonary bypass (9,10). The technique of introducing a transoesophageal probe into an intubated patient was discussed in the previous chapter. If difficulty is encountered when trying to introduce the probe blindly, then active steering or direct introduction with the aid of a laryngoscope may be helpful. With current transoesophageal transducers, high-resolution cross-sectional imaging, pulsed wave Doppler studies, and colour flow mapping studies, can be performed with a single probe. This approach does not interfere with surgery, although it may interfere with anaesthetic procedures, and there is no risk of causing a wound infection. Intraoperative transoesophageal echocardiography appears, therefore, to have definite advantages over epicardial echocardiography. The relative value of intraoperative transoesophageal echocardiography, nonetheless, compared with epicardial ultrasound, has yet to be defined.

13.1

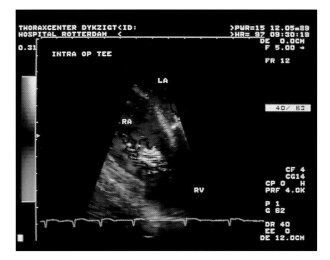

Fig. 13.1 Colour flow map obtained before cardiopulmonary bypass in a patient having surgery for tricuspid regurgitation, which appears to be no more than moderate in severity. The transoesophageal study demonstrated co-existing paraprosthetic regurgitation of the previously inserted mitral valvar prosthesis. This had not been diagnosed pre-operatively.

Transoesophageal studies during cardiac surgery should be performed before and after bypass. The study prior to cannulation aims to give the surgeon a detailed assessment of intracardiac morphology and flow patterns. It may yield additional diagnostic information, which is used to choose or to modify the surgical approach (Fig. 13.1) (11). In addition, it serves as a reference for the subsequent study, which aims to document the success of surgical repair, to assess ventricular function and volume, and to exclude significant residual lesions (11,12). All intraoperative transoesophageal studies should combine cross-sectional imaging with colour flow mapping or spectral Doppler investigations. The latter are normally restricted to pulsed wave Doppler sampling of relevant areas of interest, since facilities for continuous wave Doppler are integrated into very few types of transoesophageal probes.

In this chapter, the value of transoesophageal echocardiography in surgery for acquired and congenital heart disease is discussed, and its advantages and limitations are compared with those of intraoperative epicardial echocardiography. The use of transoesophageal echocardiography to monitor left ventricular function during general anaesthesia is discussed in *Chapter 12*.

ACQUIRED DISEASES OF THE AORTA

Aortic dissection

In an increasing number of centres, patients are now accepted directly for surgery after an acute dissection that involves the ascending aorta has been diagnosed by emergency transoesophageal echocardiography, performed as the only special investigation. Such a study may be undertaken in less than ideal circumstances, in a distressed and restless patient to whom it is impossible to give sedation because of hypotension or tamponade. Thus, it may be valuable to repeat the diagnostic study in the anaesthetic room after induction, or in the operating room. It may then be possible, during a more careful investigation, to locate entry or re-entry tears, especially when these are in the descending aorta, and to study patterns of flow in the true and false lumens. The underlying nature of a dissection can also change quite quickly; for example, a false lumen may become thrombosed between the initial study and the time of transfer to the operating room, the dissection may extend, or other new complications may develop. The information available from a repeat transoesophageal study may therefore be helpful to the cardiac surgeon. Identification of the extent of a dissection and the likely sites of intimal tears greatly influences the choice of incision and the planned surgical approach to the aorta.

The major limitation of transoesophageal echocardiography for the diagnosis of aortic dissection is just as relevant in the operating room as elsewhere. The inability of transoesophageal imaging in the transverse axis to demonstrate the upper half of the ascending aorta and the proximal part of the aortic arch (especially along its outer curvature) is a significant disadvantage. If intimal tears are present in this area, the surgeon has to determine the site of the incision without prior knowledge of their existence or site. Other preoperative investigations, such as aortography and computed tomography with contrast enhancement, may fail to identify intimal flaps, and they often cannot show the sites of tears (13,14). Furthermore, the delay involved in performing such studies or nuclear magnetic resonance imaging can be considerable.

At the Thoraxcentre, we prefer to use transoesophageal echocardiography to establish whether or not there is a dissection and, if urgent surgery is required, to take the patient straight to the operating room. The transoesophageal study determines whether or not the dissection involves the proximal ascending aorta, and whether or not there is aortic regurgitation. Usually, it also demonstrates the proximal segments of the coronary arteries and whether they are supplied

13.2

from the true or false lumen. This information is usually sufficient for the surgeon to decide if a median sternotomy is required. Thereafter, once the femoral artery has been cannulated and the chest opened, more detailed and accurate information can be obtained by direct epivascular imaging and colour flow mapping with ultrasonic probes placed on the surface of the ascending aorta (15–17). Such studies can be carried out before the pericardium is opened, although imaging of the ascending aorta and the whole of the transverse arch in a single plane is easier once the aorta has been dissected free from adjacent structures. Combined longitudinal and transverse epivascular scanning identifies any pathological changes in the segment of the thoracic aorta that is hidden from view on transoesophageal echocardiography. It may also demonstrate the origins of the major head and neck vessels.

If problems are encountered in establishing cardiopulmonary bypass, it is possible with transoesophageal echocardiography to confirm to the surgeon that femoral arterial bypass has been established into the true rather than the false lumen of a dissection that extends into the abdominal aorta and iliac arteries. It is best to do this with colour flow mapping while imaging the aortic arch, since transverse axial planes are poorly aligned for studying flow in the descending aorta. Once systemic cooling has been initiated, or the heart fibrillates, there is so much spontaneous contrast in the aorta that colour flow mapping becomes extremely difficult. Flow between the true and false lumens at the site of an intimal tear, nonetheless, may be identified by studying the pattern of motion of the particles of contrast.

Following surgery for dissection, transoesophageal echocardiography is probably the method of choice for assessing persisting abnormalities in the arch and the descending thoracic aorta, and for assessing the competence of the aortic valve. It is difficult to scan the ascending aorta, but since the structure and competence of a graft in this area is directly visible to the surgeon before the chest is closed, this is usually unnecessary. Transoesophageal echocardiography may also be useful for assessing left ventricular function, for example in the intensive care unit after surgery, because many patients will not have had coronary arteriography, although they have vascular disease and risk factors for coronary arterial disease.

Long after surgery, the distal part of a false lumen may persist, even though its proximal part and the entry tears were obliterated. Transoesophageal echocardiography can be used to assess the presence, location, or absence of residual false lumens, and the presence or absence of thrombus, spontaneous contrast, or flow within them. After successful surgery, closure rather than obliteration of a false lumen may be apparent from immediate changes in its appearance; for example, flow will be greatly reduced or absent, and the motion of the intimal flap much less. In addition, there may be prominent echocardiographic spontaneous contrast (Fig. 13.2a), or new thrombus, within the false lumen. Identification by colour flow mapping of considerable flow persisting within a false lumen, and particularly of residual turbulence (Fig. 13.2b) or jets across the intimal flap, suggests that surgery has not achieved all of its objectives. If these signs are detected by a transoesophageal or epivascular study performed in the operating room after the patient is taken off bypass, it is possible to re-operate in order to close the residual intimal tear. The interpretation of such residual abnormalities when they are found long after surgery for aortic dissection is difficult. It now appears that false lumens may persist in the majority of patients, after what is deemed by surgical and clinical criteria to have been successful surgery (18–20). More information is required from long-term follow-up of these patients in order to determine the prognosis associated with different echocardiographic features after surgery for dissection; biplane transoesophageal probes may be helpful in performing such studies. At present, it is not possible to identify any specific echocardiographic signs which imply that further surgery should be considered.

Aortic aneurysm

Imaging of aortic aneurysms from the oesophagus is restricted by the same limitations that are encountered when studying patients with dissection. Since aneurysms are usually localized and discrete, they can be inspected easily by the surgeon, and there is little to be gained by intraoperative ultrasonic imaging. If inspection reveals unexpected findings, then epivascular imaging and colour flow mapping are more useful than transoesophageal echocardiography, for example in delineating a previously unrecognized dissection. During operations for aneurysms involving the descending thoracic aorta, transoesophageal echocardiography could be used to assess the dimensions of the aorta, or the presence of thrombus within its lumen, above and below the region that has been exposed by the dissection, but the technique is of no value in operations for aneurysms of the aortic arch or the abdominal aorta.

In patients with annuloaortic ectasia, transoesophageal echocardiography is used in the operating room to assess aortic valvar function after bypass when

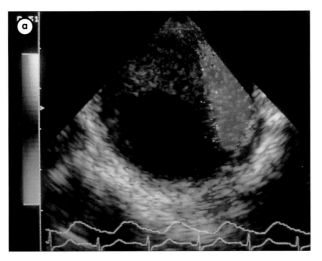 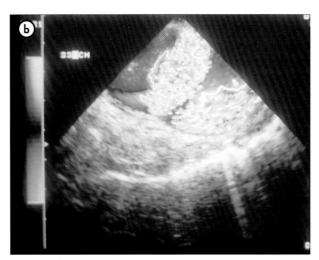

Fig. 13.2 (a) Cross-sectional image and colour flow map of the upper descending thoracic aorta in a patient who had just undergone replacement of the proximal aortic root with obliteration of the entry tear. The false lumen persists, but on colour flow mapping there is no flow apparent within it, and there is considerable spontaneous contrast which was not present before bypass. (b) Colour flow map of the distal arch of the aorta, near the upper descending thoracic aorta in another patient who had just undergone proximal aortic root replacement for a De Bakey I aortic dissection. Although the surgeon had not seen any intimal tears beyond the origin of the left subclavian artery, and he had obliterated the false lumen proximally, the echocardiogram shows that there is persistent flow and turbulence in a false lumen at this site.

the valve has been repaired or re-suspended rather than replaced. A colour M-mode recording across the left ventricular outflow tract is used to assess the significance of any residual aortic regurgitation (21), although the method has not yet been validated for the transoesophageal approach.

ACQUIRED VALVAR DISEASE

Mitral stenosis

In many countries in which rheumatic heart disease is still very prevalent, operations for acquired mitral stenosis constitute the single largest group of operations for reconstruction of a heart valve. In most countries in which intraoperative echocardiography is widely practised, however, the number of patients being treated by reconstructive surgery for mitral stenosis is falling because the disease is now relatively uncommon and because an increasing proportion of patients are treated by balloon dilatation at cardiac catheterization. As a result, surgical experience of open commissurotomy or repair of the mitral valve for rheumatic stenosis is declining, and so in the individual patient, intraoperative transoesophageal echocardiography may be quite helpful. Before cardiopulmonary bypass, transoesophageal

imaging can be used to identify that the patient is suitable for reconstruction rather than valvar replacement; for example, it will show whether or not the leaflets are sufficiently pliable (22). Unless the left atrium is very large, it should be possible using pulsed Doppler from the oesophagus to measure the peak gradient across the mitral valve without interference by aliasing. After bypass, colour flow mapping is useful for checking that a satisfactory result has been achieved, and that there is no significant residual regurgitation. If the result is unacceptable, the surgeon can re-establish cardiopulmonary bypass and replace the valve. In comparison, epicardial echocardiography is less useful for assessing residual regurgitation in patients who have calcification in the mitral leaflets or annulus, because these cause masking of flow maps in the left atrium.

Mitral regurgitation

Mitral regurgitation is one of the main indications for intraoperative echocardiography in adults, particularly since the scope and the number of reconstructive operations for regurgitation are increasing (23). Epicardial echocardiography has advantages over transverse transoesophageal imaging in the pre-bypass recognition of mitral valvar morphology, but transoesophageal

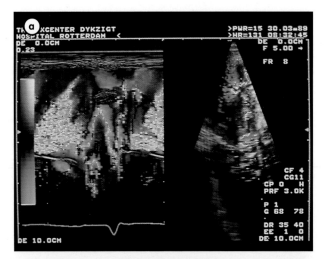

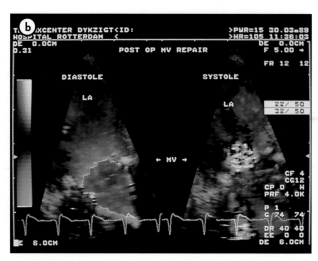

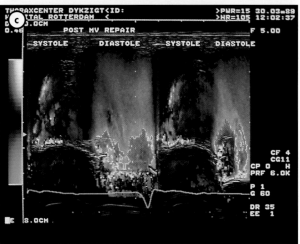

Fig. 13.3 (a) Pre-operative assessment of mitral regurgitation. The colour flow map (right side) is unclear, making it difficult to planimeter the area of the jet, but the colour M-mode display demonstrates severe pansystolic regurgitation, with the jet extending almost to the posterior wall of the left atrium. (b) Immediately after cardiopulmonary bypass and repair of the valve, there is unobstructed flow through the mitral orifice in diastole, and a small residual regurgitant jet. A mitral annular ring is clearly visible. (c) Approximately 30 minutes later, the extent of the persistent regurgitation has decreased even further, and the colour M-mode recording shows that it is restricted to the area immediately above the valvar leaflets.

echocardiography is particularly useful for assessing the severity of regurgitation before and after repair of the mitral valve, using either contrast techniques (24) or colour flow mapping (Fig. 13.3) (25). The relative strengths and weaknesses of the two approaches are summarized in Fig. 13.4.

During an epicardial echocardiographic study of the mitral valve, it is possible while scanning along the commissure to modify the position and angulation of the probe so that the imaging plane is maintained at right angles to the edges of the leaflets and the closure line of the valve. In contrast, transoesophageal echocardiographic analysis of the mitral valve in a series of transverse planes cannot demonstrate the posteromedial commissure, although it demonstrates well the middle and lateral thirds of the closure line and the leaflets at the anterolateral commissure. Longitudinal imaging allows better analysis of the posteromedial commissure and the medial third of the valve, as discussed in *Chapter 6*. Thus, in the absence of biplane transoesophageal imaging, it is difficult to be certain about pathology in this area. This is the principal reason why epicardial echocardiography is a more sensitive

technique for detecting and localizing abnormalities of the valve, which are relevant to the surgeon who is performing a repair (26). It is also easier to assess the size of the mitral annulus, as measured by surgeons, from the epicardial approach.

The diagnostic features of different patterns of mitral valvar disease, and the resulting patterns of regurgitation, are discussed in *Chapter 6*. It is possible before bypass to assess the structure and function of the valve in considerable detail, and the understanding of the mechanism of regurgitation that this gives can be used to decide what type of reconstruction is indicated (Fig. 13.5) (27). After surgery, valvar morphology should be studied again, for example to check that coaptation and normal apposition of the leaflets have been restored. If there has been a large quadrangular resection of the middle scallop of the mural leaflet of the mitral valve, then that leaflet is likely to appear immobile on subsequent echocardiograms (Fig. 13.6). Sutures can be identified in the leaflets, or in the subvalvar apparatus, for example after cordal shortening. When a mitral annular ring has been used, it will be visible, and it may prevent adequate colour flow mapping of the

Intraoperative Assessment of the Mitral Valve

	Transoesophageal echocardiography in transverse axial planes	Biplane transoesophageal echocardiography	Epicardial echocardiography
coaptation	+ +	+ + +	+ + +
apposition	+ +	+ + +	+ + +
prolapse	+	+ +	+ + +
retraction	+	+ +	+ + +
cordal rupture	+ +	+ + +	+ + +
annular size	+	+ +	+ + +
left ventricular function	+ +	+ + +	+ +
regurgitation	+ + +	+ + +	+ +
obstruction of the left ventricular outflow tract	+	+	+ + +

+ = some information but not diagnostic or quantifiable;
+ + = useful technique but some limitations; + + + = excellent technique

Fig. 13.4 Relative values of transoesophageal echocardiography and epicardial echocardiography, for studying the morphology and function of the mitral valve. For definitions of the terms used, see *Chapter 6.*

Relationship of Echocardiographic Findings with Type of Mitral Valve Repair

Apposition	Coaptation	Prolapse	Annulus	Surgery
normal	intact	no	normal enlarged	local repair (for example, for perforation) annuloplasty
normal	absent	no	enlarged	annuloplasty
abnormal	intact	AML	normal	cordal/papillary muscle shortening
		AML	enlarged	papillary shortening ± annuloplasty
		MML	enlarged	q resection MML, cordal shortening ± annuloplasty
		AML & MML	enlarged	papillary muscle shortening ± annuloplasty
abnormal	absent	MML	enlarged	q resection MML ± annuloplasty
		AML & MML	enlarged	q resection MML, cordal shortening/ re-insertion, ± annuloplasty

AML = aortic mitral leaflet; MML = mural mitral leaflet; q = quadrangular

Fig. 13.5 Relationship between morphological features of regurgitant mitral valves, and the types of reconstructive procedures that can be performed. Adapted from van Herwerden LA, Fraser AG, Gussenhoven EJ *et al* (27).

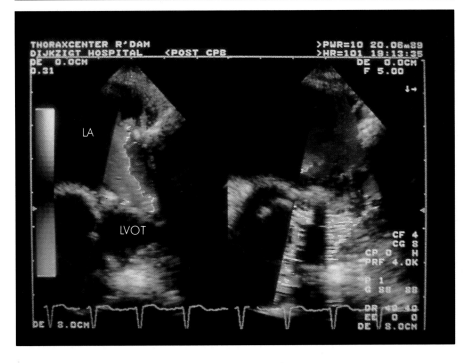

Fig. 13.6 Diastolic (on left) and systolic (on right) frames from a patient who had undergone an extensive quadrangular resection of the mural leaflet of the mitral valve. The pattern of inflow during diastole is asymmetrical because of the immobility of the mural leaflet. In systole, there is turbulent flow in the left ventricular outflow tract, but this is partly masked by the mitral annular ring that has been inserted. Epicardial echocardiography, with continuous wave Doppler studies, confirmed that the patient had developed obstruction of the left ventricular outflow tract.

left ventricular outflow tract from the oesophagus. This may be important in patients with co-existing aortic regurgitation, or when a patient develops obstruction of the left ventricular outflow tract as a complication of reconstructive mitral surgery (28). It is usually possible to recognize systolic anterior movement of the aortic leaflet and systolic turbulence in the outflow tract (Fig. 13.6) on transoesophageal imaging and colour flow mapping, but epicardial echocardiography is the preferred technique for assessing this problem. The gradient across the outflow tract can be measured noninvasively, and serially, only by using continuous wave Doppler from the ascending aorta (29).

One of the difficulties entailed in performing comparative studies of mitral regurgitant jets is that the loading conditions of the left ventricle are likely to change during any cardiac operation. There is often considerable systemic vasodilatation after cardiopulmonary bypass. Even when inotropes are used to ensure that arterial blood pressure is approximately the same as it was before bypass, the cardiac output and stroke volume may be higher. These confounding variables are likely to exaggerate the significance of any residual regurgitation that is detected by colour flow mapping. Thus, it should be realized that, even when heart rate and arterial pressure are more or less the same, comparative gradings are still prone to errors. Therefore, the colour flow map should not be used in isolation. Other factors should also be considered before a repair is deemed to have been unsuccessful and

the decision is made to go back on bypass and revise it. These include visual inspection of the valve and its competence during fluid instillation into the left ventricle, and haemodynamic variables such as left atrial pressure, heart rate, and blood pressure, although the height of recorded v waves does not correlate well with the severity of regurgitation (30).

It is impractical to perform detailed quantification of regurgitant jets in the operating room because the analyses are time-consuming. In any case, it is difficult on transoesophageal echocardiography to image the whole of the left atrium in the one image, and so it may be impossible to digitize the whole area of the left atrium for comparison with the digitized area of the regurgitant jet. Thus, more simple grading systems are usually employed; for example, the depth of the jet within the left atrium can be assessed (31), and its duration can be checked by recording a colour M-mode display (Fig. 13.7). Only pansystolic regurgitant jets are likely to be significant. It should be remembered that eccentric jets that flow along the surface of the opposite leaflet and then around the wall of the left atrium are influenced in shape by their contiguity with the solid atrial surface. Thus, they may be more significant haemodynamically than is at first apparent on the flow map (Fig. 13.8). One method of further assessing the significance of a regurgitant jet may be to study the pattern of pulmonary venous flow, as described in *Chapter 5*.

Mitral valvar replacement

When it is anticipated that the mitral valve will have to be replaced, it is unnecessary to perform a pre-bypass echocardiographic study. Similarly, if no technical difficulties are encountered, and if the surgeon has no problems in weaning the patient from cardiopulmonary bypass, then post-bypass echocardiography has little to contribute. If problems are encountered, or if the patient is in a precarious haemodynamic state as bypass is discontinued, then echocardiography may be very helpful. Epicardial imaging is not particularly useful because the prosthetic valve prevents imaging or colour flow mapping in the left atrium. Transoesophageal echocardiography is not affected by such problems, and it is usually possible to introduce a probe during surgery, as long as the surgeon and the anaesthetist allow access under the drapes at the head of the operating table. It is easy to distinguish between left ventricular dysfunction, hypovolaemia, and a malfunctioning mitral prosthesis as the cause of hypotension. Paraprosthetic regurgitant leaks are readily detected, as discussed in *Chapter 8*.

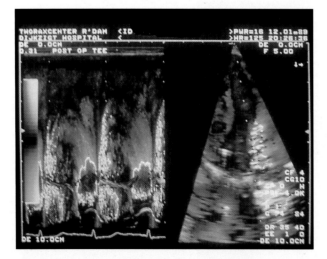

Fig. 13.7 A residual regurgitant jet that extends almost halfway into the left atrium (right-hand panel), following cardiopulmonary bypass. The colour M-mode recording demonstrates that the jet does not persist throughout systole.

Aortic valvar disease

Intraoperative transoesophageal echocardiography is unhelpful in assessing aortic stenosis. The ascending aorta and the left ventricular outflow tract are not well aligned for Doppler studies, and continuous wave Doppler is not feasible. Calcification before surgery, and of the prosthetic valve afterwards, cause considerable masking of both images and flow maps.

Transoesophageal echocardiography, however, is valuable when the primary lesion is aortic incompetence, or when a patient receives an aortic homograft or autograft. Residual regurgitation may be assessed after the aortic valve has been re-suspended. The function of the new aortic valve can be assessed after a homograft has been inserted, or after the patient's own pulmonary valve has been transferred as an autograft to the aortic position (32). In patients who have infective endocarditis and para-aortic fistulas or abscesses, which most commonly involve the posterior aortic root above the mitral curtain, colour flow mapping after bypass can confirm that any fistulas or abscesses have been closed or obliterated (Fig. 13.9).

Tricuspid valvar disease

Transoesophageal four-chamber views are useful for recording and analysing valvar regurgitation, and so intraoperative transoesophageal echocardiography can be used to assess the outcome of surgery for this lesion. After tricuspid annuloplasty, any residual regurgitation can be studied. As with mitral regurgitation, colour flow maps and colour M-mode recordings can be used in combination to identify a regurgitant jet and to assess its timing and duration. Transoesophageal imaging in the transverse axis does not allow clear study of the tricuspid leaflets, and so it cannot be used to assess their morphology in detail.

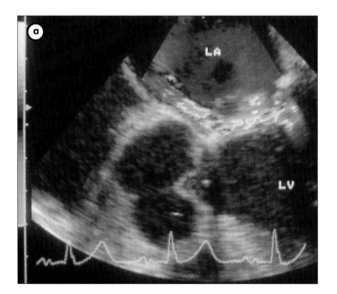
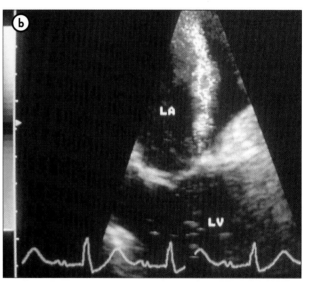

Fig. 13.8 (a) In this patient, the colour flow map obtained after discontinuation of bypass showed a turbulent eccentric regurgitant jet that adhered to the posterior surface of the aortic mitral leaflet. Detailed imaging of the closure pattern of the leaflets demonstrated that this was related to persistent asymmetrical apposition of their edges. Although the area of the jet was not large, pulmonary venous flow remained abnormal, and the patient's haemodynamic state also suggested that the result was unacceptable. (b) After a second period of bypass in which cords to the mural leaflet were shortened, this jet has disappeared. Unfortunately, however, the patient has now developed a free-standing regurgitant jet arising from the site of insertion of the mitral annular ring, suggesting that there is a small perforation in the mural leaflet. The area of turbulence may now overestimate the severity of regurgitation because it is caused by a high-velocity jet through a small orifice.

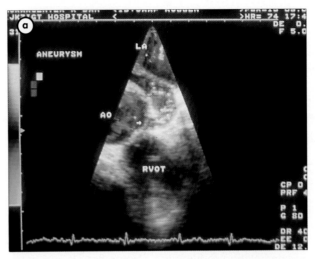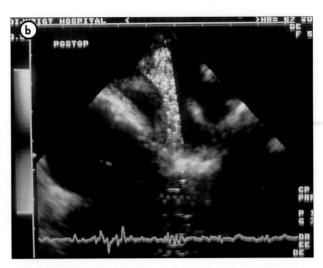

Fig. 13.9 Intraoperative transoesophageal colour flow maps (a) before and (b) after aortic valvar replacement with curettage of a posterior mycotic aneurysm in a patient with infective endocarditis. Flow into the cavity is clearly seen before the operation, but afterwards, the site of the aneurysm has been successfully excluded from the circulation.

Indications for Intraoperative Echocardiography during Surgery for Acquired Heart Disease
Transoesophageal echocardiography
mitral valvar repair
aortic dissection
valvar replacement for complicated infective endocarditis
tricuspid annuloplasty
monitoring of ventricular function (see *Chapter 12*)
Epicardial echocardiography
postinfarct ventricular septal defect
hypertrophic cardiomyopathy/myomectomy
Transoesophageal or epicardial echocardiography
homograft or autograft aortic valvar replacement
intracardiac masses
complex acquired disease (for example, fistulas)
failure to come off cardiopulmonary bypass

Fig. 13.10 Indications for intraoperative echocardiography during surgery for acquired heart disease.

OTHER ACQUIRED HEART DISEASE

Intraoperative echocardiography is useful during surgery for other types of acquired heart disease. Present indications in our institution are summarized in Fig. 13.10.

The major role of intraoperative transoesophageal echocardiography in patients with ischaemic heart disease is the assessment of ventricular function. This is discussed in *Chapter 12*. During operations for the acute complications of myocardial infarction, intraoperative echocardiography is able to define the site and morphology of ventricular septal rupture in considerable detail, but this is performed easily only from an epicardial approach.

SURGERY OF CONGENITAL HEART DISEASE

Nowadays, the majority of patients who undergo surgery for congenital cardiac malformations are infants or young children. In our own institution, approximately one-quarter of all patients undergoing total correction of congenital heart disease are younger than four months. Whereas children heavier than 20kg, and almost all adolescents and adults, can be studied with standard transoesophageal equipment (10), only the recent development of small, dedicated paediatric transoesophageal probes, with a maximal tip circumference of some 30mm, has made safe the investigation of infants down to a weight of approximately 3kg (33).

Pre-bypass transoesophageal studies

In patients with lesions involving the venous connexions, the atria, the atrial septum, or the atrioventricular junction, such as complete atrioventricular septal defects, studies before bypass can provide a better evaluation of specific morphology than may have been possible at prior precordial studies. Among some of its advantages, the technique can reliably detect multiple or fenestrated atrial septal defects, and it can definitely exclude cordal straddling of an atrioventricular valve through a ventricular septal defect. Such studies, therefore, may modify the planned surgical procedure. The clarity with which lesions at atrial or atrioventricular level are demonstrated is comparable to the information provided by the direct epicardial approach. The transoesophageal approach is better for assessing the sites of drainage of the individual pulmonary veins and their Doppler velocity profiles, so it is superior for defining abnormalities of pulmonary venous return and for monitoring their subsequent surgical repair (Fig. 13.11). In small children, nonetheless, difficulties may persist when an attempt is made clearly to define the patterns of anomalous pulmonary venous connexion. This is related to the potential interposition of the bronchial tree between the area of interest and the oesophagus, and to the relatively large artefact in the near field of some of the recently developed paediatric transducers.

The morphology of the tricuspid valve is frequently not demonstrated in detail by transoesophageal studies, as previously discussed in *Chapters 3* and *6*. Thus, in Ebstein's malformation of the tricuspid valve, which is normally associated with severe dilatation of the right heart, the transoesophageal approach is limited. If the surgeon requires detailed information about the individual leaflets, the tendinous cords, and the implantation of the papillary muscles, this is provided best by epicardial echocardiographic studies (34). Even then, complete studies may not be obtained in every case. Transoesophageal echocardiography, however, is a good method of assessing the function of the tricuspid valve.

Perimembranous ventricular septal defects, and their relationship to both atrioventricular valves and their subvalvar apparatus, are readily demonstrated by imaging before bypass. Colour flow mapping is mandatory to document small defects in the membranous septum, since echo dropout in this area may give rise to

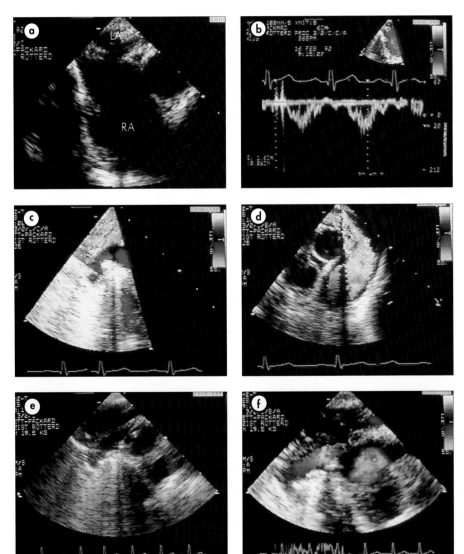

Fig. 13.11 Transoesophageal studies before and after cardiopulmonary bypass, in a child undergoing closure of a sinus venosus atrial septal defect. (a) The defect is located at the cranio-posterior aspect of the atrial septum, just inferior to the site where the superior caval vein enters the right atrium. (b) Before bypass, colour flow mapping and pulsed wave Doppler only document left-to-right shunting through the defect. (c) The right upper pulmonary vein drains into the superior caval vein, just anterior to the right pulmonary artery. Note the turbulent pattern of flow in the right pulmonary artery and the pulmonary trunk (d), which is related to the high volume of blood flowing through the lungs, rather than to any obstruction. (e) After bypass, transoesophageal echocardiography documents the site of the pericardial patch that was used to redirect the drainage of the right upper pulmonary vein and to close the defect. (f) Colour flow mapping rapidly excludes residual shunting or any obstruction to venous return.

false-positive diagnoses in older patients. Assessment of the integrity of the apical trabecular portion of the ventricular septum is unreliable using the transoesophageal approach. Even in the presence of a restrictive defect in older patients, the distance between the transducer and the area of interest is large, so that attenuation makes it impossible to obtain reliable Doppler signals. In these cases, the epicardial approach is far superior, although difficulties persist in detecting additional muscular defects in the presence of an unrestrictive defect. Demonstration of the true apex of the heart is difficult with both techniques.

With respect to the detailed assessment, before bypass, of complex congenital heart disease, including abnormalities of the ventricular outflow tracts or overriding of an arterial valve above a ventricular septal defect, the transverse transoesophageal approach has little to offer in the way of new insights. In our experience, it is clearly inferior to the epicardial approach because of the limited number of imaging planes that can be obtained.

Post-bypass transoesophageal studies

The relative values of transoesophageal and epicardial techniques for assessing the immediate outcome of surgery in patients with congenital heart disease are summarized in Fig. 13.12.

Transoesophageal studies performed at the completion of bypass, in order to document the surgical result and exclude significant residual lesions, provide only limited haemodynamic information. In particular, residual obstruction within either of the ventricular outflow tracts, such as after repair of a tetralogy of Fallot or after resection of a shelf obstructing the left ventricular outflow tract, cannot be evaluated reliably from the oesophagus because the Doppler beam is poorly aligned to the direction of flow of blood within these structures. For complete and reliable haemodynamic information, epicardial continuous wave Doppler interrogation, or invasive recordings of pressure must be used in addition. Similar considerations apply to intraoperative transoesophageal studies in infants undergoing an arterial switch procedure for complete transposition. Any obstruction across the anastomoses of the arterial trunks or the coronary arteries cannot be assessed.

All prosthetic materials used in cardiac surgery block the transmission of ultrasound to more distant structures. This causes masking both of cross-sectional images and, more importantly, of colour flow maps. In surgery of congenital malformations, prosthetic patches such as those used to close ventricular septal defects,

cause most problems, but teflon pledgets used to secure a suture line, and even the suture material itself, frequently produce artefacts in colour flow maps. Masking means that epicardial studies are limited in detecting or excluding mitral regurgitation after patch closure of a large ventricular septal defect (Fig. 13.13a), and in assessing prosthetic interatrial baffles, conduits, and prosthetic valves. Occasionally, the difficulty may be overcome by changing the position of the transducer on the epicardium, and the plane of scanning, but, more often, the transoesophageal approach helps to complete the post-bypass study. It cannot, in our experience, reliably exclude residual shunting after closure of a ventricular septal defect with a patch (Fig. 13.13b). The prosthetic material is usually interposed between the transducer and the the right ventricle, resulting in the masking of large areas of interest. The only way to circumvent this problem is to inject contrast into a left atrial line while scanning the pulmonary trunk. This technique provides reliable

Intraoperative Assessment of Surgery for Congenital Heart Disease		
	Transoesophageal	**Epicardial**
Residual lesion/procedure		
systemic venous obstruction	+	+++
pulmonary venous obstruction	+++	+
residual atrial shunting	+++	++
atrioventricular valvar regurgitation	+++	+
ventricular inflow obstruction	+++	++
prosthetic atrioventricular valvar replacement	+++	+
residual interventricular shunting	−	+++
obstruction of the ventricular outflow tract	−	+++
obstructive anastomoses great arteries	−	+++
extracardiac conduits	−(++)*	++
Mustard/Senning procedure		
baffle leaks	+++	++
baffle obstruction	+++	+
pulmonary venous obstruction	+++	+
Fontan-type procedures		
interatrial shunting	+++	++
obstruction atriopulmonary anastomoses	+++	++
obstruction atrioventricular connexions	−(++)*	++

− = unreliable; + = fair; ++ = good; +++ = excellent;
* = transoesophageal echocardiography only allows the pattern of flow into the conduit to be assessed, but this may be valuable in excluding obstruction during closure of the chest.

Fig. 13.12 Relative values of transoesophageal and epicardial echocardiography in the intraoperative exclusion of residual lesions after surgery for congenital heart disease.

quantification of any residual shunting (35), but it does not demonstrate its exact site. This information is of crucial importance when immediate revision is being considered, and it is provided by colour flow mapping performed from the epicardium.

Since residual interventricular shunts and gradients across the ventricular outflow tracts are the most common lesions to warrant immediate revision during a second period of cardiopulmonary bypass, transoesophageal echocardiography should not be used as the only intraoperative technique in patients with these problems. It should be combined with epicardial techniques in all patients who are undergoing surgical repair of lesions involving the ventricles, or else the epicardial approach alone should be used.

The intraoperative use of transoesophageal echocardiography on its own is particularly rewarding and effective in the surgery of sinus venosus defects (see *Fig. 13.11*), in the repair of atrioventricular valves (Fig. 13.14), in atrial correction procedures for

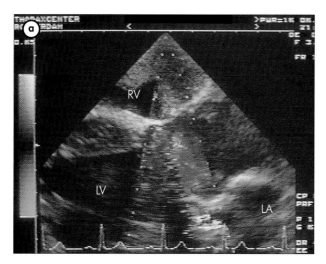
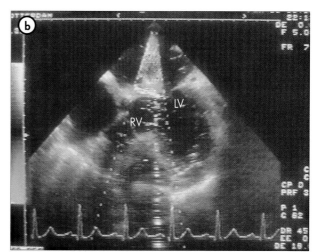

Fig. 13.13 Intraoperative echocardiographic studies performed in a patient after correction of tetralogy of Fallot and acquired mitral regurgitation. (a) The epicardial study excludes residual shunting across the ventricular septum, but it does not demonstrate the residual mitral regurgitation well. (b) The corresponding transoesophageal study clearly identifies that there is a residual regurgitant jet behind the aortic leaflet of the mitral valve, but it cannot exclude residual interventricular shunting because the prosthetic patch closing the ventricular septal defect causes a large area of flow masking in the right ventricle.

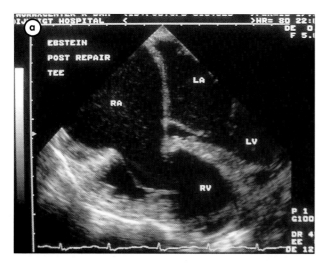
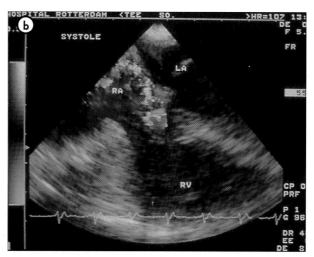

Fig. 13.14 (a) Four-chamber image obtained after repair of Ebstein's malformation. The plicated right atrioventricular junction, with narrowing of the tricuspid orifice, and the relocation of the anterosuperior leaflet, are well demonstrated. (b) In a different patient, the post-bypass colour flow map shows some residual tricuspid regurgitation that was turbulent and localized, compared with a much larger, laminar jet before the repair.

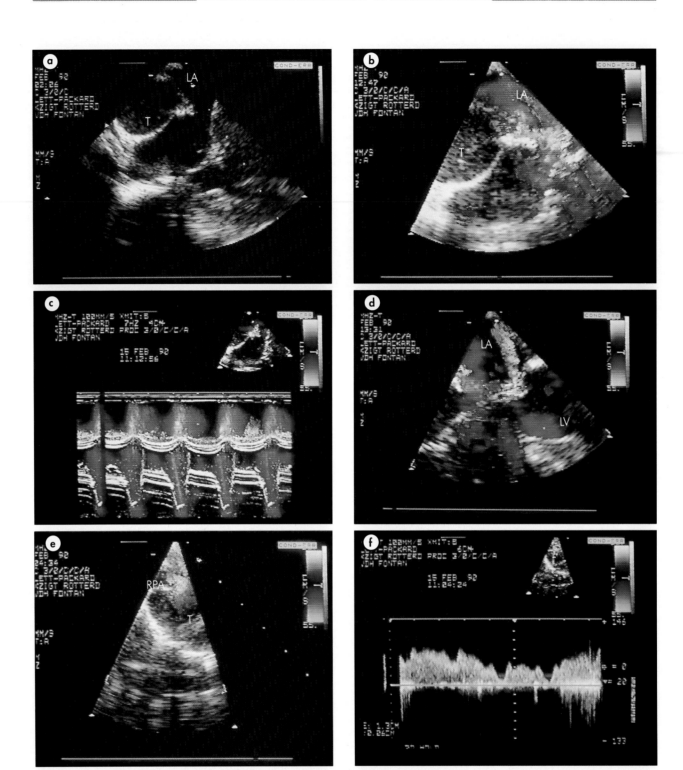

Fig. 13.15 Transoesophageal study after bypass carried out in a child who underwent a Fontan-type procedure for complex congenital heart disease (complete atrioventricular septal defect, double outlet right ventricle, and discordant ventriculoarterial connexions). (a) The morphology of the intra-atrial tunnel (T), which was created for total cavopulmonary anastomosis, is readily demonstrated on cross-sectional imaging. Although the suture line of the patch appeared to be intact, subsequent colour flow mapping revealed a moderate leak at the midportion of the suture line of the patch with the atrial septum (b). In the presence of high right atrial pressures, this results in a continuous right-to-left shunt as best documented on a colour M-mode study (c). In addition, mild regurgitation of the common atrioventricular valve is demonstrated (d). High short-axis views demonstrate the anastomosis of the 'tunnel' with the pulmonary arterial system (e). On colour flow mapping, there is mild turbulence at the site of connection with the right pulmonary artery. (f) The subsequent pulsed wave Doppler study reveals an almost continuous pattern of flow that varies considerably with respiration. This is a normal finding after such a procedure. The fact that the patterns of flow reach the baseline implies that the assumed obstruction is only minimal.

complete transposition, and in certain Fontan-type procedures for tricuspid atresia or other complex lesions.

As in adults with acquired mitral or tricuspid incompetence, transoesophageal echocardiography is useful in children with atrioventricular valvar regurgitation of congenital aetiology for assessing valvar function in detail. It is most useful after cardiopulmonary bypass for assessing residual valvar regurgitation following repair of an atrioventricular septal defect or suture of an isolated cleft of the aortic leaflet of the mitral valve. It can demonstrate the location and number of regurgitant jets clearly, but single-plane (transverse) transoesophageal imaging is not the best technique for demonstrating the morphology of these lesions because it is difficult to obtain short-axis images through the orifice of the left valve. Epicardial echocardiography is superior for this purpose. The transoesophageal approach, however, has the advantage that it can be used to assess patterns of ventricular inflow by pulsed Doppler studies, which is difficult from the epicardium. This information may be valuable after operations that have involved remodelling of either atrioventricular junction, since these can result in obstruction to ventricular inflow.

Following a Mustard or Senning procedure, the entire newly created pulmonary venous and systemic venous atria, including the anastomoses with the caval veins, can be visualized. The technique allows the detailed assessment of flow patterns within the baffle, the integrity of the suture line securing the baffle, and the morphology and function of both atrioventricular valves. Thus, pulmonary or systemic venous atrial obstruction, baffle leaks, and tricuspid valvar regurgitation, can be excluded with certainty. Furthermore, the exclusion of obstruction within individual pulmonary veins, which may be related to the placement of the suture line close to their orifices, is facilitated using the transoesophageal approach. In contrast, epicardial studies in these patients tend to be time-consuming and limited because it is difficult to align the ultrasonic beam with flow within the baffle.

Following a Fontan-type procedure (Fig. 13.15) with direct (retroaortic) anastomosis between the right atrium and the pulmonary arterial system, the site of anastomosis can be clearly visualized using transoesophageal echocardiography, in every patient. Colour flow mapping and pulsed wave Doppler studies allow the rapid exclusion of obstruction. The integrity of the interatrial septum can be documented easily, permitting the definite exclusion of residual atrial shunting. This is one of the most frequent lesions that requires early re-operation. In patients undergoing a modification of this procedure, in particular those in whom a conduit is placed anteriorly, the transoesophageal approach is limited because of the distance from the oesophagus to the conduit, and its strong reflection of ultrasound. Nevertheless, flow patterns into the conduit and within the pulmonary trunk can be monitored. This is particularly relevant while the chest is being closed, as sternal compression may cause obstruction of an anteriorly placed conduit.

ADVANTAGES AND LIMITATIONS OF TRANSOESOPHAGEAL AND EPICARDIAL ECHOCARDIOGRAPHY

Single-plane imaging in the transverse axis from the oesophagus can produce only a limited number of scan planes. In this respect, it is markedly inferior to epicardial echocardiography, which is limited only by the relatively large dimensions of standard precordial transducers, compared with the size of the sternotomy. The disparity in size makes it impossible to obtain views from the posterior and the lateral aspects of the heart and the cardiac apex. In contrast, the transoesophageal approach provides excellent information about the venous return to the heart, the atrial septum, and the function of the atrioventricular valves. It cannot, however, demonstrate much of the ventricular septum or the left ventricular apex. The limitations that result from only imaging in the transverse axis are most apparent in the assessment of specific aspects of complex congenital heart disease (such as the ventricular outflow tracts), of some aspects of acquired diseases of the atrioventricular valves (such as the posteromedial commissure of the mitral valve), and of the thoracic aorta. Thus, to provide a full range of intraoperative imaging planes from which maximal morphologic information can be derived, a combination of the transoesophageal and epicardial approaches is beneficial in selected patients.

Another drawback of the transoesophageal technique is that it does not allow a detailed haemodynamic assessment of many intracardiac lesions. Except for flow across the mitral valve, and within the pulmonary veins and the right pulmonary artery, interrogation using pulsed Doppler is generally compromised by a poor angle of incidence. Although the (semi-) quantification of residual lesions is extremely difficult immediately after cardiopulmonary bypass using any technique, it has to be attempted in order to select those patients who require immediate revision of their repair. In our experience, this can be achieved better by epicardial ultrasound, except in patients with residual atrioventricular valvar regurgitation or obstruction to ventricular inflow.

A major advantage of transoesophageal echocardiography over the precordial approach, is that it provides superior images in most adolescent and adult patients. When it is used intraoperatively, however, and compared directly with epicardial cross-sectional imaging, there is no equivalent gain. In fact, the high-frequency and short-focus precordial transducers that are used for direct epicardial scanning provide images with better definition and higher quality.

Intraoperative epicardial studies can be performed in all patients, regardless of their disease or size. In contrast, transoesophageal studies should not be attempted in patients with oesophageal disease, severe disease of the cervical spine, or a major disorder of coagulation. Unless special paediatric probes are available, we also believe that transoesophageal studies should not be attempted in children. Even when these guidelines are followed, it is unlikely that the transoesophageal probe will be introduced successfully in every patient.

The principal objective of intraoperative echocardiography is the immediate identification of residual lesions, before the chest is closed. The probe should be left within the oesophagus throughout the operation, with the machine switched off when not in use in order to prevent any thermal damage to the oesophagus, since re-insertion of the probe immediately after bypass is more difficult, and more likely to be unsuccessful or traumatic. Although large series of intraoperative transoesophageal studies have been reported without complications, there is a theoretical risk of oesophageal trauma or haemorrhage, especially while the patient is anticoagulated during cardiopulmonary bypass. These considerations are even more relevant in small children, in whom the oesophagus is more narrow relative even to the size of dedicated paediatric probes. The routine use of uncuffed endotracheal tubes in young children is another potential problem, since it produces the risk of trapping of air in the stomach when there is a probe in the oesophagus.

An epicardial echocardiographic study assesses the surgical repair and ventricular function at a specific moment, but only transoesophageal echocardiography allows continuous monitoring of patients at high risk, during weaning from cardiopulmonary bypass, during closure of the chest, and during the early period in the intensive care unit. Precordial studies performed in the intensive care unit are frequently compromised by poor windows for ultrasound and by the presence of air in the anterior mediastinum. In contrast, the transoesophageal approach is of great value in this setting for the diagnosis and management of early postoperative complications.

REFERENCES

1. Spotnitz HM, Malm JR. Two-Dimensional ultrasound and cardiac operations. *J Thorac Cardiovasc Surg* 1982;**83**:43–51.

2. Sahn DJ. Intraoperative applications of two-dimensional and contrast two-dimensional echocardiography for evaluation of congenital, acquired and coronary heart disease in open-chested humans during cardiac surgery. In: Rijsterborgh H, ed. *Echocardiology*. The Hague: Martinus Nijhoff 1981:8–23.

3. Goldman ME, Mindich BP, Teichholz LE, Burgess N *et al.* Intraoperative contrast echocardiography to evaluate mitral valve operations. *J Am Coll Cardiol* 1984;**4**:1035–40.

4. Herwerden LA, Gussenhoven WJ, Roelandt J *et al.* Intraoperative epicardial two-dimensional echocardiography. *Eur Heart J* 1986;**7**:386–95.

5. Gussenhoven EJ, van Herwerden LA, Roelandt J *et al.* Intraoperative two-dimensional echocardiography in congenital heart disease. *J Am Coll Cardiol* 1987;**9**:565–7.

6. Takamoto S, Kyo S, Adachi H *et al.* Intraoperative color flow mapping by real-time two-dimensional Doppler echocardiography for evaluation of valvular and congenital heart disease and vascular disease. *J Thorac Cardiovasc Surg* 1985;**90**:802–12.

7. Hagler DJ, Tajik AJ, Seward JB *et al.* Intraoperative two-dimensional Doppler echocardiography. *J Thorac Cardiovasc Surg* 1988;**95**:516–22.

intraoperative transoesophageal two-dimensional echocardiography. *Anesthesiology* 1987;**66**:64–8.

9. Sutherland GR, van Daele MERM, Stümper OFW *et al.* Epicardial and transoesophageal echocardiography during surgery for congenital heart disease. *Int J Cardiac Imaging* 1989;**4**:37–40.

10. Cyran SE, Kimball TR, Meyer RA *et al.* Efficacy of intraoperative transesophageal echocardiography in children with congenital heart disease. *Am J Cardiol* 1989;**63**:594–8.

11. Sheikh KH, de Bruijn NP, Rankin JS *et al.* The utility of transesophageal echocardiography and Doppler color flow imaging in patients undergoing cardiac surgery. *J Am Coll Cardiol* 1990;**15**:363–72.

12. Kyo S, Takamoto S, Matsumura M *et al.* Early postoperative evaluation of results of cardiac surgery by transesophageal two-dimensional Doppler echocardiography. *Circulation* 1987;**76** (suppl V):V113–21.

13. Shuford WH, Sybers RG, Weens HS. Problems in the aortographic diagnosis of dissecting aneurysm of the aorta. *N Eng J Med* 1969;**280**:225–31.

14. White RD, Lipton MJ, Higgins CB *et al.* Noninvasive evaluation of suspected thoracic aortic disease by contrast-enhanced computed tomography. *Am J Cardiol* 1986;**57**:282–90.

15. Goldman ME, Guarino T, Mindich BP. Localization of aortic

dissection intimal flap by intraoperative two-dimensional echocardiography. *J Am Coll Cardiol* 1985;**6**:1155–9.

16. Schippers OA, Gussenhoven WJ, van Herwerden LA *et al*. The role of intraoperative two-dimensional echocardiography in the assessment of thoracic aorta pathology. *Thorac Cardiovasc Surg* 1988;**36**:208–13.

17. Fraser AG, Geuskens R, van Herwerden LA *et al*. Transesophageal and intraoperative echocardiography in aortic dissection and aneurysm [Abstract]. *Circulation* 1989;**80**:II-2.

18. Mohr-Kahaly S, Erbel R, Rennollet H *et al*. Ambulatory follow-up of aortic dissection by transesophageal two-dimensional and color-coded Doppler echocardiography. *Circulation* 1989;**80**:24–33.

19. Iwasaki M, Suzuki S, Takayama Y *et al*. The usefulness of two-dimensional transesophageal echocardiography in follow-up studies of dissecting aortic aneurysm. *Nippon Kyobu Geka Gakkai Zasshi* 1989;**37**:622–30.

20. Erbel R, Engberding R, Daniel R *et al*. Follow-up of aortic dissection by TEE — A cooperative study [Abstract]. *Circulation* 1989; **80**:II-2.

21. Perry GJ, Helmcke F, Nanda NC *et al*. Evaluation of aortic insufficiency by Doppler color flow mapping. *J Am Coll Cardiol* 1987;**9**:952–9.

22. Antunes MJ. *Mitral valve repair*. Kempfenhausen am Starnberger See: RS Schulz, 1989.

23. Cosgrove DM, Stewart WJ. Mitral valvuloplasty. *Curr Prob in Cardiol* 1989;**14**:353–416.

24. Dahm M, Iversen S, Schmid FX *et al*. Intraoperative evaluation of reconstruction of the atrioventricular valves by transesophageal echocardiography. *Thorac Cardiovasc Surg* 1987;**35**:140–2.

25. Kleinman JP, Czer LS, DeRobertis M *et al*. A quantitative comparison of transesophageal and epicardial color Doppler echocardiography in the intraoperative assessment of mitral regurgitation. *Am J Cardiol* 1989;**64**:1168–72.

26. Fraser AG, van Herwerden LA, van Daele MERM, Sutherland GR. Is a combination of epicardial and transoesophageal echocardiography the best technique to monitor mitral valve repair? [Abstract]. *Eur Heart J* 1989;**10** (suppl):33.

27. van Herwerden LA, Fraser AG, Gussenhoven EJ *et al*. Echocardiographic analysis of regurgitant mitral valves: intraoperative functional anatomy and its relation to valve reconstruction. In: *Epicardial Echocardiography* [MD Thesis]. Rotterdam: Erasmus University, 1990.

28. Mihaileanu S, Marino JP, Chauvaud S *et al*. Left ventricular outflow obstruction after mitral valve repair (Carpentier's technique). Proposed mechanisms of disease. *Circulation* 1988;**78**:I-78–I-84.

29. van Herwerden LA, Fraser AG, Bos E. Left ventricular outflow tract obstruction after mitral valve repair assessed with intraoperative echocardiography: non-interventional treatment. *J Thorac Cardiovasc Surg*; (in press).

30. Fuchs RM, Heuser RR, Yin FCP, Brinker JA. Limitations of pulmonary wedge v waves in diagnosing mitral regurgitation. *Am J Cardiol* 1982;**49**:849–54.

31. Miyatake K, Izumi S, Okamoto M *et al*. Semiquantitative grading of severity of mitral regurgitation by real-time two-dimensional Doppler flow imaging technique. *J Am Coll Cardiol* 1986;**7**:82–8.

32. Ross D. Pulmonary valve autotransplantation (The Ross operation). *J Cardiac Surg* 1988;**3**:313–20.

33. Kyo S, Koike K, Takanawa E *et al*. Impact of transesophageal Doppler echocardiography on pediatric cardiac surgery. *Int J Card Imaging* 1989;**4**:41–2.

34. Quaegebeur JM, Sreeram N, Fraser AG *et al*. Surgery for Ebstein's anomaly: the clinical and echocardiographic evaluation of a new technique. *J Am Coll Cardiol*; (in press).

35. Stümper O, Fraser AG, Elzenga NJ *et al*. Assessment of ventricular septal defect closure by intraoperative epicardial ultrasound. *J Am Coll Cardiol* 1990;**16**:1672–9.

14

Congenital heart disease in adolescents and adults

Oliver F W Stümper
George R Sutherland

INTRODUCTION

A complete assessment of intracardiac morphology and related haemodynamic changes is required for the optimal management of every patient with congenital heart disease, particularly when surgical correction is being considered. This is routinely performed in infants or children by means of precordial ultrasonic investigations, either in combination with cardiac catheterization or, increasingly, by ultrasound alone. Whereas the precordial approach can provide diagnostic information in the vast majority of cases in the younger age group, it is frequently limited when congenital heart malformations are studied in adolescents and adults. Imaging from the precordium becomes more difficult with increasing age due to the increase in size of the chest and heart, and to the natural reduction of the transthoracic windows for cardiac ultrasound. This is a common problem in patients with congenital heart malformations who have undergone previous intracardiac surgery via a midline sternotomy, since acquired fibrous adhesions further restrict the precordial window. In addition, complex malformations of the heart are frequently present when the heart is itself abnormally positioned and, hence, is completely or partially obscured by the sternum or the lungs, or is in the presence of significant abnormalities of the spinal or thoracic cage, which make precordial ultrasonic examination difficult. Finally, with the dramatic

improvements in cardiac surgical techniques, a number of older patients with complex congenital malformations who have previously been designated as being inoperable, may nowadays be considered as being suitable for total correction. Frequently, in this group of patients, neither combined precordial studies nor cardiac catheterization can provide the full range of morphologic and haemodynamic information required for the exact planning of the surgical repair.

The major advantage of transoesophageal echocardiography in this group of patients, is that a superior image quality can be obtained, which, in turn, allows a more detailed insight into the underlying morphology of many cardiac malformations. Thus, the use of transoesophageal echocardiography in adolescents and adults with congenital heart disease might be expected to be highly rewarding, both in the primary pre-operative diagnosis and in the long-term follow-up of complex lesions. Despite this, there are, to date, only a few reports in the literature on the potential value of transoesophageal echocardiography in congenital heart disease (1–4). The relative neglect of this fascinating application of transoesophageal ultrasound is, in part, related to the relatively small number of adolescents and adults with congenital heart disease compared to the total number of cardiac patients requiring transoesophageal examinations (although it is steadily increasing), and to the fact that transoesophageal ultrasound is still considered to be an investigative

Sequential Scheme for Transoesophageal Studies of Congenital Malformations of the Heart	
i)	complete atrial scan, including the definition of the anatomy of both atrial appendages
ii)	demonstration of the pattern of both systemic and pulmonary venous connexions, including a hepatic scan for documentation of hepatic venous drainage
iii)	documentation of the integrity of the atrial septum
iv)	definition of the mode and morphology of the atrioventricular connexion
v)	assessment of the morphology and function of both atrioventricular valves
vi)	examination of the integrity of the ventricular septum
vii)	demonstration of the morphology of the ventricular outflow tracts
viii)	definition of ventriculoarterial connexions and exclusion of pathology affecting the arterial valves
ix)	assessment of the pulmonary trunk and its branches
x)	demonstration of the morphology of the thoracic aorta

Fig. 14.1 The routine scheme adopted for transoesophageal studies of congenital malformations of the heart.

Standard examination planes	Visualization of cardiac structures	Examples of pathology visualized
Transgastric planes	ventricular morphology ventricular relations	supero/inferior ventricles ventricular dominance
	ventricular function cordal apparatus MV inferior caval vein hepatic veins atrioventricular valves	parachute MV interruption individual drainage common valvar orifice
Lower oesophagus	coronary sinus	unroofed coronary sinus dilated coronary sinus muscular inlet VSD
	tricuspid valve	Ebstein tricuspid atresia
	four-chamber view	offset atrioventricular valves atrioventricular septal defects perimembranous VSD
Mid-oesophagus	mitral valve	valvar regurgitation endocarditis
	atrial septum	patent oval foramen deficiencies of the oval fossa
	pulmonary veins atrial chambers	anomalous connexion atrial arrangement Mustard baffles divided left atrium
	LV outflow tract	membranes fibrous continuity arterial override
Basal views	aortic valve atrial septum	valvar aortic stenosis sinus venosus defect juxtaposition
	VA junction superior caval vein	concordance/discordance persistent left anomalous drainage RUPV
	RV outflow tract pulmonary trunk	Fallot patent arterial duct supravalvar stenosis
	pulmonary arteries	palliative shunts peripheral stenosis
Thoracic aorta	aortic arch descending aorta	coarctation arterial duct collaterals

Fig. 14.2 Summary of the sequence of imaging planes (and the lesions that they image) used during transoesophageal echocardiographic investigations in children, adolescents, and adults with congenital heart disease.

technique solely for the adult patient with acquired cardiac lesions.

In this chapter, our approach to the assessment of congenital heart disease in adolescents and adults is described, based on our own recent experience at the Thoraxcentre of some 230 cases studied on an outpatient basis.

Since the tolerance of the patient towards transoesophageal studies in the adolescent age group is often relatively poor, the use of appropriate sedation for these investigations should be a standard procedure. Oximetric monitoring should also be a routine precaution in cyanotic patients. The standard procedure for investigation, however, is essentially the same as that described in *Chapter 3*. Due to the complexity of some congenital heart lesions, or of the surgical procedures performed in their repair, the echocardiographic studies in adults and adolescents with congenital heart disease will largely focus on specific aspects and, therefore, will tend to be more time consuming.

OVERALL ASSESSMENT OF CONGENITAL MALFORMATIONS OF THE HEART

Transoesophageal investigations in patients with congenital heart disease, irrespective of their age, should follow a predetermined standardized protocol, which will allow a complete assessment of both the underlying morphologic changes and the resulting haemodynamic features. In our experience, the scheme shown in Fig. 14.1 has proved to be satisfactory. It is based on the sequential chamber analysis required in the diagnosis and classification of congenital malformations of the heart (5).

The guidelines listed in Fig. 14.2 are discussed further in this chapter, which describes the information concerning congenital cardiac malformations that can be obtained by transoesophageal echocardiography. The same guidelines are followed in *Chapter 15* on the use of transoesophageal echocardiography in children, highlighting the major differences between the studies as performed in children and adults.

LOCATION OF THE HEART

Whereas the precordial approach is often limited in patients with an abnormally located or rotated heart (midline or in the right chest), these abnormalities do not present any limitations to the transoesophageal approach. In essence, they simply require a different series of manipulations of the transducer, which are

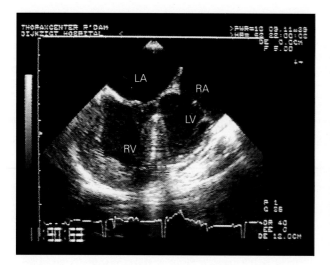

Fig. 14.3 Transoesophageal four-chamber view in a patient with mirror-image atrial arrangement (situs inversus), a right-sided heart, and discordant atrioventricular and ventriculoarterial connexions (congenitally corrected transposition). The left-sided morphologically right atrium drains into the morphologically left ventricle (fine trabeculations and no septal attachments of the atrioventricular valve cords). The right-sided morphologically left atrium drains into the morphologically right ventricle (coarse trabeculations and septal attachments of the atrioventricular valve cords), which is hypertrophied. The ventriculoarterial connexions are demonstrated by scanning a series of high transoesophageal views.

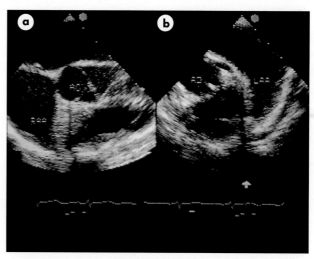

Fig. 14.4 The morphology of the appendages in a patient with usual atrial arrangement. (a) The right atrial appendage is demonstrated to have a blunt triangular shape; the junction between the appendage and the venous component of the atrium is wide. (b) The left atrial appendage is readily identified by its narrow lumen and the narrow junction with the atrial cavity.

relatively easy to learn; for example, in patients with a right-sided heart (dextrocardia), the sequence of manipulations is a mirror image of those required for studies in patients with a normally positioned left-sided heart. With experience, complete studies can be obtained in every patient (Fig. 14.3) and, indeed, minor degrees of abnormal position may even go unappreciated by the operator when the examination is conducted from the oesophagus.

ATRIA AND ATRIAL APPENDAGES

One of the major advantages of transoesophageal echocardiography is that the technique allows direct visualization of both atrial appendages, with cross-sectional imaging allowing the identification of their unique morphologic characteristics. The morphologically right atrial appendage is shown to have a blunt triangular shape, with a wide cavity and a broad junction with the venous component of the atrium (Fig. 14.4a). In contrast, the morphologically left atrial appendage is demonstrated as a long, crescentic and crenellated structure, with a narrow lumen and a narrow junction with the atrium (Fig. 14.4b). The appearance of both

appendages can consistently be differentiated one from the other. Thus, the technique allows the direct diagnosis of the arrangement of the atria (atrial situs) in every patient studied (6). Transoesophageal echocardiography, therefore, may be anticipated to become the most reliable technique for the determination of atrial arrangement in unoperated patients. Studies should be performed in those cases where ambiguity still persists after appropriate combined precordial echocardiographic and radiographic investigations (7,8). Juxtaposition of the atrial appendages is readily diagnosed by transoesophageal imaging. In the left juxtaposition, there is a characteristic deviation of the atrial septum into a more frontal plane when scanning a four-chamber view, and in its anterosuperior position is then demonstrated to form the floor and the posterior wall of the morphologically right atrium.

Both atrial cavities should be assessed by a series of short-axis cuts so as to rule out any abnormalities such as grossly enlarged valves of the venous orifices, Chiari networks, partitions within the atrial chambers (cor triatriatum), or supramitral stenosis. Transoesophageal echocardiography can provide additional relevant information, such as the exact site of insertion and the extent of these obstructive partitions, particularly in patients with divided atria, and in those with supravalvar mitral stenosis (2). Pulsed wave Doppler sampling then allows the assessment of any resulting gradient across these obstructive lesions. Whereas a continuous pattern of flow will be found in patients with partitioned atrial chambers, phasic patterns of flow are encountered over a supramitral stenosis (9).

SYSTEMIC VENOUS CONNEXIONS

The site of connexion of the inferior caval vein with the right atrium is readily demonstrated in every patient studied. The size of its venous valve (the Eustachian valve), in rare cases, may cause turbulent patterns of flow within the right atrium on colour flow mapping studies. When the inferior caval vein is studied, further advancement of the probe, together with clockwise rotation, allows the demonstration of its infradiaphragmatic portion, and, if present, documentation of a common hepatic venous confluence; this is of particular importance in patients with isomerism of the atrial appendages and visceral heterotaxy. This step of the investigation, however, is frequently poorly tolerated in unsedated patients.

The drainage of the superior caval vein is demonstrated by withdrawing the probe and imaging towards the right-hand side of the patient. A distal segment of this vessel can routinely be visualized before the right main bronchus precludes imaging of its midportion. Infrequently, in adolescents, the proximal portion can be demonstrated, together with the drainage of the azygos vein. Any assessment of patterns of flow within either caval vein by means of pulsed wave Doppler sampling is limited, since the angle of incidence is almost always at 90° to the stream when using imaging planes in the transverse axis.

Abnormalities of systemic venous connexions, such as a persistent left superior caval vein draining either directly into the roof of the left atrium or via the coronary sinus into the right atrium (see *Fig. 15.6*), or interruption of the inferior caval vein, can all be demonstrated. The combination of cross-sectional imaging and colour flow mapping facilitates the documentation of the course of these vessels and allows for the rapid exclusion of any obstruction to systemic venous return.

PULMONARY VENOUS CONNEXIONS

The documentation of the site of drainage of the individual pulmonary veins is greatly facilitated by the oesophageal approach when compared to precordial ultrasonic investigations (10). Demonstration of the connexion of all four pulmonary veins will be achieved in approximately 75% of cases using cross-sectional imaging and colour flow mapping. The right lower pulmonary vein remains the most difficult to visualize, and Doppler alignment to the flow patterns is generally poor.

The existence of anomalous pulmonary venous connexions, either partial or total, must be ruled out in any patient with congenital heart disease. Whereas the transoesophageal window provides substantially more information on supradiaphragmatic anomalous pulmonary venous connexions when compared with the precordial approach, the identification of partial infradiaphragmatic anomalous pulmonary connexions remains a problem. Partial anomalous connexions must be suspected in every case where all four pulmonary veins cannot be demonstrated to connect into one atrium. The right upper pulmonary vein, by far the most common vessel involved, must be systematically located just posterior of the connexion of the superior caval vein and caudal to the right pulmonary artery (see *Fig 15.5*). Although the abnormal drainage of the vessel can be demonstrated in almost every case, the inability to scan the entire superior caval vein, using transverse planes on their own, precludes the demonstration of drainage into its middle segment.

THE ATRIAL SEPTUM

The integrity of the interatrial septum is readily demonstrated in a series of short-axis cuts through the atrial chambers. The oval fossa must be closely inspected in order to rule out any patency, which, if present, will be demonstrated as a two-layer structure. Some flow may be detected on colour flow mapping between these layers thus indicating probe patency. Interatrial shunting may occur and is not necessarily demonstrated with a turbulent pattern of flow. Aneurysms of the interatrial septum, which are readily demonstrated on cross-sectional imaging, are described in *Chapter 4*.

The exact number, size and location of defects within the oval fossa ('secundum' defects) can be assessed by a combination of cross-sectional imaging and colour flow mapping (Fig. 14.5). The use of colour M-mode tracings will rapidly document the direction of the resultant flow, and allow the demonstration of transient right-to-left shunting, which, in the majority of patients, occurs at the onset of systole.

Sinus venosus defects, and their related patterns of anomalous pulmonary venous connexion, are best demonstrated when using high views of the right

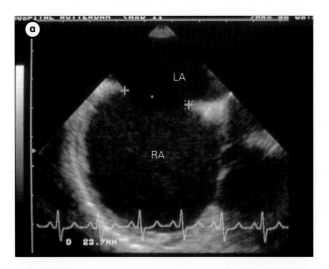
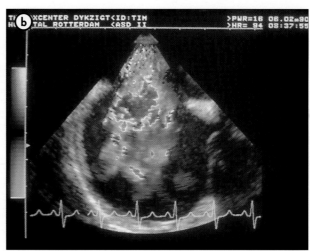

Fig. 14.5 Atrial septal defect within the oval fossa (so-called secundum defect). (a) The interatrial septum is demonstrated in an almost horizontal plane. The size and exact localization of the defect are visualized in close detail. (b) The subsequent colour flow mapping study documents the predominant left-to-right shunt.

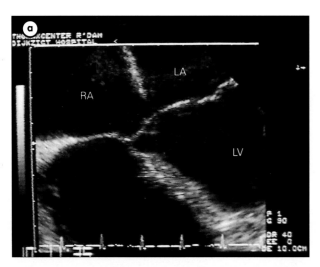
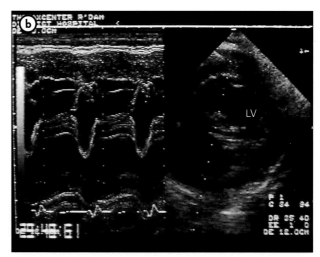

Fig. 14.6 A partial atrioventricular defect. (a) Transoesophageal view of an atrioventricular septal defect with only interatrial shunting ('primum defect'). Both atrioventricular valves are attached on the same level. (b) The transgastric view allows for the documentation of the trifoliate arrangement of the left atrioventricular valve that is usually encountered. The M-mode study reveals a failure of coaptation at this site, resulting in valvar regurgitation.

atrium and its junction with the superior caval vein. Colour flow mapping facilitates the identification of the individual vessels and the related haemodynamic changes produced by these defects (see *Fig. 13.11*). The rare types of inferior sinus venosus defects that involve the inferior caval vein and the right lower pulmonary vein, can be demonstrated in the planes used for scanning the junction of the inferior caval vein with the atrium.

Defects of the atrioventricular septum with only interatrial shunting ('primum' defect) must be excluded in all patients in whom the atrioventricular valves are

inserted at the same level. Any such defect and its related interatrial shunt are demonstrated with more clarity than is obtained by precordial studies (Fig. 14.6). The demonstration of an atrioventricular septal defect with separate valvar orifices and interatrial shunting only requires the detailed assessment of the morphology and function of both atrioventricular valves. In particular, the trifoliate arrangement of the left valve ('cleft' mitral valve) has to be excluded; if present, it is best demonstrated by transgastric short-axis views (Fig. 14.6b).

The potential for shunting across the atrioventricular septal defect at ventricular level presages a different

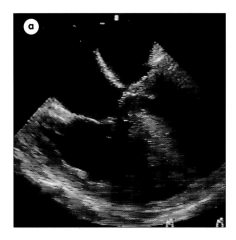
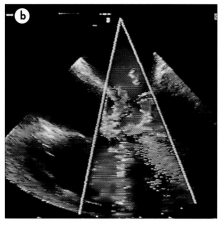

Fig. 14.7 Atrioventricular septal defect with both interatrial and interventricular shunting. (a) The individual components of the common atrioventricular valve are readily demonstrated on a series of four-chamber views, as are their cordal attachments. (b) The close-packed cords of the bridging leaflets cause the mild restriction of the interventricular shunt, which is shown by colour flow mapping.

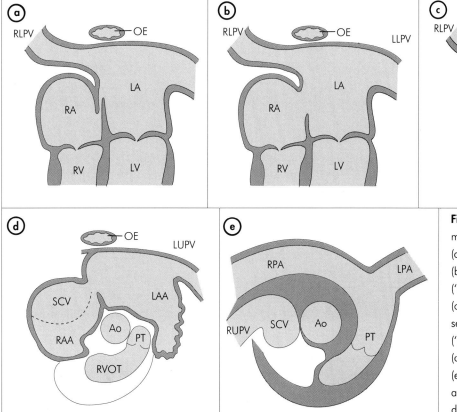
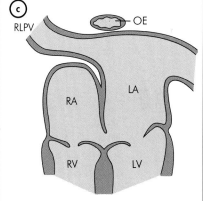

Fig. 14.8 Synopsis of the malformations of the interatrial septum.
(a) Patent oval foramen.
(b) Deficiency of the oval fossa ('secundum' defect).
(c) Atrioventricular septal defect with separate atrioventricular valves ('primum' defect).
(d) Sinus venosus defect.
(e) Anomalous drainage of the RUPV associated with the sinus venosus defect.

natural history and requires different surgical management. The morphology of the common atrioventricular valve found with a complete atrioventricular septal defect can best be assessed using a combination of transgastric and four-chamber views; these latter scans are particularly helpful in documenting any valvar regurgitation (Fig. 14.7). An attempt should be made in all patients with a complete atrioventricular septal defect to define precisely the size and the cordal insertions of the bridging leaflets of the common valve. Exact definition of the ventricular component of these defects requires the use of colour flow mapping or spectral Doppler for assessment of the related patterns of flow.

The mere demonstration of dropout of echoes in the inlet portion of the ventricular septum is by no means sufficient for diagnosis and documentation of the various forms of atrioventricular septal defects.

Defects of the atrioventricular portion of the membranous septum, with otherwise normal atrioventricular valve septation, lesions resulting in shunting from the left ventricle to the right atrium (so-called Gerbode defects), are difficult to appreciate on cross-sectional imaging alone. Colour flow mapping studies, however, will clearly reveal these defects and allow the precise differentiation from any co-existing tricuspid regurgitation. Such defects or shunts are occasionally encountered following surgical closure of perimembranous ventricular septal defects with reattachment of the septal leaflet of the tricuspid valve.

A synopsis of the salient features of the more common interatrial communications is shown in Fig. 14.8.

ATRIOVENTRICULAR JUNCTION

Since the detailed investigation of the atrioventricular valves has been discussed in *Chapter 6*, and the assessment of atrioventricular septal defects has been reviewed above, this section will concentrate on the morphology of the atrioventricular junction, that is, with the identification of the different types and modes of atrioventricular connexion.

In patients with an intact interventricular septum, the presence of concordant or discordant atrioventricular connexions can be determined fairly easily by observing the offsetting of the septal attachment of the atrioventricular valves, with the tricuspid valve inserting more apically (see *Fig. 14.2*). A more accurate criterion for the morphology of the ventricles, however, which can routinely be demonstrated by transoesophageal imaging, is cordal insertion of the tricuspid valve to the inlet component of the morphologically right ventricle. This is normally associated with the existence of fibrous continuity of the atrioventricular and arterial valves in the morphologically left ventricle. These features, particularly the first, are most important in patients with perimembranous ventricular septal defects opening between the ventricular inlets, since, in such patients, the septal attachments of the atrioventricular valves are inserted at the same level. Features such as the trabecular pattern of the ventricle, and the existence of a moderator band within the morphologically right ventricular chamber, are only inconstantly depicted with transoesophageal studies. These features, nonetheless, when taken together, permit the demonstration of ventricular topology in those patients with isomerism of the atrial appendages and a biventricular, but ambiguous, atrioventricular connexion.

Absence of an atrioventricular connexion is readily demonstrated by the fibro-fatty (sulcus) tissue of the atrioventricular groove, which separates the floor of the blind-ending atrium from the ventricular mass. This feature can consistently be differentiated from an imperforate atrioventricular valve, which is sometimes difficult to achieve by precordial investigations (see *Fig. 15.8*).

Double-inlet ventricles are also well demonstrated by transoesophageal cross-sectional imaging, the morphology and relationship of dominant and incomplete ventricles being clearly shown. In particular, the subvalvar apparatus can be assessed with much more clarity than can usually be obtained by precordial studies in older patients. Using a combination of four-chamber and transgastric views, all papillary muscles and the cords to the corresponding atrioventricular valves, as well as the implantation of cords into the crest of the ventricular septum, can be consistently documented (Fig. 14.9). In our experience, transoesophageal imaging would appear to be the technique of choice for exclusion of cordal straddling.

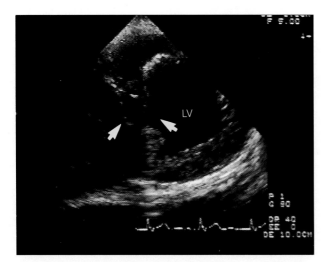

Fig. 14.9 Low transoesophageal view of the atrioventricular valves in a patient with double-outlet right ventricle. The precordial study in this patient failed to demonstrate the precise cordal attachments of the atrioventricular valves. Cordal straddling in the presence of a perimembranous ventricular septal defect, which extended into the muscular inlet portion, could be definitely excluded during the transoesophageal study. Although some minor cords were found to be attached to the crest of the interventricular septum, a complete repair could be performed.

THE VENTRICULAR SEPTUM

Precordial ultrasound has proved to be remarkably accurate in the assessment of ventricular septal defects. Problems persist only in the detection of multiple muscular defects, even when using colour flow mapping (11,12). In contrast to this, the transoesophageal approach in older patients allows only poor visualization of the anterior and the apical portion of the trabecular part of the interventricular septum. The distances between the oesophagus and these areas of interest are too great to allow satisfactory information to be obtained with colour Doppler. Transoesophageal echocardiography, therefore, has little additional information to offer in the diagnosis or definite exclusion of muscular ventricular septal defects. In fact, only defects of the perimembranous area and those opening to the outlet of the right ventricle can consistently be imaged. Doppler investigations are essential, nonetheless, since a dropout of echoes, particularly in the area of the membranous septum between the inlets may give false-positive results.

VENTRICULAR OUTFLOW TRACTS

The ventricular outflow tracts are frequently involved in congenital cardiac malformations. Demonstration of the precise morphology and function of either outflow tract is therefore a crucial part of every investigation. The excellent insight that is obtained by transoesophageal cross-sectional imaging of the morphology of the left ventricular outflow tract has already been described in detail in *Chapter 7*. It is noteworthy that any involvement of the mitral valvar apparatus can be clearly identified in these lesions. In contrast, the assessment of the right ventricular outflow tract in older patients with concordant ventriculoarterial connexions remains a problem during the transoesophageal study. It is frequently not possible to demonstrate the entire anterior free wall of the right ventricular outflow tract, nor the morphology of the pulmonary valve. This is particularly true in patients with long-standing volume overload of the right ventricle, such as that which occurs as the consequence of an atrial septal defect. The relatively large oesophageal ultrasonic window also decreases with age. Thus, in older patients, it will be the exception, rather than the rule, to get a good view of this particular area. Furthermore, the planes that can be obtained by transoesophageal imaging in the transverse axis remain unsatisfactory in assessing the right ventricular outflow tract. If demonstrated, the right ventricular outflow tract and the pulmonary valve are cut obliquely (see *Fig. 15.10*). The information to be obtained, therefore, is strictly limited.

ARTERIAL VALVES AND GREAT VESSELS

The transoesophageal evaluation of congenital abnormalities of either arterial valve remains difficult and most often unsatisfactory since the sections obtained produce oblique images of the valve leaflets, limiting the assessment of their finer details. The commissures of the aortic valve, with the exception of that between the right and noncoronary leaflets, are only poorly demonstrated. It is frequently not possible to rule out with certainty, the presence of a (functionally) bicuspid aortic valve. Lesions such as endocarditic vegetations,

nonetheless, are clearly demonstrated (see *Chapter 9*). The pulmonary valve is only infrequently visualized in adolescents and adults.

Only the proximal third or half of the ascending aorta is demonstrated by transverse-axis imaging. Pathologic changes, such as dilatation of the aortic root and the ascending aorta in Marfan's syndrome (see *Chapter 10*), or supravalvar aortic stenosis, nonetheless, can clearly be demonstrated. Whereas the orifice of the right coronary artery is difficult to visualize, the left coronary artery can routinely be demonstrated. In particular, the circumflex artery can be followed for a long distance. The finding of a dilated coronary artery should dictate thorough investigations for exclusion of a coronary arterial fistula, the course and drainage of which can routinely be identified by combined imaging and colour flow mapping studies (see *Fig. 15.13*).

Single-plane transoesophageal imaging remains a poor technique in the assessment of coarctation of the aorta; only localized ring-like lesions can be demonstrated with clarity. The approach remains incomplete in cases with more complex forms of coarctation. The technique does not allow a reliable documentation of collateral vessels, nor can the head and neck vessels routinely be demonstrated. The assessment of the pulmonary arterial system remains incomplete in most adolescents and adults. This is due to the interposition of both main bronchi between the oesophagus and the branches of the pulmonary trunk. The left pulmonary artery, in particular, can only be visualized at the site of the bifurcation of the pulmonary trunk, since the left main bronchus runs directly posterior to this vessel. In contrast, the right pulmonary artery can almost always be identified at the site where it crosses the superior caval vein.

EXAMINATION OF THE POSTOPERATIVE PATIENT

The majority of patients with congenital heart disease who will be seen by the adult cardiologist will be those who have undergone surgical correction in childhood. With the dramatic improvement of cardiac surgical techniques, the total number of these patients who attend the adult cardiologic out-patient clinic will be ever increasing. Unfortunately, a large proportion of such patients will present with residual haemodynamic lesions. The detection of these lesions, together with a complete assessment of the intracardiac morphology and the surgical repair performed, will challenge the diagnostic armamentarium of any cardiologist. Precordial studies are extremely cumbersome in these patients since the transthoracic windows are largely compromised by fibrous tissue adhesions that follow sternotomy. In our opinion, transoesophageal echocardiographic studies, therefore, should be carried out in all postoperative patients with suspected lesions at either the atrial or atrioventricular level, in whom precordial ultrasound cannot provide the full range of information required. The technique is widely available nowadays, must be considered noninvasive in the adult patient group, and is likely to contribute significant information on a variety of lesions.

REPAIR AND REPLACEMENT OF ATRIOVENTRICULAR VALVES

Following surgical repair of congenital abnormalities of the atrioventricular valves, a large proportion of patients will present either early, or late, during the follow-up period, with residual lesions such as valvar stenosis or regurgitation. Surprisingly, only a few patients suffer from endocarditic lesions, even when residual intracardiac shunts persist. The investigation of patients with suspected or proven atrioventricular valvar malfunction by transoesophageal echocardiography is extremely rewarding due to the detailed morphologic insights that can be obtained. In particular, the evaluation of valvar function after repair of the various types of atrioventricular septal defects allows a complete assessment of the valvar morphology and the subvalvar apparatus, and the precise determination of the site and mechanism of valvar regurgitation (Fig. 14.10). Limitations of transverse-axis imaging on its own in the

assessment of the entire line of coaptation of the leaflets (see *Chapter 6*) are less pronounced in patients with atrioventricular septal defects. The functional septal commissure (the 'cleft') of the left valve in partial atrioventricular septal defects, or the zone of coaptation of a former common valve in complete atrioventricular septal defects, can be examined in great detail. In all of these patients, the left ventricular outflow tract has to be carefully visualized for the exclusion of any co-existing obstruction. Left ventricular to right atrial shunts, which may be related to the imperfect placement of the surgical sutures, are readily excluded by colour flow mapping studies. The demonstration of convergence zones on the left ventricular side permits differentiation from any (co-existing) eccentric tricuspid regurgitation. Frequently, in this group of patients, sufficient information is obtained by a thorough transoesophageal study so that appropriate surgical therapy can be planned without prior cardiac catheterization.

In a small group of patients with congenital abnormalities of the atrioventricular valves, valvar replacement is performed as a desperate means to improve long-term prognosis. When this is carried out at an early age, the patient is likely to develop dysfunction of the prosthetic valve, which will frequently become too small. By the time these patients present to the adult cardiologist, the majority will have already undergone repeat valvar replacement and cardiac catheterization. Transoesophageal echocardiography would appear to be the diagnostic approach of choice (see *Chapter 8*). Since mechanical prostheses are preferred in younger

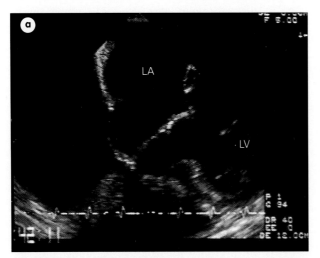
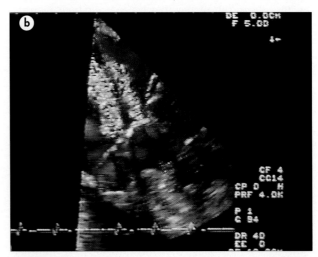

Fig. 14.10 Transoesophageal study in a patient after repair of an atrioventricular septal defect.
(a) The cross-sectional imaging study demonstrates the bulging towards the right side of the pericardial patch used in the repair. The right-sided component of the common atrioventricular valve is relatively small when compared with the left component. (b) On the subsequent colour flow mapping study, two regurgitant jets are demonstrated across the left-sided valve. One is centrally located, and the second results from malapposition of the superior and inferior bridging leaflets.

patients (13), however, a complete assessment of valvar function can frequently only be obtained when precordial and transoesophageal studies are combined.

FONTAN CIRCULATION

The Fontan procedure and its various modifications, became a standard surgical technique for 'correction' of tricuspid atresia, double-inlet ventricles, and other forms of complex congenital heart disease (14). The systemic venous blood is re-routed to drain entirely into the pulmonary circulation. This is achieved by establishing direct connexions between the right atrium and the pulmonary arterial system, or by using valved or nonvalved conduits. The principle goal of these procedures is to establish normal arterial blood saturations and to prevent the adverse effects of left ventricular volume overload. The majority of patients thus treated, however, will become symptomatic during their long-term postoperative period (15,16). More frequent haemodynamic lesions include residual intracardiac shunting, systemic atrioventricular valvar regurgitation, and obstructions to pulmonary blood flow (17).

Transoesophageal echocardiography, in our experience, gives a detailed insight into the Fontan circulation in the majority of patients (Fig. 14.11). Its use, therefore, may be expected to reduce the need for repeat cardiac catheterization in these high-risk patients. In particular, the pathologic changes to be found in the right atrial cavity (Fig. 14.12), the systemic and pulmonary venous connexions, and the function of the (left) atrioventricular valve, can all be assessed with more clarity than is usually possible using precordial ultrasound. The pulmonary arteries are particularly well demonstrated in patients who have undergone a direct

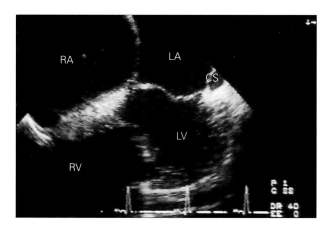

Fig. 14.11 Postoperative study in a patient with a Fontan circulation for tricuspid atresia (absent right connexion with the left atrium connected to a dominant left ventricle). The right atrial chamber is massively dilated, as is the coronary sinus (CS) that drains into the right atrium. Note the dense tissue of the atrioventricular groove, which extends to the crux, and the existence of a rudimentary and incomplete right ventricle.

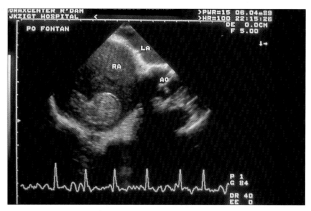

Fig. 14.12 Right atrial thrombus in a patient with the Fontan circulation. The large thrombus was found anterior to a prominent Eustachian valve, and extended far into the right atrial cavity.

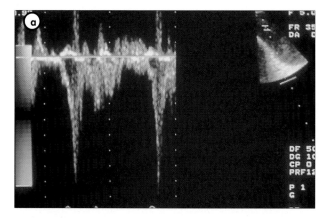

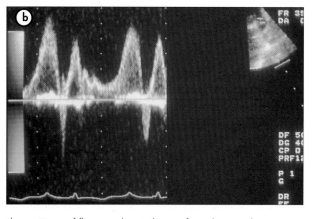

Fig. 14.13 Pulsed wave Doppler studies in a patient with a right-sided Glenn anastomosis and a direct connexion between the right atrium and the left pulmonary artery. (a) The right upper pulmonary vein drains in an almost posterior–anterior direction, thus patterns of flow are directed away from the transducer.
(b) The patterns of flow are, nevertheless, comparable to those that are obtained when sampling in the left upper pulmonary vein.

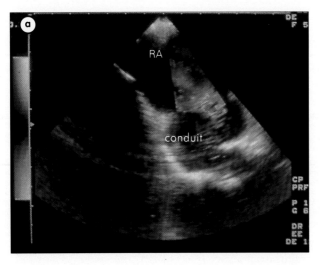

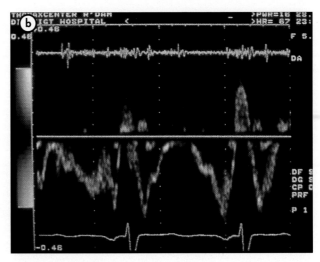

Fig. 14.14 The transoesphageal appearances of a direct atriopulmonary Fontan connexion in a patient with an absent right atrioventricular connexion. (a) Colour flow mapping study in a patient with an anterior conduit connexion between the right atrium and the pulmonary trunk. (b) Although the conduit itself appears to be irregular and narrow in shape on this section, the inflow patterns are found to be laminar and biphasic.

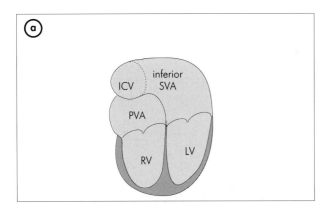

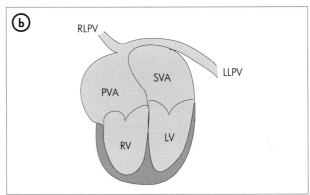

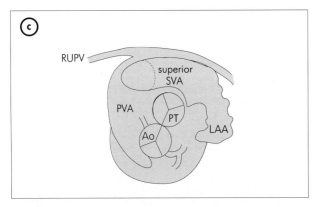

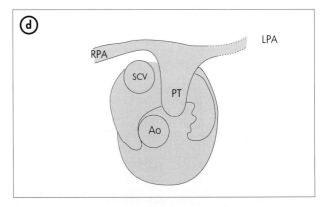

Fig. 14.15 Synopsis of the relevant cross sections of an atrial baffle, assessed by transoesophageal echocardiography.
(a) Low four-chamber view demonstrating the inferior limb of the systemic venous atrium (SVA). Anteriorly, the supratricuspid portion of the pulmonary venous atrium is routinely demonstrated. Posteriorly, both inferior pulmonary veins will be detected when the probe is rotated. The site of drainage of the inferior caval vein can be demonstrated by further introduction of the probe and slight clockwise rotation. (b) Standard four-chamber view in a patient with an interatrial baffle. The common portion of the SVA is demonstrated as is the mitral valve and the entire pulmonary venous atrium (PVA). (c) Further slight withdrawal of the probe and clockwise rotation demonstrates the superior limb of the SVA as well as both upper pulmonary veins and the posterior portion of the PVA. Both arterial valves will be sectioned in the same plane. (d) Final section through the pulmonary trunk and its bifurcation, demonstrating the distal portion of the superior caval vein .

atriopulmonary anastomosis (see *Fig. 13.15*). Transoesophageal studies allow for the precise documentation of patterns of flow within the pulmonary arteries, which, in combination with the patterns of pulmonary venous (Fig. 14.13) and mitral valvar flow, provide a detailed insight into the characteristic haemodynamic features of this circulation, which is largely dependent on the function of the left ventricle. The patency and unobstructed patterns of flow of a Glenn anastomosis can be readily assessed. In patients who were corrected by the use of an anteriorly placed conduit, or in whom the rudimentary right ventricle was used in the repair, the transoesophageal studies are limited to the documentation of conduit inflow patterns (Fig. 14.14), which, in combination with flow patterns within the pulmonary arteries and the pulmonary veins, represent an indicator of conduit function.

MUSTARD OR SENNING CIRCULATION

The evaluation of suspected baffle dysfunction, following atrial redirection procedures for complete transposition (Mustard or Senning procedures), is frequently limited from the precordial windows. Although the supramitral portion of the systemic venous atrium and the entire pulmonary venous atrium can consistently be visualized from the precordium, the individual limbs of the systemic venous pathways and the anastomotic sites of the baffle are almost inaccessible. Furthermore, the demonstration of individual pulmonary veins, and subsequent pulsed wave Doppler sampling, meet with the severest difficulties not only in adolescents and adults.

Transoesophageal echocardiography, in contrast, allows the complete assessment of both the entire systemic and pulmonary venous atria, and the demonstration of all four pulmonary veins in all patients studied (18). The relevant views that can, and should, be obtained in every patient by transoesophageal imaging in the transverse axis, are summarized in Fig. 14.15. The major advantages of the technique include consistent visualization of the site of the anastomosis of the superior caval vein with the interatrial baffle and the proximal portion of its superior limb. This allows the definite exclusion, or the detailed demonstration, of any stenosis within the superior limb, irrespective of its site within the baffle (Fig. 14.16); the same applies for the inferior limb of the systemic venous pathway. This latter step of the investigation, however, requires a scan across the liver to trace the inferior caval vein into the atrium and to check its anastomosis carefully. It is noteworthy that leaks across the baffle are frequently found

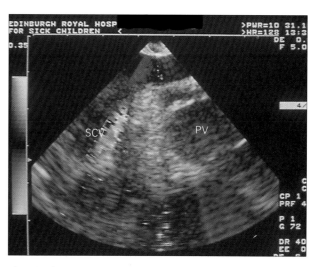

Fig 14.16 Severe obstruction of the superior limb of the systemic venous atrium. The echo-dense structure is situated at the area of the remnant of the interatrial septum that has to be resected during the subsequent repair.

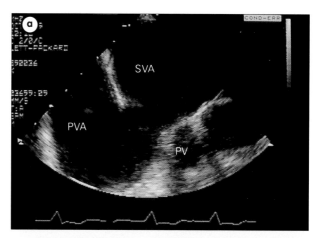

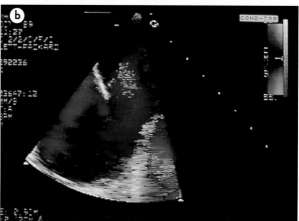

Fig. 14.17 The transoesophageal echo appearances of a large anterior atrial baffle leak. (a) Cross-sectional image of a large atrial baffle leak in a patient after a Mustard procedure. The suture line of the patch is disrupted from its anterior attachment on the level of the pulmonary valve (PV). (b) The subsequent colour flow mapping study revealed bidirectional, but predominant right-to-left, shunting.

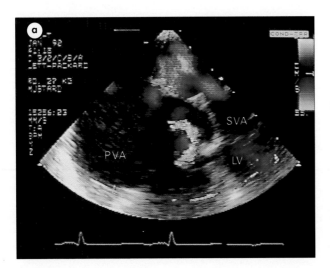

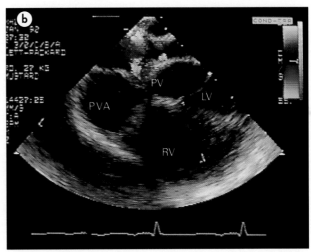

Fig. 14.18 The transoesophageal echo appearances of a large posterior atrial baffle leak. (a) Large baffle leak at the posterior attachment of the interatrial baffle to the crest of tissue separating the left-sided pulmonary veins. (b) Additional small baffle leak at the anterior suture line of the superior limb.

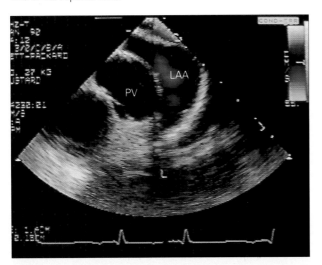

Fig. 14.19 Demonstration of the left-sided portion of the superior limb of the systemic venous atrium. The baffle is attached to the crest separating the left atrial appendage and the left upper pulmonary vein. Pulsed wave Doppler sampling of the patterns of flow within the left-sided pulmonary veins is essential for exclusion of individual pulmonary venous obstruction.

Fig. 14.20 Pseudoaneurysm formation of the perimembranous septum (arrowed) in a patient after a Mustard procedure that resulted in left ventricular outflow obstruction.

at this site; they must, therefore, be sought routinely. Other sites of leaks across the baffle, of which some may be detected on cross-sectional imaging alone, include the area where the baffle is sutured to the remnant of the interatrial septum (Fig. 14.17) and the lateral site of the anastomosis with the superior caval vein. In this latter area, however, dropout of echoes frequently poses difficulties in interpretation of the cross-sectional images. Colour flow mapping studies and pulsed wave Doppler interrogation have to be carried out to establish the diagnosis of leakage at this site. A thorough investigation of the entire baffle suture line,

by combined cross-sectional imaging and colour flow mapping, will allow the detection of multiple leaks or those in other, less-frequent positions (Fig. 14.18).

The pulmonary venous atrium is assessed just as well by the transoesophageal approach as it is by the precordial approach. Stenoses, which are less frequent than obstructions of the systemic venous pathways, are most frequently located in the midportion of the pulmonary venous atrium. Imaging in isolation, nonetheless, must be considered inadequate in providing all the information required. In contrast to the excellent assessment of the pulmonary venous atrium by both precordial and transoesophageal ultrasound, it is only the transoesophageal approach that allows the definite exclusion of obstruction of individual pulmonary veins in every patient studied. These lesions more frequently involve the left-sided veins, and are related to suturing the interatrial baffle onto the crest of tissue separating the left atrial appendage from the left upper pulmonary vein (Fig. 14.19).

The evaluation of haemodynamic lesions in symptomatic patients, following either a Mustard or Senning procedure, is highly rewarding using transoesophageal colour flow mapping and pulsed wave Doppler studies. Colour flow mapping on its own, however, may be misleading since turbulent intra-atrial or baffle flow is a frequent finding, even in the absence of haemodynamically significant lesions. Only careful studies using pulsed wave Doppler will allow a definite judgment to be made concerning the existence of obstructive lesions. The common feature of these lesions is a continuous turbulent pattern of flow distal to the stenosis. As the angle of incidence for Doppler interrogation of the systemic venous pathway is generally poor, the detection of high-velocity patterns of flow remains exceptional. The haemodynamic assessment of the pulmonary venous pathway should commence with pulsed wave Doppler sampling in individual pulmonary veins. This excludes any stenotic lesion and permits assessment of the severity of any co-existing tricuspid valvar regurgitation. Further sites of sampling have to include the midportion of the pulmonary venous atrium and the tricuspid valve.

In addition to the complete assessment of atrial baffle morphology and function, the transoesophageal technique is of great additional value in the assessment of ventricular function and in the documentation of any co-existing lesions, such as left ventricular outflow obstruction (Fig. 14.20).

MISCELLANEOUS PROCEDURES

Transoesophageal echocardiography is a poor diagnostic technique in the follow-up of patients who have undergone (prosthetic) patch closure of ventricular septal defects, since flow-masking properties of the synthetic material preclude reliable colour flow mapping information to be obtained in the exclusion of residual interventricular shunting (see *Fig. 13b*). The same problem arises following surgical correction of tetralogy of Fallot but, in addition, precludes the exclusion of residual right ventricular obstruction of the outflow tract. Thus, the clinician may be advised not to resort to transoesophageal studies in these groups of patients. Similar problems arise when an attempt is undertaken to evaluate the morphology and function of anteriorly placed conduits such as in the Rastelli procedure. Cardiac catheterization or magnetic resonance imaging remains the investigative technique of choice, if precordial ultrasound studies do not provide the required information in such cases. Follow-up investigations of patients who have undergone surgical correction of aortic coarctation are other less-rewarding areas for transoesophageal imaging in the transverse axis. Although narrowing of the lumen of the descending aorta can be identified in most cases where it is present, complex forms of re-coarctations are not reliably identified.

CONCLUSION

Transoesophageal echocardiography in adolescents and adults with congenital heart disease is of great value in pre-operative diagnosis, as well as in postoperative follow-up and management. It is a relatively new imaging technique in the field of congenital heart disease where it has the potential to contribute significant detail in a variety of lesions. In face of the ever increasing number of adolescents and adults with congenital heart disease, and the limitations of precordial ultrasound that are encountered in such patients, the role of transoesophageal echocardiography in this interdisciplinary field will increase rapidly.

REFERENCES

1. Hanrath P, Schlüter M, Langenstein BA *et al*. Detection of ostium secundum atrial septal defects by transoesophageal cross-sectional echocardiography. *Br Heart J* 1983;**49**:350–84.

2. Schlüter M, Langenstein BA, Thier W *et al*. Transesophageal two-dimensional echocardiography in the diagnosis of cor triatriatum in the adult. *J Am Coll Cardiol* 1983;**2**:1011–5.

3. Reifart N, Strohm WD, Classen M. Detection of atrial and ventricular septum defects by transoesophageal two-dimensional echocardiography with a mechanical sectorscanner. *Scand J Gastroenterol Suppl* 1984;**94**:101–6.

4. Sutherland GR, Geuskens R, Taams M *et al*. The role of transoesophageal echocardiography in adolescents and adults with congenital heart disease [Abstract]. *Circulation* 1989;**80**:II-474.

5. Tynan MJ, Becker AE, Macartney FJ *et al*. Nomenclature and classification of congenital heart disease. *Br Heart J* 1979;**41**:544–53.

6. Stümper O, Sreeram N, Elzenga NJ, Sutherland GR. The diagnosis of atrial situs by transesophageal echocardiography. *J Am Coll Cardiol* 1990; **16**:442–6.

7. Deanfield JE, Leanage R, Stroobant J *et al*. Use of high kilovoltage filtered beam radiographs for detection of bronchial situs in infants and young children. *Br Heart J* 1980;**44**:577–83.

8. Huhta JC, Smallhorn JF, Macartney FJ. Two dimensional echocardiographic diagnosis of situs. *Br Heart J* 1982;**48**:97–108.

9. Ostman-Smith I, Silverman NH, Oldershaw P *et al*. Cor triatriatum sinistrum. *Br Heart J* 1984;**51**:211–7.

10. Weigl TJ, Seward JB, Hagler DJ. Transesophageal echocardiography in anomalous pulmonary and systemic venous connections. *Circulation* 1989;**80**:II-339.

11. Ludomirsky A, Huhta JC, Vick GW *et al*. Color Doppler detection of multiple ventricular septal defects. *Circulation* 1986;**74**:1317–22.

12. Sutherland GR, Smyllie JH, Ogilvie BC, Keeton BR. Colour flow mapping in the diagnosis of multiple ventricular septal defects. *Br Heart J* 1989;**62**:43–9.

13. Carpentier A, Congenital malformations of the mitral valve. In: Stark J, deLeval M, eds. *Surgery for congenital heart defects*. London: Grune and Stratton Inc, 1983:467–82.

14. Stellin G, Mazzucco A, Bortolotti U *et al*. Tricuspid atresia versus other complex lesions. *J Thorac Cardiovasc Surg* 1988;**96**:204–11.

15. Ottenkamp J, Rohmer J, Quaegebeur JM *et al*. Nine years' experience of physiological correction of tricuspid atresia: long-term results and current surgical approach. *Thorax* 1982;**37**:718–26.

16. de Vivie ER, Rupprath G. Long-term results after Fontan procedure and its modifications. *J Thorac Cardiovasc Surg* 1986;**91**:690–7.

17. Leung MP, Benson LN, Smallhorn JF *et al*. Abnormal cardiac signs after Fontan type of operation: indicators of residua and sequelae. *Br Heart J* 1989;**61**:52–8.

18. Kaulitz R, Stümper O, Geuskens R *et al*. The comparative values of the precordial and transesophageal approaches in the ultrasound evaluation of atrial baffle function following atrial correction procedures. *J Am Coll Cardiol* 1990; **16**: 686–94.

15

Congenital heart disease in children

Oliver F W Stümper
George R Sutherland

INTRODUCTION

The precordial ultrasound approach yields diagnostic information in the vast majority of young children with congenital heart disease. Limitations to the information gained from this approach, however, are frequently encountered in children who have undergone previous intracardiac surgery, in those who have chest-wall abnormalities, or in those with an abnormally positioned heart. Furthermore, specific structures are frequently only poorly visualized from the precordium; these include the pulmonary veins, the atrial cavities, both atrial appendages, and the cordal implantations of either atrioventricular valve. Thus, when used in selected children, transoesophageal echocardiography might be expected to be of complementary value to the routine precordial approach when attempting a complete ultrasonic assessment of specific aspects of congenital malformations of the heart.

Although the investigation of children with standard adult transoesophageal probes (tip circumference of more than 50mm) has been reported to be a safe procedure in those with a body weight of more than 20kg (1,2), the routine use of such probes must be considered to be potentially hazardous in children. The recent development of small, dedicated paediatric transoesophageal probes, with a maximal tip circumference of approximately 30mm (that is, 7 x 8mm or 5 x 10mm), has made possible the safe investigation of

children down to a body weight of 4kg (3,4). These paediatric probes are constructed using either a paediatric bronchoscope or a gastroscope as a carrying device. The probes have diameters of some 7mm and steering facilities that are restricted to produce only anterior and posterior angulation of the tip. The miniaturization required for the construction of such probes has initially been achieved by significantly decreasing the number of ultrasound crystals mounted at the tip. This, in turn, has resulted in a reduction in quality of the image when compared to the standard 5MHz probes designed for use in adults, which have 48–64 element transducers. A second generation of phased-array paediatric probes (Fig. 15.1), however, has been

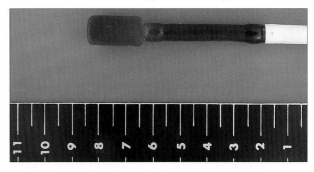

Fig. 15.1 Tip of a phased-array paediatric transoesophageal probe. The use of this probe allows the safe investigation of children down to some 4kg body weight. The dimensions of the tip are 5 x 10mm, and the diameter of the shaft is 7mm. Steering facilities are limited to anteroposterior angulation.

constructed for use in children; these probes contain 48 elements, thus providing a much improved quality of image. Secondly, the Doppler penetration of this second-generation phased-array probe (both for colour flow mapping and pulsed wave Doppler sampling) is much improved, so that this probe can allow diagnostic studies in patients up to a body weight of 50kg. In addition, the near-field artefact of these transoesophageal probes, which was once a problem in the initial phase, has been much reduced, thus providing diagnostic studies in even small children. The technical developments in the field of dedicated paediatric transoesophageal probes is dramatic. Annular-array transoesophageal probes, which will allow for continuous wave Doppler interrogation in children, will soon be introduced. Furthermore, 7-MHz, 64-element phased-array probes are under design.

In young children, diagnostic transoesophageal studies will normally be carried out under general anaesthesia during cardiac catheterization, or else in the perioperative period (see *Chapter 13*). Such studies are inappropriate in the out-patient clinic but, in older children, they can be performed safely on a day-care basis when carried out under heavy sedation in combination with local anaesthesia of the hypopharynx to abolish the gag reflex. This latter possibility becomes the more important as paediatric transoesophageal echocardiography evolves to become an investigative method of choice in the long-term follow-up of specific lesions (such as surgical correction at atrial level). Based on our experience with more than 170 studies at the Thoraxcentre, transoesophageal studies in paediatric patients should be considered to be a safe technique. In particular, we have not encountered signs of either oesophageal bleeding or any other probe-induced trauma. Transoesophageal studies could be performed successfully in all children of more than a body weight of 4kg; studies may well be performed in even smaller children. In our opinion, however, the diagnostic indication for transoesophageal studies in the unoperated neonate and infant remains questionable.

The morphologic and haemodynamic information

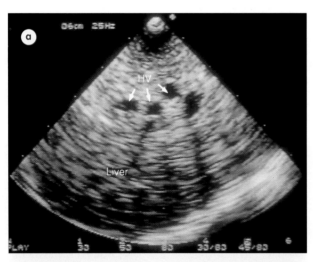

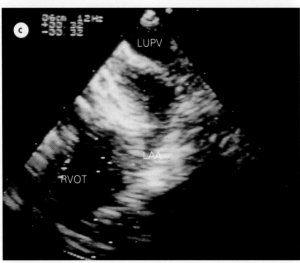

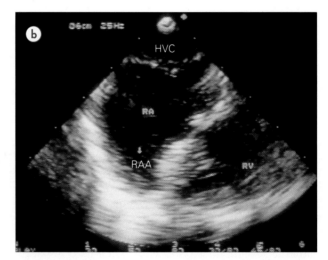

Fig. 15.2 Left atrial isomerism suspected in this 9-kg child after precordial investigation. The transoesophageal study showed (a) interruption of the inferior caval vein and a common confluence of the hepatic veins (HV) on the hepatic scan. Withdrawal of the probe and slight anticlockwise rotation demonstrated (b) the drainage of the hepatic vein confluence (HVC) at its normal position, a moderately enlarged Eustachian valve, and a right-sided appendage of morphologically right pattern (arrowed). Note the blunt ending of the appendage and its broad junction with the atrial cavity. (c) After demonstration of the left upper pulmonary vein (LUPV), the left-sided atrial appendage could also be visualized. The narrow junction with the left atrium, the crenellation and the long narrow lumen of this appendage confirmed it to be of left morphology — usual atrial arrangement (atrial situs solitus) was thus documented.

that can be obtained from single-plane (transverse-axis) transoesophageal echocardiography in children with congenital heart disease are outlined in this chapter. Relevant differences in the transoesophageal assessment of congenital heart disease in adolescents and adults are also discussed, in addition to some specific aspects of congenital heart disease seen in children.

ATRIA AND VENOUS CONNEXIONS

Transoesophageal echocardiography consistently allows the visualization of the unique morphologic details of both atrial appendages (see *Fig. 14.2*). This feature is the most reliable means of determining the arrangement of the atrial chambers. Direct ultrasonic visualization of morphology of the appendages should be performed in every patient with congenital heart disease (Fig. 15.2). The technique should prove particularly valuable in those rare cases where ambiguity concerning atrial arrangement persists, even after a combination of precordial ultrasonic investigations and the radiographic determination of bronchial arrangement using high kilovoltage filter films.

The morphology of the interatrial septum is similarly demonstrated in great detail when scanning a series of four-chamber planes. The region of the oval fossa is easily visualized, and its patency is readily identified by a typical two-layered appearance. Colour flow mapping of flows within the atria allows the rapid exclusion of any left-to-right shunting (Fig. 15.3). In cases where

doubt exists about interatrial shunting, the addition of a contrast injection via a venous line may be used to test for septal patency. The exact morphology of deficiencies of the oval fossa (secundum defects), sinus venosus, or the various forms of atrioventricular septal defects, is documented with ease using the transoesophageal approach; the echocardiographic features of such deficiences have been described in *Chapter 14*. In particular, the relationship of the individual sites of connexion of the systemic and pulmonary veins, with respect to a sinus venosus defect (see *Fig. 13.11*), can be assessed with much more clarity than is routinely possible from the precordial approach (5). Colour flow mapping is most useful in documenting the presence of interatrial shunting, but colour M-mode scans allow the best evaluation of the direction and duration of any such shunting, while pulsed wave Doppler interrogation provides the most reliable information concerning interatrial pressure gradients. Transoesophageal colour flow mapping is also a very sensitive technique for the detection, or definitive exclusion, of the multiple defects found when the floor of the oval fossa is fenestrated.

In children, the superior caval vein (sectioned in short axis) can be followed cranially for a greater distance than is routinely possible in adults. Frequently, even the drainage of the azygos vein will be identified. Partial anomalous pulmonary venous connexion of the right upper pulmonary vein to this vessel can be demonstrated in the majority of patients in whom this occurs. The exception to this is when the anomalous vein is connected to the site where the right bronchus is interposed between the oesophagus and the superior caval vein, thus precluding visualization of the midportion of the vessel. Further advancement of the probe to the lower oesophagus demonstrates the entire right atrial cavity and the orifice of the inferior caval vein. A high transgastric hepatic scan will then allow the visualization of the infradiaphragmatic portion of the inferior caval vein, together with the confluence of the hepatic veins (see *Fig. 15.2a*). This latter scan should routinely be performed in all patients with congenital heart disease since it allows assessment of inferior caval venous abnormalities and the exclusion of abnormal hepatic venous drainage. When the probe is withdrawn slightly from this position and rotated slightly in an anticlockwise fashion, the drainage of the inferior caval vein into the right atrium is demonstrated (see *Fig. 15.2b*). These scans are mandatory in patients who have previously undergone an atrial correction procedure for complete transposition so as to exclude any obstruction of the inferior caval venous pathway within the systemic venous atrium. They are also required for exclusion of baffle leaks, these being most frequently

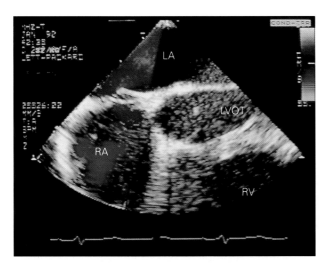

Fig. 15.3 Transverse-axis transoesophageal scan of a patent oval foramen. On colour flow mapping, there is evidence of flow between the two layers of the flap. On cardiac catheterization, the left atrium can be reached routinely through such foramens.

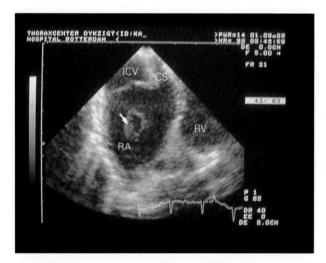

Fig. 15.4 Low-transverse axis view in a child with pulmonary atresia with intact ventricular septum. Normal drainage of the inferior caval vein and the coronary sinus is demonstrated. Note the redundant tissue of the venous valve in the right atrium, forming a prominent mobile mass (arrowed).

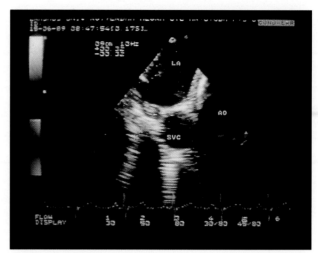

Fig. 15.5 High right atrial view for detection of the right upper pulmonary vein just posterior to the superior caval vein . When this vessel cannot be found at this site, an anomalous connexion of the right upper pulmonary vein must be suspected. Usually, scans of the superior caval vein will then demonstrate the site of drainage.

encountered at the suture line of the baffle at the inferior caval vein.

When scanning the orifice of the inferior caval vein in younger children, a remnant of the Eustachian valve is usually seen within the right atrial cavity. This structure tends to be particularly prominent in patients with tricuspid atresia. These valves at the venous orifices will be seen to cross the posterior aspect of the right atrium almost in a frontal plane. Redundant tissue of such valves may form a moving mass within the right atrial cavity and can be demonstrated in great detail — a feature of major importance in the differential diagnosis of atrial masses (Fig. 15.4).

The normal site of connexion of individual pulmonary veins can be demonstrated either by transoesophageal cross-sectional imaging, or by identifying, by means of colour flow mapping, the individual sites of venous return to the atrium. In contrast to investigations in adults and adolescents with congenital heart disease, the precise connexion of at least three pulmonary veins can routinely be documented in some 90% of cases, with identification of only the right lower pulmonary vein being problematic. The right upper pulmonary vein is usually located immediately posterior to the site of connexion of the superior caval vein to the right atrium and inferior to the right pulmonary artery. In cases where it cannot be visualized at this site (Fig. 15.5), partial anomalous connexion must be assumed, and subsequent scanning of the superior caval vein should be carried out. The left upper pulmonary vein is seen when scanning the cranial aspect of the left atrium; it is best found by identifying the left atrial appendage and scanning posterolateral to that structure. This should bring the left upper pulmonary vein into view, separated by a crest of tissue from the atrial appendage. Slight advancement of the probe, combined with anticlockwise rotation, will then identify the site of connexion of the left lower pulmonary vein. Pulsed wave Doppler sampling of the flow patterns within individual pulmonary veins should be routinely carried out; this is particularly important when individual pulmonary venous obstruction, or obstruction within the pulmonary venous atrium, is suspected. These can reliably be diagnosed by the detection of a continuous turbulent flow pattern on pulsed wave Doppler examinations. In patients with a variety of cardiac abnormalities, including the Fontan circulation, Mustard or Senning baffles, or a range of problems in the left heart such as obstruction of the left ventricular outflow tract or hypertrophic cardiomyopathies, the analysis of the flow patterns of pulmonary venous return can allow important new insights into the systolic and diastolic ventricular function and the severity of systemic atrioventricular valvar regurgitation (see *Chapter 5*). The patterns of pulmonary venous flow in children with congenital heart disease are, however, much more complex than in patients with acquired heart disease. Not only do traces vary with the heart rate, the volume status, and the site of sampling within the pulmonary veins, they are also altered dramatically by the existence and amount of any interatrial or interventricular shunting and the amount of the

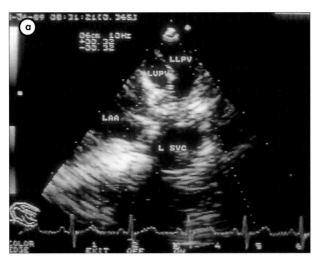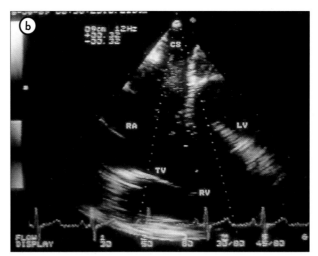

Fig. 15.6 The transoesophageal appearances of a left superior caval vein draining to coronary sinus. (a) Demonstration of the persistent left superior caval vein. The vessel is interposed between the left upper pulmonary vein and the left atrial appendage. The visualization of the left lower pulmonary vein in the same plane is the exception rather than the rule. (b) Colour flow mapping showed that the left superior caval vein drained into the dilated coronary sinus.

corresponding perfusion of the lungs (palliative shunts, pulmonary arterial stenoses).

In patients who are suspected to have a persistent left superior caval vein, the vessel will be found interposed between the left atrial appendage and the left upper pulmonary vein (Fig. 15.6a). In all cases, this abnormal vessel can be followed caudally and most often will be found to drain into a dilated coronary sinus (Fig. 15.6b). Other sites of connexion, and in particular connexion with a pulmonary vein, are more difficult to document. By using a combination of colour flow mapping and pulsed Doppler interrogation, however, this diagnosis should routinely be made using transoesophageal echocardiography.

The site of connexion of the coronary sinus within the right atrium can be demonstrated in every patient. Due to the rapid movement of the heart in small children, however, interrogation of flow patterns within the coronary sinus using pulsed wave Doppler is only rarely successful.

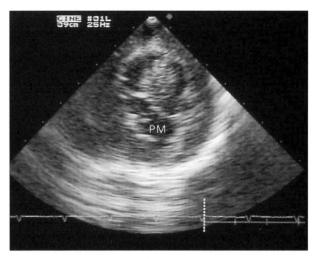

Fig. 15.7 Transgastric short-axis view of a parachute mitral valve showing the single papillary muscle.

ATRIOVENTRICULAR VALVES

Both atrioventricular valves and their subvalvar apparatus are best assessed by using a combination of four-chamber and transgastric short-axis views. These views will allow a detailed demonstration of any mitral valvar abnormality such as an additional septal commissure ('cleft' mitral valve). They also show the precise morphology of the common atrioventricular valve in the presence of a complete atrioventricular septal defect, or the single papillary muscle of a parachute mitral valve (Fig. 15.7). Although such morphology is readily demonstrated, the measurement of the diameter of the annulus of either atrioventricular valve is unreliable using four-chamber views because of its elliptical shape. High transgastric views allow for a potentially better assessment of these data. The transoesophageal approach is also ideal for demonstrating the exact underlying morphology of tricuspid atresia. Absence of the right atrioventricular connexion can be differentiated with ease from an imperforate tricuspid valve (Fig. 15.8). Although this finding does not influence the surgical approach to these patients, it contributes to a better understanding of the complex pathologic mechanisms in these lesions. The insertion of the tensor apparatus of either atrioventricular valve is better demonstrated

using the transoesophageal approach than by any other investigative technique. In our opinion, cordal straddling can be excluded with certainty in every suspected case. This has proved to be of utmost value in patients with complex abnormalities of the atrioventricular junction. The technique may become the ultimate diagnostic investigation, for example, in those patients with double-inlet left ventricles in whom ventricular septation is being considered.

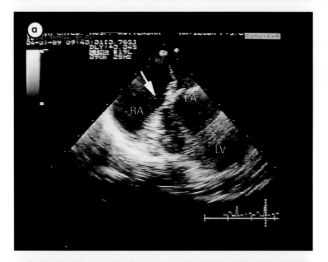

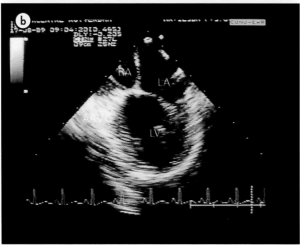

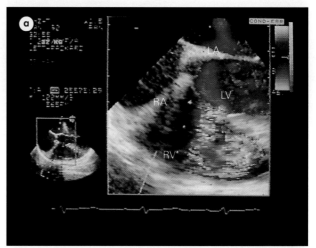

Fig. 15.8 Tricuspid atresia: imperforate membrane or absent connexion? (a) Four-chamber view in a patient with tricuspid atresia. The precordial study in this patient had suggested absence of the right atrioventricular connexion. The transoesophageal study, however, clearly defines an imperforate tricuspid valve (arrowed). Note the small right ventricular cavity and the attachment of both the imperforate valve and the mitral valve at the same level in the roof of a perimembranous ventricular septal defect opening to the inlet of the right ventricle. (b) In contrast, in patients with absence of the right atrioventricular connexion, ('classical' tricuspid atresia) the tissue of the atrioventricular groove extends to the crux cordis.

Fig. 15.9 (a) Transverse-axis view of a perimembranous ventricular septal defect opening to the outlet of the right ventricle with resulting right-to-left shunting demonstrated on colour flow mapping. Using a series of views, the exact relationship of these defects to either atrioventricular valve, to either ventricular outflow tract, and to the aortic valve, can be demonstrated.
(b) Demonstration of a small, muscular, outlet ventricular septal defect on colour flow mapping. Four-chamber views documented the normal offsetting of both atrioventricular valves, reflecting the integrity of the membranous septum. A precordial study in this patient suggested the existence of a doubly committed defect. The transoesophageal study, however, demonstrated a muscle bar separating the attachments of the leaflets of the arterial valves (arrowed).

VENTRICULAR SEPTAL DEFECTS

The fibrous continuity between the aortic and tricuspid leaflets, the hallmark of a perimembranous ventricular septal defect, is readily demonstrated using appropriate four-chamber views, as is the relationship of such defects to the components of the ventricles and the aortic root. The false-positive appearance of such a defect on cross-sectional imaging as a consequence of ultrasound shadows in the region of the crux cordis, is much less common in children than in adults. Colour flow mapping studies of restrictive defects, and pulsed wave Doppler interrogation of nonrestrictive defects, should be used to confirm the presence and site of flow across the septum (Fig. 15.9). Tissue tags and pseudoaneurysmal formations derived from the leaflets of the tricuspid valve, frequently encountered in patients with perimembranous defects opening to the inlet of the right ventricle, are easily demonstrated. Transoesophageal imaging in children can also clearly delineate the exact morphology of those doubly committed ventricular septal defects, characterized by fibrous continuity between the leaflets of the aortic and pulmonary valves. This should allow the definite differentiation from those defects opening to the outlet of the right ventricle with completely muscular rims. The additional information provided by transoesophageal studies in turn may be helpful in exact planning of the surgical correction. In contrast, the transoesophageal assessment of ventricular septal defects located in other areas, particularly in the apical trabecular portion of the muscular septum, is difficult and remains unreliable. Although restrictive trabecular muscular defects will be detected by transoesophageal studies in children, we consider the precordial ultrasound approach to be superior. In addition, only the precordial approach currently allows the provision of reliable haemodynamic data on ventricular septal defects.

VENTRICULAR OUTFLOW TRACTS

The assessment of either ventricular outflow tract by transoesophageal imaging in a single plane is much more easily effected in children when compared with similar studies in adolescents and adults. Nevertheless, even in small children, the evaluation of the right ventricular outflow tract remains problematic, since, although the infundibular portion, the anterior right ventricular free wall, and the pulmonary valve, can routinely be demonstrated, the scan planes in the transverse axis remain unsatisfactory (Fig. 15.10); only the use of imaging planes providing longitudinal sections

will solve this problem. Our limited experience with such a biplane transoesophageal probe has shown that the planes in the long axis provide superb demonstration of the entire right ventricular outflow tract (6). Although transoesophageal imaging in the transverse axis yields a more detailed insight into the underlying morphology of obstruction within the left ventricular

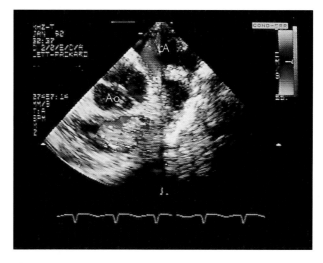

Fig. 15.10 Transverse-axis imaging of the right ventricular outflow tract in a patient with tetralogy of Fallot. The exact morphology of the infundibular stenosis, however, cannot be assessed in detail using sections in the transverse axis. Mostly turbulent patterns of flow are documented on colour flow mapping. Doppler interrogation remains unsatisfactory as the direction of flow is almost always perpendicular to the Doppler beam.

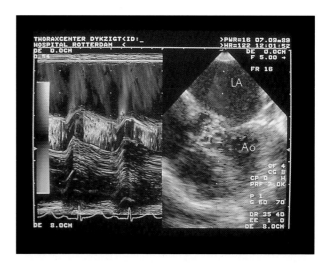

Fig. 15.11 Colour flow mapping of an obstructed left ventricular outflow tract. The transoesophageal approach allows a detailed insight into the underlying morphology of such a lesion but the haemodynamic evaluation is difficult. Aortic valvar regurgitation has to be excluded using colour M-mode studies.

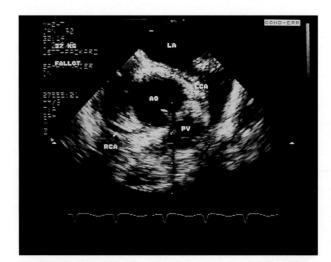

Fig. 15.12 Demonstration of the coronary arterial anatomy in a patient with tetralogy of Fallot and normal origins of both the right and left coronary arteries. Visualization of the branching pattern of the main stem of the left coronary artery allowed the exclusion of an infundibular artery, which is an important surgical consideration.

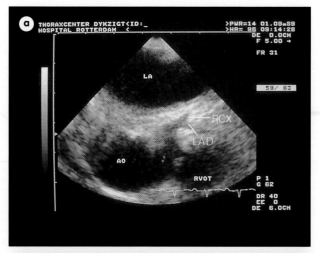

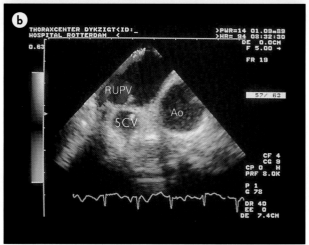

Fig. 15.13 (a) A dilated left coronary artery and circumflex artery in an 8-kg child, suggesting a coronary arterial fistula. (b) On subsequent colour flow mapping, a fistula was demonstrated between the circumflex artery and the left atrium, and the exact site of its drainage was documented. Note the (normal) drainage of the right upper pulmonary vein just posterior to the superior caval vein.

outflow tract than does precordial imaging, it has little to offer in the haemodynamic evaluation of such lesions. This is because the interrogating Doppler beam can only be aligned poorly to the direction of flow (Fig. 15.11). Both ventricular outflow tracts are frequently better assessed in children by using transgastric views with cranial angulation of the tip, rather than by scanning these structures from within the oesophagus. This is particularly so in patients with discordant ventriculoarterial connexions. The resulting distance from the transducer to the point of interest, however, is too far to allow any meaningful pulsed wave Doppler interrogation of obstructive lesions within either ventricular outflow tract.

CORONARY ARTERIES AND GREAT VESSELS

The origin and the course of the proximal left coronary artery, with its bifurcation into the anterior descending and circumflex arteries, can be visualized with ease in every patient studied. In contrast, the orifice of the right coronary artery is frequently difficult to visualize and, most often, only a short segment can be demonstrated. Visualization of the coronary arteries, nonetheless, should be attempted in every patient studied, especially in those with tetralogy of Fallot with pulmonary stenosis or atresia, who have a high incidence of abnormal coronary arterial anatomy (Fig. 15.12). The finding of dilated proximal coronary arteries may suggest the presence of a fistulous connexion of the coronary arteries, the course and drainage of which can normally be identified using colour flow mapping (Fig. 15.13). Furthermore, in patients with pulmonary atresia and an intact ventricular septum, fistulous communications from the coronary arteries to the right ventricle are readily demonstrated, as are the majority of coronary arterial aneurysms in patients with Kawasaki's disease. In this latter group of patients, transoesophageal echocardiography may become particularly useful in serial follow-up studies when aneurysms of proximal coronary arteries have been identified, or when diagnostic ambiguity persists after high-quality precordial ultrasound studies.

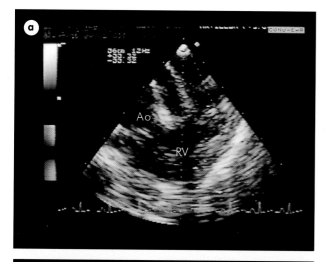

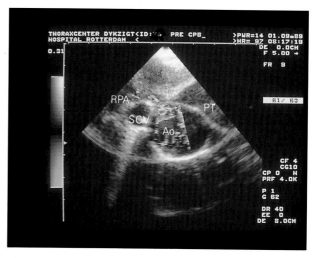

Fig. 15.15 Total obstruction of the right pulmonary artery in a child with a long-standing Waterston shunt. The exact morphology of the communication, the related patterns of arterial flow and the right pulmonary branch can all be documented with ease in children when using these high cuts in the short axis.

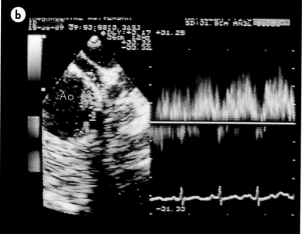

Fig. 15.14 Transoesophageal studies in two patients with atretic pulmonary outflow tracts. (a) Underneath the imperforate pulmonary valve, there is a moderate-sized right ventricular chamber. The imperforate valve moved during the cardiac cycle. (b) The typical 'seagull' appearance of the central pulmonary arteries is well demonstrated in this patient with an atretic infundibulum. Pulsed wave Doppler interrogation documents the pattern of flow in the right pulmonary artery in the presence of a left-sided Blalock shunt.

The central pulmonary arterial system can be examined more easily in children than in adults. The extent of visualization of these arteries is largely dependent on a combination of features, including the size of the patient, the underlying cardiac malformation, the overall cardiac dimensions, and the existence of ventricular hypertrophy. Nevertheless, the visualization of the central pulmonary arteries, and the assessment of flow patterns within the pulmonary arteries by combined colour flow mapping and pulsed wave Doppler studies, should be a routine part of every study. The precise definition of the underlying morphology of an atretic pulmonary outflow tract (imperforate valve versus atretic

infundibulum) is routinely possible (Fig. 15.14). The pulmonary trunk and its bifurcation are easily seen when present, and pulsed wave Doppler investigations of the characteristics of pulmonary arterial flow can be carried out with an accurate angle of incidence to the interrogating Doppler beam. In almost every case, the right pulmonary artery can be followed to just distal to the point where it crosses the superior caval vein, permitting visualization of its first peripheral branch point (Fig. 15.15). In contrast, the left pulmonary artery can only be seen in infants, as it is partially obscured in older children by the left main bronchus. When this occurs, the vessel will only be demonstrated proximally at its origin and distally where it lies anterior to the descending aorta. Again, pulsed wave Doppler interrogation can be performed with a reasonable angle of incidence in the distal segment of this vessel. Thus, transoesophageal echocardiography would appear to be a valuable investigative technique in children for the evaluation of suspected stenosis of the branch pulmonary arteries.

The patency of systemic to pulmonary shunts is readily documented on pulsed wave Doppler studies by confirming continuous flow within the relevant branch of the pulmonary trunk, as are stenoses and obstructions within the pulmonary arterial system proximal to these shunts. The site of anastomosis of long-standing Blalock shunts, however, is only infrequently visualized since, in such cases, the pulmonary artery receiving the shunt will normally be displaced cranially and, thus, will be obscured by the bronchus and the lung. In contrast, the exact site, the morphology of the anastomoses, and the function of Waterston shunts or central interposition shunts, can be easily demonstrated (Fig. 15.15).

As previously discussed in *Chapter 14*, transoesophageal imaging in the transverse axis has a limited role in the evaluation of most forms of aortic coarctation; this is especially true in the neonate or infant with complex forms of coarctation. In addition, the origin and morphology of brachiocephalic vessels, or the existence of collateral arteries, will not routinely be appreciated with transoesophageal imaging in the transverse axis. Even simple coarctations in patients with a right-sided arch may not be visualized as most often in these circumstances, there will only be poor contact between the oesophagus and the descending aorta. The technique should provide, nonetheless, a definite diagnosis of interruption of the aortic arch, and is of value in the assessment of recoarctation after previous surgical repair or angioplasty. In these latter conditions, transoesophageal imaging routinely allows the exclusion of pseudoaneurysmal formation, and colour flow mapping will reliably detect any intimal tears. In patients suspected of having multiple systemic-to-pulmonary collateral arteries in tetralogy of Fallot with pulmonary atresia, the transthoracic ultrasonic approach from the suprasternal notch provides more detailed information in infants, while angiography and/or magnetic resonance imaging remain the techniques of first choice in older patients. Similar limitations are encountered when an attempt is made to assess patency of the arterial duct, or the morphology and function of vascular rings by transoesophageal imaging.

LIMITATIONS

The morphologic areas that remain problematic for transoesophageal investigations in children are the right ventricular outflow tract, the apical muscular interventricular septum, the upper segment of the ascending aorta, and the left pulmonary artery. Using transverse-axis imaging planes, the precise morphology of any right ventricular outflow obstruction cannot be fully demonstrated. The assessment of the degree of any override of either arterial valve above a ventricular septal defect remains unreliable. Although restrictive defects of the antero-apical trabecular portion of the muscular ventricular septum can be demonstrated by transoesophageal colour flow mapping studies in smaller children, the precordial approach must be considered routinely to provide superior diagnostic information.

The haemodynamic assessment of congenital heart disease from within the oesophagus is limited to the evaluation of flow patterns within the pulmonary veins, flow across either atrioventricular valve, and the patterns of blood flow in the pulmonary trunk and the pulmonary arterial branches. All other areas of interest can only be interrogated with the Doppler beam having a large angle of incidence relative to the direction of blood flow. Furthermore, transoesophageal probes do not usually provide facilities for continuous wave Doppler interrogation, precluding the reliable assessment of the jets of high-velocity flow encountered in obstruction of either ventricular outflow tract or in the presence of atrioventricular valvar regurgitation. When one considers, however, the oblique scan planes of either ventricular outflow tract, which are obtained by transoesophageal imaging in the transverse axis, the additional value of continuous wave Doppler facilities in the assessment of lesions involving these cardiac levels remains questionable.

Transoesophageal echocardiography has proved to be a versatile technique for intraoperative monitoring, and some centres recommend its routine use in surgery for congenital heart disease. Due to the limited haemodynamic information provided, together with the restricted range of views that can be obtained from within the oesophagus, the technique cannot entirely replace epicardial intraoperative echocardiography. The latter technique allows a more complete morphologic and haemodynamic assessment of almost all aspects of the underlying congenital lesion and the surgical repair performed. One of the most relevant limitations of intraoperative transoesophageal echocardiography is that the technique does not allow the definite exclusion of residual shunting following closure of ventricular septal defects by means of a prosthetic patch; the synthetic material will inevitably result in a large area of masking in the anterior right ventricle (see *Chapter 13*).

INDICATIONS

Currently, there are three principal areas where transoesophageal echocardiography can be used to provide unique diagnostic information in children with congenital heart disease: firstly, in primary diagnosis, secondly, in the perioperative period, and thirdly, for long-term follow-up after intracardiac repair. The indication for a transoesophageal study in a small child must be clearcut and appropriate, since the technique is semi-invasive, requires either anaesthesia or heavy sedation, and complications are possible. Thus, transoesophageal echocardiography should be performed if important additional information is required for the management of the patient, and if it is considered that this is the imaging technique likely to yield this new information. Studies can be performed during routine scheduled cardiac catheterization, without delaying the procedure, and without requiring additional anaesthesia. Alternatively, studies can be performed on a day-care basis under heavy sedation in older children.

Based on the limitations of the technique outlined above, and the potential information provided by transoesophageal echocardiography, it should be clear that only a lack of information concerning specific areas of congenital heart disease will justify the use of transoesophageal echocardiography in the primary diagnosis. The most important primary diagnostic areas will be the exclusion of cordal straddling, exclusion of anomalies of either systemic or pulmonary venous connexion, the morphologic assessment of obstruction within the left ventricular outflow tract (7), or the detection of stenoses in the pulmonary arteries (Fig. 15.16). Transoesophageal studies can then be planned to take place prior to any scheduled cardiac catheterization.

In contrast to the limited role of transoesophageal echocardiography as a diagnostic tool in the initial evaluation of congenital heart disease, its use as a perioperative monitoring technique is highly rewarding, in particular its use in the intensive-care unit for prolonged monitoring of children at high risk and in the diagnosis and management of early postoperative complications. These areas may well become the standard indications for transoesophageal studies in children. Another area where transoesophageal echocardiographic studies are likely to become a standard part of the diagnostic armamentarium of the paediatric cardiologist is in the postoperative long-term follow-up of specific congenital cardiac lesions subsequent to surgical correction; for example, we have found the transoesophageal evaluation of the morphology and function of the atrial baffle following a Mustard or Senning procedure for complete transposition to be superior in many cases when compared to findings obtained during cardiac catheterization (8). Both the entire systemic and pulmonary venous pathways, including the individual pulmonary veins, can be assessed much more completely than is achieved from precordial studies. Following replacement of atrioventricular valves in infancy and childhood, the impact of transoesophageal echocardiography in the diagnosis and management of symptomatic patients is comparable to that in adult cardiologic practice. In particular, dysfunction of a mechanical valve can be assessed with more ease than by the precordial approach. The role of transoesophageal echocardiography in patients with a Fontan circulation remains yet to be defined. Whereas

complete diagnostic information is obtained in virtually every patient with a direct atriopulmonary anastomosis, severe difficulties are encountered when the Fontan circulation is established by means of an anteriorly placed conduit. These conduits can rarely be visualized in their entire course using the transoesophageal approach. The documentation of the patterns of flow into the conduit and within the pulmonary arteries, however, may yield important clues in the assessment of the function of the conduit. Sampling of patterns of flow of individual pulmonary veins allows the reliable detection of gross perfusion abnormalities of either lungs in all patients.

Finally, the use of transoesophageal echocardiography as a technique for monitoring and guidance during interventional cardiac catheterization, should be extremely helpful. The detailed demonstration of, for example, the interatrial septum should prove to be of

Indications for Transoesophageal Echocardiography in Children with Congenital Heart Disease	
Primary diagnosis	
atrial arrangement	direct diagnosis of atrial morphology
systemic venous connexions	abnormal drainage, obstruction
pulmonary venous connexions	abnormal drainage, obstruction
interatrial septum	sinus venosus defects
atrioventricular valves	morphology valvar and subvalvar apparatus – exclusion of cordal straddling – complete atrioventricular septal defects
left ventricular outflow tract	morphology of obstructive lesions – discrete fibromuscular membrane – tunnel-like lesions
central pulmonary arteries	central/peripheral stenosis pulmonary atresia central systemic-to-pulmonary shunts
Perioperative	
prior to repair after repair	detailed morphologic diagnosis monitoring of ventricular function assessment of surgical repair exclusion of residual lesions
intensive care unit	prolonged monitoring diagnosis/management of early postoperative complications
Follow-up	
poor precordial ultrasound windows	
Mustard/Senning procedures	morphology and function of atrial baffles systemic and pulmonary venous pathways tricuspid regurgitation valve dysfunction/paravalvar leaks
Valve repair/ replacement	prosthetic valvar endocarditis direct atriopulmonary connexions
Fontan circulation	Glenn anastomosis residual atrial septal defects right atrial pathology

Fig. 15.16 Indications for transoesophageal echocardiography studies in children with congenital heart disease.

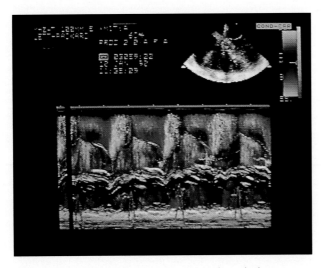

Fig. 15.17 Transoesophageal colour M-mode study during balloon valvoplasty of the aortic valve in an 18-kg child with severe aortic stenosis. Any valvar regurgitation can be excluded immediately after each inflation of the balloon. Transgastric views also allow the continuous monitoring of left ventricular function during the period of recovery.

value for closure of atrial septal defects using an umbrella. The technique should provide detailed morphologic information on the exact location and size of the defect, would allow monitoring of the exact positioning of the device, and could document the immediate results. The same would apply for balloon dilatation of obstructed interatrial baffles and the branches of the pulmonary arteries; not only could the exact positioning of the balloons be monitored but the immediate results could also be assessed. In addition, following Mustard baffle dilatation, the immediate exclusion of baffle leaks becomes feasible without resorting to additional angiocardiographic studies. Continuous monitoring of left ventricular function and exclusion of valvar regurgitation by transoesophageal echocardiographic techniques, have proved to be extremely helpful during balloon valvotomies of stenotic aortic or mitral valves (9); not only does it allow the immediate exclusion of complications after every balloon inflation, but it also helps to reduce the amount of radiation and contrast agent during these procedures (Fig. 15.17).

PERSPECTIVES

Future equipment developed for transoesophageal echocardiography in children must concentrate on improving the quality of cross-sectional images. The creation of even smaller probes must, in our opinion, be considered a secondary goal. A further increase in the number of transducer elements, without enlargement of the total dimension of the transducer, would appear to be most desirable. Alternatively, an increase of ultrasound frequency to 7.5MHz may be feasible, but may result in a much-reduced Doppler penetration. The incorporation of lateral steering facilities of the probe may be expected to be beneficial in various instances in the complete assessment of congenital heart disease.

Based on initial experience in adults, the introduction of biplane transoesophageal imaging may be expected to be of substantial additional value in children. This would allow a much-improved assessment of the morphology of the right ventricular outflow tract, documentation of the degree of arterial override, and assessment of extracardiac conduits and complex congenital lesions (for example, criss-cross hearts, or hearts with double-outlet ventriculoarterial connexions). To date, however, biplane imaging can only be realized at the expense of the number of ultrasound crystals and, thus, the quality of the images obtained. The construction of probes permitting imaging in the longitudinal axis, and providing high-quality images, may be more appropriate. Studies could then be performed using either, or, subsequently, both transducers, depending on the clinical question. Ultimately, rotational tip probes may be developed.

The incorporation of facilities for continuous wave Doppler may be expected to provide little additional haemodynamic information in children with congenital heart disease. This is due to the poor alignment that can usually be obtained when performing transoesophageal Doppler studies, and to the fact that the precordial ultrasound windows are almost always large enough to allow the acquisition of the relevant high-velocity Doppler signals. The exception to this would appear to be in the assessment of obstruction of the branches of the pulmonary arteries.

REFERENCES

1. Cyran SE, Kimball TR, Meyer RA *et al.* Efficacy of intraoperative transesophageal echocardiography in children with congenital heart disease. *Am J Cardiol* 1989;**63**:594–8.

2. Lam J, vd Burg B, Basart DCG *et al.* Feasibility and value of transesophageal echocardiography in anesthetized children. In: Erbel R *et al*, eds. *Transesophageal echocardiography.* Springer–Verlag, 1989:293–8.

3. Kyo S, Koike K, Takanawa E *et al.* Impact of transesophageal Doppler echocardiography on pediatric cardiac surgery. *Int J Card Imag* 1989;**4**:41–2.

4. Stümper O, Elzenga NJ, Hess J, Sutherland GR. Transesophageal echocardiography in children with congenital heart disease. *J Am Coll of Cardiol,* 1990; **16**:433–41.

5. Weigel TJ, Seward JB, Hagler DJ. Transesophageal echocardiography in anomalous pulmonary and systemic venous connections. *Circulation* 1989;**80**:II-339.

6. Stümper O, Fraser AG, Ho SY *et al.* Transoesophageal imaging in the longitudinal axis: a correlative echocardiographic — anatomical study and its clinical implications. *Br Heart J* 1990;**64**:282–8.

7. Stümper O, Elzenga NJ, Sutherland GR. Left ventricular outflow obstruction in childhood — improved diagnosis by transoesophageal echocardiography. *Int J Cardiol* 1990;**28**:107–9.

8. Kaulitz R, Stümper O, Geuskens R *et al.* The comparative values of the precordial and transesophageal approaches in the ultrasound evaluation of atrial baffle function following an atrial correction procedure. *J Am Coll of Cardiol* 1990;**16**:686–94.

9. Cyran S E, Kemball T R, Schwartz D C *et al.* Evaluation of balloon aortic valvuloplasty with transesophageal echocardiography. *Am Heart J* 1988;**115**:460–2.

INDEX

abscesses
  endocarditis 9.2–5, 13.8
  para-aortic 3.16
  prosthetic endocarditis 8.5
AIDS 3.2
air, intracardiac 12.8
air embolization, paradoxical 4.8, 12.8
anaesthesia
  children 15.2
  general 3.4, 12.2
  local 3.3–4
  see also sedation
aneurysms
  aortic 3.30, 10.3–4, 13.3–4
  atrial septal 4.2, 4.9–10
  biplane views 3.30
  coronary artery 11.3–5
  mycotic 9.2–5
  pseudoaneurysms 4.4, 11.10–11
angiosarcoma of right atrium and ventricle 4.13
annular phased-array transducers 2.5, 15.2
annuloaortic ectasia 10.2–3, 13.3–4
antibiotic prophylaxis 3.3, 9.8
anticoagulant therapy 4.4, 4.11
aorta
  acquired diseases 13.2–4
  imaging 3.22–4
  para-aortic abscesses 3.16
  para-aortic fistulas 13.8
  thoracic, diseases of 10.1–15
aortic aneurysm 3.30, 10.3–4, 13.3–4
aortic autograft 13.8
aortic coarctation 14.8, 15.9
  balloon dilatation 10.13
  correction of 14.14
aortic dissection 10.4–12, 13.2–3
  biplane views 3.30, 10.7
  complications 10.11–12
  De Bakey classification 10.5–7
  hypotension 10.5
  intimal flaps 10.9–10
  intimal tears 10.7–9
  postoperative monitoring 10.12
  sedation of patient 3.3
  spiral 10.10
aortic homograft 13.8
aortic regurgitation 5.14–15, 7.3–9, 10.12, 13.8
aortic stenosis 7.1–3, 5.15, 13.8
  calcific 7.2
  supravalvar 14.8
aortic transection 10.12–13
aortic valve 3.17–18, 7.1–3
  bicuspid 14.8
  calcific stenosis 7.6
  coaptation of leaflets 3.18, 14.8
  congenital malformations 7.4
  disease 10.3, 13.8
  endocarditis 9.4–5
  leaflets 3.17–18
  prosthetic 8.3, 9.4–6
  stenosis 7.6
  valvuloplasty 7.3
arrhythmias 4.6–8, 5.10
arterial valves 14.8
arteries see coronary arteries; pulmonary arteries
atheromatous aneurysms, coronary arteries 11.3–5

atherosclerosis, thoracic aorta 10.2
atria 3.13–15
  congenital heart disease 14.3–4
  divided 14.3
  spontaneous contrast 4.2–5, 6.5
  see also left atrium; right atrium
atrial appendages 3.20–21
  children 15.3
  congenital heart disease 14.3–4
  thrombus detection 3.20, 4.7
  see also left atrial appendage
atrial arrangement (situs) 3.20
atrial arrhythmias 4.6–8
atrial baffle 15.11
atrial fibrillation 5.10
atrial flutter 4.6, 5.10
atrial lesions 4.1–14
atrial myxoma 4.12
atrial pacing 11.7–8
atrial septal aneurysm 4.2, 4.9–10
atrial septal defects 5.16, 14.4–6
  and atrial septal aneurysm 4.9
  caused by transseptal puncture 6.7
  paradoxical air embolization 4.8, 12.8
  pre-bypass studies 13.10–11
atrial septum 3.13–15, 14.4–6
atrial thrombus
  complication of mitral prostheses 8.5
  deep vein thrombosis 4.11
atriopulmonary anastomosis 14.10
atrioventricular defects 14.4–6
atrioventricular junction, congenital heart disease 14.7
atrioventricular septal defects 14.9, 15.3
  shunts 14.5–6
atrioventricular valves
  children with congenital heart disease 15.5–7
  left see mitral valve
  prosthetic 8.2, 14.9, 15.11
  regurgitation of congenital aetiology 13.14, 15.4
  repair 13.12, 14.9
  right see tricuspid valve
  see also mitral valve; tricuspid valve

bacteraemia (bacteriaemia) 3.3, 9.8
baffle leaks 14.12–14, 15.4
balloon dilatation of coarctation 10.13
balloon valvotomy, mitral stenosis 6.5–6
basal transverse-axis images 3.16–22
bicuspid aortic valve 14.8
biopsy of tumour 4.13
biplane imaging
  aortic dissection 3.30, 10.7
  aortic aneurysms 3.30
  children 15.7, 15.12
  endocarditis 9.6
  mapping of mitral regurgitant jets 6.15
  mitral valve 6.5, 6.9, 13.5
  prosthetic regurgitation 8.8
  thoracic aorta 10.1–2
biplane probes 2.3–4, 3.6, 3.24–30, 4.10, 11.1, 15.7
Blalock shunt 5.16, 15.9

calcific aortic stenosis 7.2, 7.6
calcified subaortic fibromuscular shelf 7.6
calcium deposits 4.4, 11.3
cardiac arrhythmias 4.6–8, 5.10